Animal Behavior and Management

Animal Behavior and Management

Edited by **Kenneth Hayes**

SYRAWOOD
PUBLISHING HOUSE
New York

Published by Syrawood Publishing House,
750 Third Avenue, 9th Floor,
New York, NY 10017, USA
www.syrawoodpublishinghouse.com

Animal Behavior and Management
Edited by Kenneth Hayes

International Standard Book Number: 978-1-68286-236-0 (Hardback)

Printed in China.

Contents

Preface

Behavior is an essential component of animal life. The study of behavior has given us remarkable insights into understanding the reactions of animals. This book is a complete source of knowledge on animal behavior and is a collective contribution of internationally renowned experts. It is a vital tool for all researching or studying zoology or veterinary science as it gives incredible insights into emerging trends and concepts of animal behavior and management. The text discusses in detail the psychological responses of animals to humans and their environment. It also presents some studies on rehabilitation of animals. From theories to research to practical applications, case studies related to all contemporary topics of relevance to this field have been included in this book.

All of the data presented henceforth, was collaborated in the wake of recent advancements in the field. The aim of this book is to present the diversified developments from across the globe in a comprehensible manner. The opinions expressed in each chapter belong solely to the contributing authors. Their interpretations of the topics are the integral part of this book, which I have carefully compiled for a better understanding of the readers.

At the end, I would like to thank all those who dedicated their time and efforts for the successful completion of this book. I also wish to convey my gratitude towards my friends and family who supported me at every step.

Editor

1

Dogs' Body Language Relevant to Learning Achievement

Masashi Hasegawa †, Nobuyo Ohtani * and Mitsuaki Ohta

Azabu University School of Veterinary Medicine, 1-17-71, Fuchinobe, Chuo-ku, Sagamihara, Kanagawa 252-5201, Japan; E-Mail: mohta@azabu-u.ac.jp

† Current affiliation: Animal Life Solutions, Inc., 16-6, Ibukino, Midori-ku, Yokohama, Kanagawa 226-0028, Japan; E-Mail: hasegawa@animallifesolutions.com.

* Author to whom correspondence should be addressed; E-Mail: ohtani@azabu-u.ac.jp.

Simple Summary: For humans and dogs to live together amiably, dog training is required, and a lack of obedience training is significantly related to the prevalence of certain behavioral problems. To train efficiently, it is important that the trainer/owner ascertains the learning level of the dog. Understanding the dog's body language helps humans understand the animal's emotions. This study evaluated the posture of certain dog body parts during operant conditioning. Our findings suggest that certain postures were related to the dog's learning level during operant conditioning. Being aware of these postures could be helpful to understand canine emotion during learning.

Abstract: The facial expressions and body postures of dogs can give helpful information about their moods and emotional states. People can more effectively obedience train their dogs if we can identify the mannerisms associated with learning in dogs. The aim of this study was to clarify the dog's body language during operant conditioning to predict achievement in the test that followed by measuring the duration of behaviors. Forty-six untrained dogs (17 males and 26 females) of various breeds were used. Each session consisted of 5 minutes of training with a treat reward followed by 3 minutes of rest and finally an operant conditioning test that consisted of 20 "hand motion" cues. The operant tests were conducted a total of nine times over three consecutive days, and the success numbers were counted. The duration of the dog's behavior, focusing on the dog's eyes, mouth, ears, tail and tail-wagging, was recorded during the operant conditioning sessions before the test. Particular behaviors, including wide-eyes, closed mouth, erect ears, and forward and high tail carriage, without wagging or with short and quick wagging, related to high achievement results. It is concluded that dogs' body language during operant conditioning was related to their success rate.

Keywords: body language; *Canis familiaris*; learning; operant conditioning; training

---

1. Introduction

Dogs, which were probably the first domesticated animals, have shared a common environment with humans for over ten thousand years [1]. Hare's 2002 study did not support the predictions of either the canid generalization hypothesis, which states that dogs have inherited their skills from wolves, or the human exposure hypothesis, which states that dogs are skillful because they experience intense exposure to humans through their lives [2]. Instead, the study provided support for the domestication hypothesis: that dogs acquired their social-communicative skills with humans during the process of domestication [3–5]. Dogs and humans are capable of a unique interspecies communication, and understanding, and share basic emotions [6]. Over the last decade, many studies have shown that dogs respond to human actions, which might be an effect of domestication [7–11]. These reports have demonstrated that dogs understand and responded to human gestures and cues, such as pointing, head turning, gazing and nodding, to locate hidden food items.

Dogs have three main methods of communicating with others: auditory, visual and olfactory [12]. The visual communication methods, including postures and facial expressions, are known to be descended from those of wolves, their ancestor [13]. However, the selection by humans for particular physical features has hampered the dog's abilities to use certain structures for visual communication [14,15]. For example, drooping ears and/or docked tails may be less able to signal the dog's status than more wolf-like conformations [12]. There are more than 400 canine breeds differing in external morphology and behavior [16–18]. Furthermore, there is a great deal of variability in the social behavior towards humans and the communicative behavior due to the breeds [19,20]. For example, it is much easier to teach a Labrador than a Great Pyrenees to retrieve [21]. However, no dog is immune to the principles of learning.

In Japan, nearly 24% of households have pet dogs, resulting in a total of over 10 million dogs, and this is almost the same as the number of children under 14 years of age [22,23]. The more humans that have close ties to dogs, the more dog behavioral problems become a serious issue. Many of the problem behaviors arise from the types of relationships people have with their dogs [24,25]. Obedience training is usually recommended for dogs displaying overexcitement [19,26]. Additionally, the timing of meals and sleeping arrangements, as well as the owners' prior experiences with dogs and their reasons for acquiring a dog, are all significantly related to the prevalence of certain behavioral problems [27]. Thus, we need to increase the awareness of the importance of appropriate dog obedience training in Japan.

The obedience training of domestic dogs, and indeed other animals, to perform behaviors on command is well established using operant conditioning and Pavlovian conditioning techniques [28,29].

Many trainers utilize the method of luring a dog by hand into a position using food or toys, marking the behavior with a clicker or voice cue, and offering a reward for learning a new obedience behavior, such as sitting [30]. The percentage of dog owners using the reward method for sit training was identified as 75% through questionnaires [31].

For effective training, it is necessary that the dog is highly motivated and concentrating to enable it to learn, and that the owner has the appropriate training skills. Dog owners may not have the time or ability to acquire the skills of a dog trainer. However, the owners can perform more effective dog training if they can read, by some kind of method, the dog's emotional and motivational states as well as their attention span for learning.

In humans, the importance of non-verbal signals during verbal exchanges is widely recognized [32]. Although emotion recognition includes expressions and gestures, facial expressions are uniquely relevant, and the correct interpretations of facial expressions are needed for appropriate emotional reactions and appropriate behavior in social situations [33]. A number of studies indicated that perceivers were more influenced by visual cues, particularly the facial expressions of humans, than by a vocal component [34–36]. Thus, it is natural that we humans try to understand dog emotions through their visual cues. On the other hand, although some studies have shown the meaning of various facial expressions and body postures of canids [13,37,38], there is little information on the relationship between body language and learning level.

Thus, the aim of this study was to elucidate the common body language in a variety of breeds relevant to learning achievement by operant conditioning. Our results may establish a relationship between body language and learning achievement in dogs.

2. Experimental Section

2.1. Ethics

All of the procedures were approved by the Animal Experiments Ethics Committee of Azabu University in accordance with the World Medical Association Declaration of Helsinki.

2.2. Subjects

Forty-six dogs (17 males and 26 females) of various breeds, kept at the World Ranch in Osaka, Japan, participated in this study (Table 1). All of the dogs were sexually intact and between 12 to 79 months of age (average 35.9 months, not including three dogs whose ages were unknown). They were housed in individual 120 cm × 200 cm metal cages from 17:00 to 9:00 away from human contact and provided with commercial dog food (Adult Maintenance, Nutro Products Inc., Victorville, CA, USA), according to the industry recommendations. Food was given twice a day, at 8:00 in the morning and at 17:00 in the evening. Furthermore, all of the dogs were released outside at the same facility from 9:00 to 17:00 in an exercise yard, which was surrounded by a 200 cm × 300 cm metal fence for at least one year. They had been socialized through interactions with people of various ages that visited the ranch.

Additionally, the kennel staff confirmed that the dogs had not been trained nor did they respond to a verbal sit command or the associated hand motion. As a result, dogs that did not respond to either stimuli became experimental subjects.

Table 1. Characteristics of dogs *(Canis familiaris)* used in the present study.

Breed	Sex	Age (months)		Breed	Sex	Age (months)
Australian Terrier	♂	62		*Irish Setter*	♂	49
Australian Cattle Dog	♂	54		*Irish Wolfhound*	♂	66
Australian Kelpie	♂	67		*Irish Wolfhound*	♀	79
Basset Hound	♀	49		*Japanese Spitz*	♀	12
Beagle	♂	12		*Miniature Pinscher*	♀	12
Beagle	♀	12		*Miniature Schnauzer*	♂	27
Border Collie	♀	12		*Newfoundland*	♀	30
Boxer	♀	25		*Newfoundland*	♂	77
Boxer	♂	36		*Newfoundland*	♀	30
Bulldog	♀	48		*Norfolk Terrier*	♂	12
Chihuahua	♀	66		*Papillon*	♀	13
Chihuahua	♀	12		*Papillon*	♀	12
Clumber Spaniel	♀	12		*Pug*	♀	54
Dandie Dinmont Terrier	♂	UN		*Pug*	♀	24
English Cocker Spaniel	♀	17		*Saint Bernard*	♀	55
English Cocker Spaniel	♂	45		*Schipperke*	♂	UN
English Setter	♀	41		*Shar pei*	♂	25
English Springer Spaniel	♀	40		*Shetland Sheepdog*	♀	49
French Bulldog	♀	17		*Vizsla*	♂	39
French Bulldog	♂	24		*West Highland White Terrier*	♀	12
Greyhound	♀	73		*Yorkshire Terrier*	♂	36
Ibizan Hound	♀	UN				UN: Unknown

2.3. Training Procedure

The training and experiments were conducted in the dog's familiar exercise yard by a handler (male, 28 years old, accustomed to working with dogs). The exercise yard was 150 cm × 200 cm and distracting smells were eliminated by cleaning as much as possible. The experiments were not affected by visual and auditory stimuli. The dogs and the handler had never met before the first training session. The treat used was a multi-balanced dog food (330 kcal/100 g, Nisshin Co.), stored in a bag kept at a constant humidity and temperature. The handler ascertained that all the dogs followed the hand with the treat before the training sessions began.

In the 5 min training of the dogs, the handler, holding one piece of food between his thumb and forefinger, lead the dog to sniff his hand in situations where the dog was free in the exercise yard. With the dog's nose on the handler's fingers, the handler slowly moved his hand up and over the dog's head. The operant conditioning was repeated as much as possible during the 5 min training sessions. The handler conditioned the dog to follow the hand motion. Thus, a hand motion from the dog's nose to overhead became a discriminative stimulus and induced sitting behavior as an operant response. However, to avoid associating any irrelevant motion with the sitting behavior, the handler did not start the hand motion if the dog was not interested in his hand. Thus, the hand motion was only performed when the dog was likely to follow the hand and experience success.

During each operant conditioning test, the dog was given the same discriminative stimuli (the hand motion) 20 times, and the number of successes was counted. Since the food might be the visual prompt for the dogs to sit, and prompt must be gradually be eliminated so that the animal learns to perform the behavior without the prompting [39], the handler did not have the food in his hands when he tested the dogs. In the test, we ascertained that just the hand motion was the discriminative stimulus to sit.

Continuous reinforcement was performed in all of the 5 min training sessions *and the test*, and a partial or intermittent reinforcement schedule was never used to avoid extinction. Thus, we carefully performed the operant conditioning sessions and the test to avoid extinction by rewarding every instance of sitting in response to the hand cue during training and test conditions.

One session consisted of 5 min of training with the treat reward and an operant conditioning test that consisted of 20 "hand motion" cues followed after 3 min of rest. Dogs had three sessions per a day, with 3 minutes of rest in between each session. This training schedule of a day (Table 2) was repeated for three consecutive days (leading to nine sessions per dog) in the afternoon prior to the evening feeding time.

Table 2. The daily training schedule.

	Session 1		
Time	5 min	3 min	hand motion 20 times
Detail	Training with treat	Resting	Operant conditioning test

2.4. Behavioral Evaluation

We conducted pre-experiments on 10 other dogs before this main experiment. This pre-experiment was carried out for three days with training schedules that were exactly the same as the main experiment. The sessions were recorded using a digital video camera (DCR-HC90, Sony, Japan). We categorized the body language of the dogs using the videos and many references [12,40–43]. Body languages were frequently observed in the videos and were given simple classifications that a dog owner could recognize. Eyes (Ey) and Ears (Ea) were divided into three categories based on their appearance. In addition, the types of ears were broadly classified into drop ear and prick ear. Mouth (M) appearance was divided into five categories. The Tail (T) category recorded tail height from the lowest to highest position. Tail-Wagging (TW) was also classified based on the visual records. The behavioral categories are shown in Figures 1–4 and Table 3.

Figure 1. Categories of eyes (Ey) in dogs during their training.

Eyes:	Ey-1	Eyes open wide
	Ey-2	Eyes open normally
	Ey-3	Eyes narrow

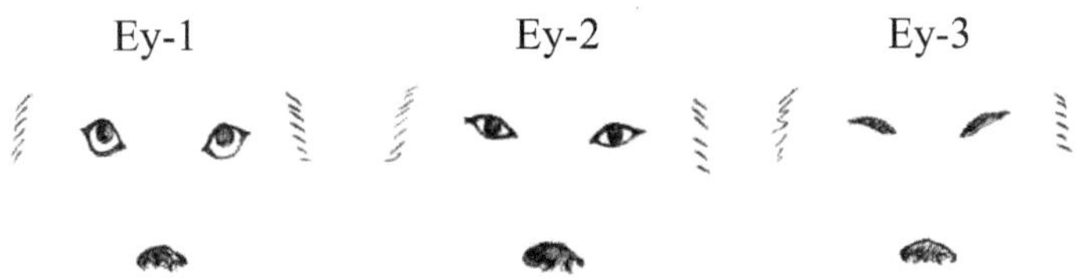

Figure 2. Categories of mouth (M) expressions in dogs during their training.

	M-1	Mouth shut
	M-2	Mouth slightly open
Mouth:	M-3	Mouth opens wide and the tongue is visible
	M-4	Mouth opens, the teeth are visible, and the cheek muscles look firm
	M-5	The front and back teeth are visible, and the look is obviously aggressive

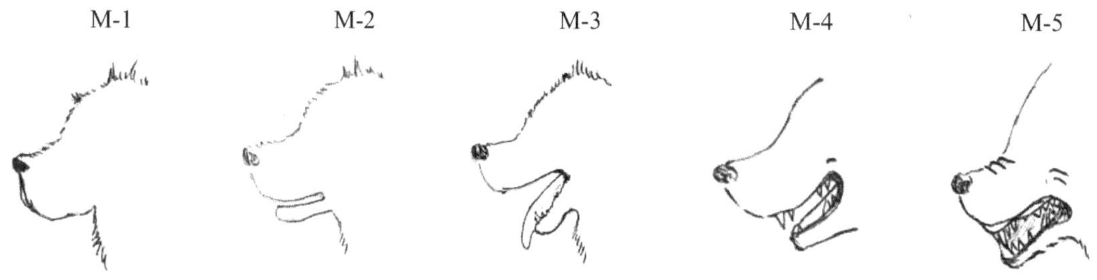

Figure 3. Categories of ear (Ea) appearances in dogs during their training.

	Ea-1	Ears are turned forward
Ears:	Ea-2	Ears are slightly turned back
	Ea-3	Ears are turned back

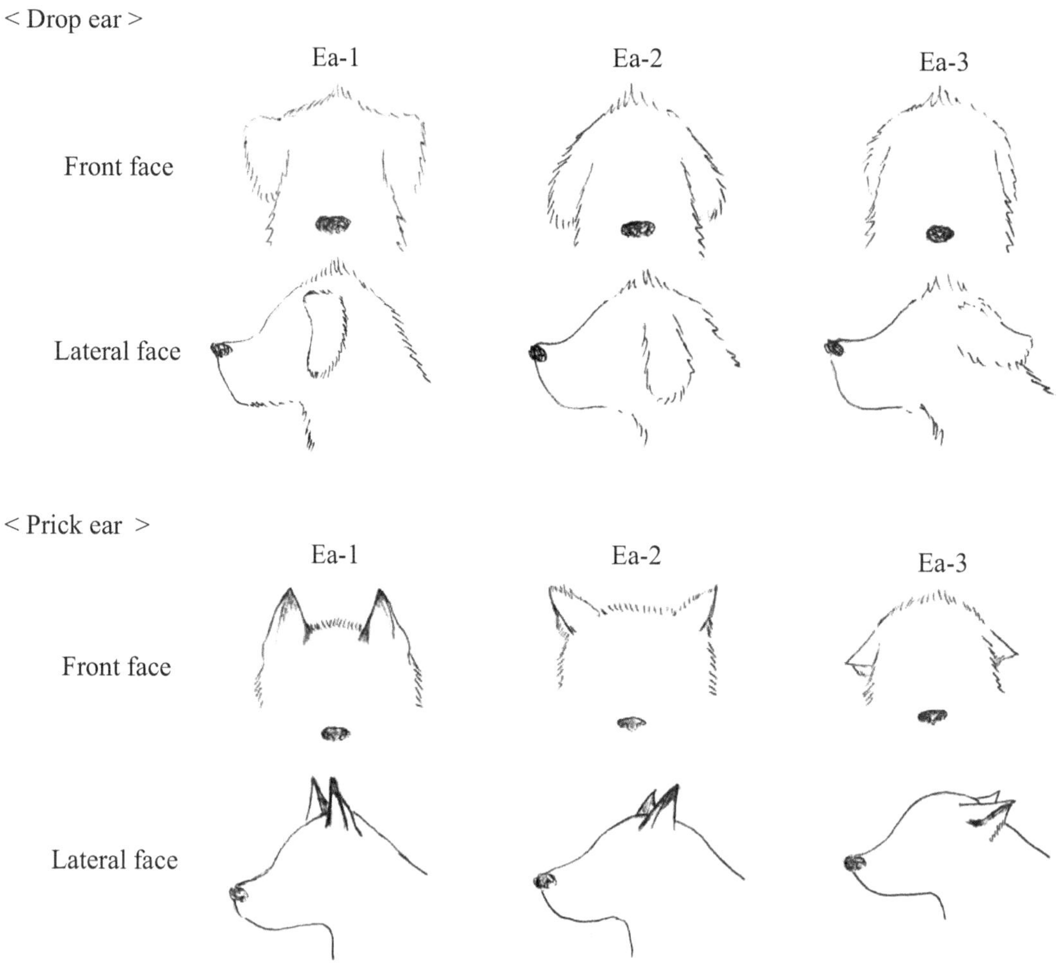

Figure 4. Categories of tail (T) body language in dogs during their training.

Tail:	T-1	Tail is between the legs
	T-2	Tail is hanging down
	T-3	Tip of the tail is lower than the height of the back
	T-4	Tail is parallel to the back
	T-5	Tail is higher than the height of the back
	T-6	Tail is up almost vertically

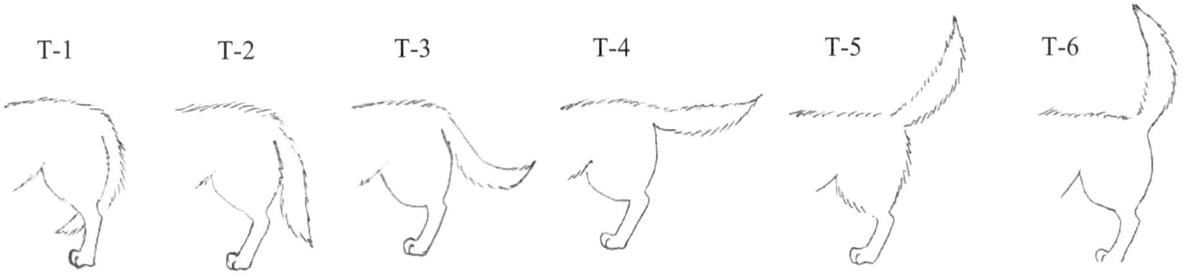

Table 3. Categories of dog tail-wagging (TW) during operant conditioning training.

Tail-Wagging:	TW-1	Tail is not wagging
	TW-2	Only the tip of the tail is wagging
	TW-3	Tail is wagging shortly and slowly
	TW-4	Tail is wagging shortly and quickly
	TW-5	Tail is wagging widely and slowly
	TW-6	Tail is wagging widely and quickly
	TW-7	Tail is wagging with wiggling at the hip and waist
	TW-8	Tail is spinning around

In the main experiment, three experimenters recorded observations independently for each behavioral category, Eyes (Ey), Mouth (M), Ears (Ea), Tail (T) and Tail-Wagging (TW), during the nine training sessions excluding the operant conditioning tests. The three observers had been trained in the methods of behavioral evaluations of dogs. The behavioral assessments were performed by analyzing slow motion replays of the 5 min of taped training. These evaluations lasted approximately 25 min. However, we have excluded from the records of the tail movements that could not be evaluated, such as those of the Pugs.

2.5. Statistical Analysis

The number of the operant conditioning events during the 5 min training sessions, and of the successful operant responses after the conditioning, were counted. It was necessary to identify any correlation between the conditioning number in the training and the success number in the test. Since the age of subject dogs ranged from 1 to 6.5 years old in this experiment, there could be age-dependent differences in the learning acquisition rate. Therefore, the correlation between the conditioning number and success number, and the test results and the dogs' ages, were analyzed using Spearman's rank correlation coefficient.

Additionally, the three experimenters recorded the duration of the body language categories, thus the inter-experimenter reliability was established using Cronbach's alpha analysis.

This study was done to clarify the body language of dogs that performed well during operant conditioning. Therefore, a stepwise multiple regression analysis was performed to determine whether the duration of each of the behavioral categories was a good predictor for high achievement during the operant conditioning test. The high achievement dogs showed more than the median split number of successful operant responses. And the stepwise multiple regression was used to avoid problems of multicollinearity. In this analysis, the significant variables were selected using backwards elimination, and the categories of body language were independent variables and learning achievement in the operant conditioning test was the dependent variable. The statistical analysis was performed using the computing software R (http://www.r-project.org).

3. Results

There was a significant positive correlation between the number of conditioning events and the success number of the test (rs = 0.7, $p < 0.05$). There were no statistical correlation between the age of dogs and results of operant conditioning test (rs = −0.31, $p = -0.35$). Moreover, inter-experimenter reliability was confirmed using Cronbach's alpha analysis ($\alpha = 0.83$).

The median split number of success responses in the test was 9. The stepwise multiple regression analysis is shown in Table 4. The results indicated that the significant traits were Ey open wide (standard partial regression coefficient = 0.14, $P < 0.05$), M shut (standard partial regression coefficient = 0.48, $P < 0.001$), Ea turned forward (standard partial regression coefficient = 0.19, $P < 0.01$), T is hanging down (standard partial regression coefficient = −0.16, $P < 0.05$), T is up almost vertically (standard partial regression coefficient = 0.18, $P < 0.01$), TW is not wagging (standard partial regression coefficient = 0.34, $P < 0.001$), and TW is wagging short and quick (standard partial regression coefficient = 0.33, $P < 0.001$).

Table 4. Statistical results on the duration of each behavioral category as good predictors of the achievement rate in the operant conditioning tests (Stepwise multiple regression analysis).

Variables		***β***	**t**
Eyes	Ey-1	0.14 *	2.01
Mouth	M-1	0.48 ***	7.15
Ears	Ea-1	0.19 **	2.58
Tail	T-2	-0.16 *	2.1
	T-6	0.18 **	2.44
Tail-Wagging	TW-1	0.34 ***	3.79
	TW-4	0.33 ***	4.79

* $P < 0.05$, ** $P < 0.01$, *** $P < 0.001$.

4. Discussion

To clarify the body language of dogs with high learning performances, we recorded the duration of each behavioral category during nine training sessions over three consecutive days. This study revealed, by detailed behavioral evaluation and statistical analysis, that some of the dog's body language correlated with high achievement in the operant conditioning tests. Wide eyes and upright ears have been observed in dogs that are expressing aggression or dominance, and in those that feel challenged or threatened [40]. In this study, the wide-open eyes were linked with high learning results, which suggests that some of the dogs were expressing dominance over humans. A dominant dog shows a self-assured gait, a large, confident body posture, raised head, raised ears, large eyes, curled lips, and carries the tails high with a slight wag [40]. However, the body language categories linked to a high learning performance were closed mouths, forward ears, and high tail carriage without wagging. This is similar to the body language of dominant dogs, but was different in the categories of mouths (lips) and tail-wagging, which suggests that the dogs that recorded high results in the test were not dominant over the experimenter.

Humans learn many things by eyesight, and eye contact is essential for developing social skills [44]; however, in dogs, staring eye-to-eye means opposition [40]. Submissive dogs avoid direct eye contact with the dominant dog, and it has been suggested that the relative status of the dogs is determined by this visual communication [14]. In this study, wide eyes were observed mostly when the dogs looked up at the handler's face. The tendency of dogs to have periods of face/eye contact with people longer than socialized wolves in the food task was observed [45]. Thus, dogs naturally do not watch other dog's eyes; however, it is thought that an effect of domestication is that dogs will watch a person's eyes. Furthermore, while face/eye contact indicated the superior and inferior relationship between dogs [40], looking up at a human face and making eye contact can be categorized as body language focusing or expectation on a human.

Although the dog's body language that was linked to a high learning performance included the category of closed mouth in this study, as the training period progressed, in general, dogs start panting to maintain their body temperature. Additionally, even if the dog was socialized, the experimenter was a stranger to the dogs in the exercise yard. Since excessive stress may induce dogs to perform thermoregulatory behavior like panting [46], it may be that dog's panting was started by stress of the stranger. Therefore, it may be difficult to discriminate how much dogs are focusing on people just by watching their mouths.

The duration of the ears pointing forward was relevant to a high learning performance. The normal body language of a dog when greeting a human or another dog includes the movement of its ears up and down [40]. However, a forward ear position is associated with a state of heightened attention [47], motivation, confidence, and/or aggression; whereas, a backward ear position is often associated with submission and/or fear [40]. These results suggest that while the dogs are focused on the handler, their ears point towards them.

In the category of the tail height, the duration of the tail being held straight up was linked with the dog's high response during the test. In the category of tail wagging, it was revealed that a non-wagging tail or a tail wagging shortly and quickly could predict a high learning performance during the training. It may be suggested that the position and wagging of the tail represent the motivation status of the dog.

However, the shapes and sizes of the tails differ in all breeds and there are breeds that cannot bring their tails up straight [40]. Thus, such an index can only be used for dog breeds that are able to bring their tails up straight and may not apply to some breeds that have specific types of tails. However, the combination of the position and motion of a domestic dog's tail still provides information regarding the dog's state, including friendly, playful, fearful, submissive, dominant and aggressive [12,42,48–50]. Therefore, a study that focuses on only the tail position and wagging should be conducted in each breed. Quaranta *et al.* studied the asymmetric tail-wagging responses of dogs to different emotive stimuli [51]. In their study, the brain activity occurring when the dog's tail was wagged to the left or right was discussed. Although we did not analyze the direction of tail wagging in our study, further studies may be able to explain the brain activity during training.

One question that remains is what it was about the low achieving dogs that caused them to learn more slowly. All of the dogs were given treats in the 5 minutes of training and the operant conditioning test using continuous reinforcement. Thus, the training and test conditions were not to extinction. However, in the test, the handler gave the same hand motion 20 times as a discriminative stimuli to the dogs, regardless of their learning, when the dogs looked at the handler's hand. We believe that these dogs are displaying learned irrelevance. Learned irrelevance, learning to ignore things that are of no importance [39], is a particularly efficient way of learning. Therefore, it might take more time for the low achievement dogs in the test to learn that the hand motion was a discriminative stimulus to sit cue. In other words, the low achievement dogs might have needed to increase the frequency of training.

Additionally, there might be other causes of the slow learning in dogs that recorded low achievement numbers, such as breed differences/behavior, and changes in motivation due to satiation (treats). Hart and Hart examined the breed behavior profiles of 56 breeds of dogs using 13 behavioral traits, and elucidated that the obedience training performance was affected by the dog's breed [19]. We had 33 breeds in our experiment, and it is possible that there might be a difference in learning performance between these breeds. However, there were too few of each dog breed to perform a statistical analysis that would ascertain the ability for training between dog breeds. Additionally, we gave each dog one treat for each event during the operant conditioning. The treat size was standard and not based the size of the dog. Thus, we did not change the size of the treat to account for the dog's feeling of satiation. The total number of operant conditioning events for the Newfoundland was 130, the Papillion was 194, and the Chihuahua was 141 in this experiment. It appears that the number of operant conditioning events was unaffected by the size of the treats. However, to conduct a more detailed experiment and be able to do a statistical analysis, it will be necessary to increase the number of dogs per breed to investigate the relationship between dog breed and learning performance.

Body language shows the dog's status, such as dominant and submissive [40]. In this study, an unknown handler trained dogs that had not lived with human owners. Thus, they probably they had various emotional responses to the handler, and their body language may differ from the general home dog. However, using these body language parameters in our dog school for pet dogs, the learning results were improved. To evaluate the usefulness of these traits, it would be necessary to perform the same evaluation of dogs living with their owners.

The body language of dogs linked with high test results was very similar to the body language of a dominant dog. However, there were differences in the categories of mouths (lips) and tail-wagging. The dominant dog watches other dog closely [14], and the dogs that recorded high learning results were also looking up at the human face/eyes. Thus, it may be that the categories of eyes open wide and ears turned forward, without the categories of mouths (lips), tail and tail-wagging, mean attention to others.

Thus, wide eyes and forward ear positions, which were the categorized body language in this study, determined the common body language in a variety of breeds relevant to learning achievement during the operant conditioning. This body language will become the key to understanding the level of motivation and attention in the operant conditioning of dogs. However, in the dog's body language each emotion is expressed using the whole body. Thus, elucidation of the entire body language, not just those related to the eyes and ear position, is required, especially the dog's tail position/wagging in each breed.

5. Conclusions

During dog training, the common dog body language among some breeds that predicted high learning achievement was wide-open eyes, ears erect and having a forward tail position. These traits could aid in the efficient training of dogs. Additionally, the mouth appearance was affected by temperature and stress, and the category of the tail needs to be examined in a breed-based manner.

Acknowledgments

This research was supported by a Grant-in-Aid for Matching Fund Subsidy for Private Universities from The Promotion and Mutual Aid Corporation for Private Schools of Japan.

Author Contributions

M. Hasegawa designed and carried out experiments and drafted the manuscript. M. Ohta and N. Ohtani helped with analysis, and contributed to writing the manuscript.

Conflicts of Interest

The authors declare no conflict of interest.

References

1. Udell, M.A.; Wynne, C.D. A review of domestic dogs' (*Canis Familiaris*) human-like behaviors: Or why behavior analysts should stop worrying and love their dogs. *J. Exp. Anal. Behav.* **2008**, *89*, 247–261.
2. Hare, B.; Brown, M.; Williamson, C.; Tomasello, M. The domestication of social cognition in dogs. *Science* **2002**, *298*, 1634–1636.
3. Range, F.; Viranyi, Z. The effect of domestication on cognitive abilities of dogs. *J. Vet. Behav. Clin. Appl. Res.* **2012**, *7*, e14.
4. Gosling, S.D.; Kwan, V.S.; John, O.P. A dog's got personality: A cross-species comparative approach to personality judgments in dogs and humans. *J. Pers. Soc. Psychol.* **2003**, *85*, 1161–1169.

5. Hare, B.; Rosati, A.; Kaminski, J.; Bräuer, J.; Call, J.; Tomasello, M. The domestication hypothesis for dogs' skills with human communication: a response to and. *Anim. Behav.* **2010**, *79*, e1–e6.
6. Panksepp, J. *Affective Neuroscience: The Foundations of Human and Animal Emotions*; Oxford University Press: New York, NY, USA, 1998.
7. Miklósi, Á.; Polgárdi, R.; Topál, J.; Csányi, V. Use of experimenter-given cues in dogs. *Anim. Cogn.* **1998**, *1*, 113–121.
8. Hare, B.; Tomasello, M. Domestic dogs (*Canis familiaris*) use human and conspecific social cues to locate hidden food. *J. Comp. Psychol.* **1999**, *113*, 173–177.
9. Soproni, K.; Miklósi, Á.; Topál, J.; Csányi, V. Comprehension of human communicative signs in pet dogs (*Canis familiaris*). *J. Comp. Psychol.* **2001**, *115*, 122–126.
10. Soproni, K.; Miklósi, Á.; Topál, J.; Csányi, V. Dogs' (*Canis familaris*) responsiveness to human pointing gestures. *J. Comp. Psychol.* **2002**, *116*, 27–34.
11. Udell, M.A.; Giglio, R.F.; Wynne, C.D. Domestic dogs (*Canis familiaris*) use human gestures but not nonhuman tokens to find hidden food. *J. Comp. Psychol.* **2008**, *122*, 84–93.
12. Bradshaw, J.; Nott, H. Social and communication behaviour of companion dog. In *The Domestic Dog: Its Evolution, Behaviour and Interactions with People*; Serpell, J., Ed.; Cambridge University Press: Cambridge, UK, 1995; pp. 115–130.
13. Fox, M.W. A comparative study of the development of facial expressions in canids; wolf, coyote and foxes. *Behaviour* **1970**, *36*, 49–73.
14. Beaver, B. Distance-increasing postures of dogs. *Vet. Med. Small Anim. Clin.* **1982**, *77*, 1023–1024.
15. Blackshaw, J. Human and animal inter-relationships. Review series: 3. Normal behaviour patterns of dogs. Part 1. *Austr. Vet. Pract.* **1985**, *15*, 110–112.
16. Hart, B.L.; Hart, L.A. *Canine and Feline Behavioral Therapy*; Lea & Febiger: Philadelphia, PA, USA, 1985; pp. 133–145.
17. Bradshaw, J.; Goodwin, D.; Lea, A.; Whitehead, S. A survey of the behavioural characteristics of pure-bred dogs in the United Kingdom. *Vet. Rec.* **1996**, *139*, 465–468.
18. Svartberg, K. Breed-typical behaviour in dogs—Historical remnants or recent constructs? *Appl. Anim. Behav. Sci.* **2006**, *96*, 293–313.
19. Hart, B.L.; Hart, L.A. Selecting pet dogs on the basis of cluster analysis of breed behavior profiles and gender. *J. Am. Vet. Med. Assoc.* **1985**, *186*, 1181–1185.
20. Feddersen-Petersen, D. Behaviour problems in dogs, and factors in breeding, keeping and training that are responsible. *Prakt. Tierarzt* **1990**, *71*, 18–28.
21. Alexander, M.C. *Click for Joy! Questions and Answers from Clicker Trainers and Their Dogs*; Sunshine Books, Inc.: Waltham, MA, USA, 2003; pp. 4–5.
22. Omoe, T.H.; Omoe, K. Social environment and control status of companion animal-borne zoonoses in Japan. *Animals* **2012**, *2*, 38–54.
23. *Statistical Handbook of Japan 2013*; Ministry of Internal Affairs and Communications: Tokyo, Japan, 2013; Available online: http://www.stat.go.jp/english/data/handbook/pdf/2013all.pdf (accessed on 21 February 2014).

24. Voith, V.L. Attachment between people and their pets: behavior problems of pets that arise from the relationship between pets and people. In *Interrelations between People and Pets*; Fogle, B., Ed.; Charles C. Thomas: Springfield, IL, USA, 1981; pp. 271–294.
25. Mugford, R.A. Attachment *vs.* dominance: Alternative views of man-dog relationship. In *The Human-Pet Relationship*; the Austrian Academy of Sciences by IEMT-Institute for Interdisciplinary Research on the Human-Pet Relationship: Vienna, Austria, 1985; pp. 157–165.
26. Myles, S. Trainers and chokers. How dog trainers affect behavior problems in dogs. *Vet. Clin. North Am. Small Anim. Pract.* **1991**, *21*, 239–246.
27. Jagoe, A.; Serpell, J. Owner characteristics and interactions and the prevalence of canine behaviour problems. *Appl. Anim. Behav. Sci.* **1996**, *47*, 31–42.
28. Pryor, K. *Don't Shoot the Dog! The New Art of Teaching and Training*; Bantam Books: New York, NY, USA, 1999.
29. Chance, P. *Learning and Behavior*, 6th ed.; Brooks/Cole Publishing Company: Belmont, CA, USA, 2008.
30. Alexander, M.B.; Friend, T.; Haug, L. Obedience training effects on search dog performance. *Appl. Anim. Behav. Sci.* **2011**, *132*, 152–159.
31. Hiby, E.F.; Rooney, N.J.; Bradshaw, J. Dog training methods: their use, effectiveness and interaction with behavior and welfare. *Anim. Welfare* **2004**, *13*, 63–69.
32. Burgoon, J.K.; Buller, D.B.; Woodall, W.G. *Nonverbal Communication: the Unspoken Dialogue*; McGraw-Hill: New York, NY, USA, 1996.
33. Stetina, B.U.; Turner, K.; Burger, E.; Glenk, L.M.; McElheney, J.C.; Handlos, U.; Kothgassner, O.D. Learning emotion recognition from canines? Two for the road. *J. Vet. Behav. Clin. Appl. Res.* **2011**, *6*, 108–114.
34. Mehrabian, A.; Ferris, S.R. Inference of attitudes from nonverbal communication in two channels. *J. Consult. Psychol.* **1967**, *31*, 248–252.
35. Bugental, D.E.; Kaswan, J.W.; Love, L.R. Perception of contradictory meanings conveyed by verbal and nonverbal channels. *J. Pers. Soc. Psychol.* **1970**, *16*, 647–655.
36. DePaulo, B.M. Decoding discrepant nonverbal cues. *J. Pers. Soc. Psychol.* **1978**, *36*, 313–323.
37. Schenkel, R. Submission: Its features and function in the wolf and dog. *Am. Zool.* **1967**, *7*, 319–329.
38. Abrantes, R. The expression of emotions in man and canid. *J. Small Anim. Pract.* **1987**, *28*, 1030–1036.
39. Pamela, J.R. *Excel-Erated Learning*; James & Kenneth Publishers: Berkeley, CA, USA, 1996.
40. Abrantes, R. *Dog Language: An Encyclopedia of Canine Behaviour*; Wakan Tanka Publishers: Wenatchee, WA, USA, 1997; pp. 92–251.
41. Coren, S. *The Intelligence of Dogs: A Guide to the Thoughts, Emotions, and Inner Lives of Our Canine Companions*; Simon and Schuster, Inc.: New York, NY, USA, 2005.
42. Coren, S. *How to Speak Dog: Mastering the art of Dog-Human Communication*; Simon and Schuster, Inc.: New York, NY, USA, 2010.
43. Overall, K.L. *Clinical Behavioral Medicine for Small Animals*; Mosby, Inc.: St. Louis, MO, USA, 1997; pp. 9–44.

44. Farroni, T.; Csibra, G.; Simion, F.; Johnson, M.H. Eye contact detection in humans from birth. *Proc. Natl. Acad. Sci. USA* **2002**, *99*, 9602–9605.
45. Miklósi, Á.; Kubinyi, E.; Topál, J.; Gácsi, M.; Virányi, Z.; Csányi, V. A simple reason for a big difference: Wolves do not look back at humans, but dogs do. *Curr. Biol.* **2003**, *13*, 763–766.
46. Beerda, B.; Schilder, M.B.; van Hooff, J.A.; de Vries, H.W. Manifestations of chronic and acute stress in dogs. *Appl. Anim. Behav. Sci.* **1997**, *52*, 307–319.
47. De Palma, C.; Viggiano, E.; Barillari, E.; Palme, R.; Dufour, A.B.; Fantini, C.; Natoli, E. Evaluating the temperament in shelter dogs. *Behaviour* **2005**, *142*, 1307–1328.
48. Fox, M.W. The anatomy of aggression and its ritualization in Canidae: A developmental and comparative study. *Behaviour* **1969**, *35*, 242–258.
49. Morton, D. Docking of dogs: practical and ethical aspects. *Vet. Rec.* **1992**, *131*, 301–306.
50. Wansbrough, R.K. Cosmetic tail docking of dogs. *Aust. Vet. J.* **1996**, *74*, 59–63.
51. Quaranta, A.; Siniscalchi, M.; Vallortigara, G. Asymmetric tail-wagging responses by dogs to different emotive stimuli. *Curr. Biol.* **2007**, *17*, R199–R201.

2

No Pet or Their Person Left Behind: Increasing the Disaster Resilience of Vulnerable Groups through Animal Attachment, Activities and Networks

Kirrilly Thompson [1,*], Danielle Every [1], Sophia Rainbird [1], Victoria Cornell [2], Bradley Smith [1] and Joshua Trigg [1]

[1] Appleton Institute, Central Queensland University, 44 Greenhill Road, Wayville, Adelaide, SA 5034, Australia; E-Mails: d.every@cqu.edu.au (D.E.); s.rainbird@cqu.edu.au (S.R.); b.p.smith@cqu.edu.au (B.S.); j.trigg@cqu.edu.au (J.T.)

[2] Faculty of Medicine, Nursing and Health Sciences, Flinders University, Adelaide, SA 5001, Australia; E-Mail: victoria.cornell@flinders.edu.au

* Author to whom correspondence should be addressed; E-Mail: kirrilly.thompson@cqu.edu.au.

Simple Summary: The potential for reconfiguring pet ownership from a risk factor to a protective factor for natural disaster survival has been recently proposed. But how might this resilience-building proposition apply to members of the community who are already considered vulnerable? This article addresses this important question by synthesizing information about what makes seven particular groups vulnerable, the challenges to increasing their resilience and how animals figure in their lives. It concludes that animal attachment could provide a novel conduit for accessing, communicating with and motivating vulnerable people to engage in resilience building behaviors that promote survival and facilitate recovery.

Abstract: Increased vulnerability to natural disasters has been associated with particular groups in the community. This includes those who are considered *de facto* vulnerable (children, older people, those with disabilities *etc.*) and those who own pets (not to mention pets themselves). The potential for reconfiguring pet ownership from a risk factor to a protective factor for natural disaster survival has been recently proposed. But how might this resilience-building proposition apply to vulnerable members of the community who own pets or other animals? This article addresses this important question by synthesizing information about what makes particular groups vulnerable, the challenges to increasing their resilience and how animals figure in their lives. Despite different vulnerabilities, animals were found to be important to the disaster resilience of seven vulnerable groups in Australia. Animal attachment and animal-related activities and networks are identified as underexplored devices for disseminating or 'piggybacking' disaster-related information and engaging vulnerable people in resilience building behaviors (in addition to including animals in disaster planning initiatives in general). Animals may provide the kind of innovative approach required to overcome the challenges in accessing and engaging vulnerable groups. As the survival of humans and animals are so often intertwined, the benefits of increasing the resilience of vulnerable communities through animal attachment is twofold: human and animal lives can be saved together.

Keywords: pets; animal attachment; natural disasters; vulnerability; resilience; protective factors; risk factors; preparedness; response and recovery

---

1. Introduction

Humans form strong attachments to pets and other animals. The complex interdependency of human and animal survival has been demonstrated during natural disasters when people risk their own lives to save those of animals [1,2] or lose their lives trying. However, rather than see animal attachment as a risk factor for human survival, there is significant potential for using animal-attachment to motivate disaster preparedness, early evacuation and survival [3]. That is, animal attachment can be used to motivate actions that improve survival and increase disaster resilience. However, resilience is not evenly distributed across the community [4] (p. 2), leaving some groups more vulnerable than others. The Australian National Strategy for Disaster Resilience [4] warns that the level of exposure to disaster risk, understanding of risk, and ability to respond and recover from disasters vary. Factors such as remoteness, mobility, age and speaking English as a second language can all play a role in the vulnerability of individuals to disasters. As animal attachment can be seen as an additional factor, there is a need to understand how animals and pet ownership impact the disaster resilience of vulnerable people.

In Australia, five groups are commonly described as 'vulnerable': Indigenous Australians, culturally and linguistically diverse communities (CALD), children and youth, the elderly and people with disabilities [5]. Two other groups also warrant consideration: the homeless and people with mental health issues. The difficulties in engaging vulnerable groups in disaster resilience initiatives include access, resonance, motivation, communication and language. That is, how do we find them, why should they care, what would make them act, how can we contact them and what form should our communications, warnings and messaging take? As vulnerable people can often be socially isolated and not always literate, innovative engagement strategies are required. Engaging vulnerable people in disaster resilience strategies through their desire to save pets and animals could be one effective approach. We use the term 'vulnerable' as a term of convenience and imply that these groups are under a higher level of risk (or 'at risk'), but appreciate that not all members within a group have the same potential to be resilient and resourceful.

As discussed below, pets and animals are important to vulnerable people for practical and personal reasons. It follows that pets and animals impact the emergency behavior and disaster resilience of those vulnerable people who own or care for them. For instance, vulnerable people may be reluctant to evacuate without their animals, may decline emergency accommodation if their animal is unwelcome, and may struggle more than others to cope with recovery and rebuilding without them. This article suggests that animal attachment and animal-related activities could be successful vehicles for disseminating information and engaging vulnerable people in strategies designed to increase resilience. As argued in relation to the general population [3], encouraging vulnerable groups to think about emergency planning for their pet or animal could motivate them to prepare for themselves. In addition, where there is a need for an innovative approach that resonates strongly with a target audience—as is the case with vulnerable groups—animal attachment could be particularly effective in engaging animal owners and guardians in disaster resilience behaviors. That is, pet and animal-related activities and social networks could be used as conduits for disseminating disaster resilience information and engaging pet and animal owners in disaster resilience building behaviors.

This success of 'piggybacking' one message onto another can be seen in the promotion of dog walking as a public health strategy to increase human activity [6]. Such opportunistic messaging also underpins comments in the guide to Vulnerable Persons Registers. For example,

> *If someone calls for themselves or a family member or friend, this is a good opportunity to provide someone with information about emergency planning resources and to encourage them to undertake some planning activities or to prompt the person they are calling about to connect with local community or personal networks* [7].

Similarly, incorporating disaster resilience materials and strategies in existing animal-related motivations, activities and social networks could serve to increase disaster awareness, preparedness and resilience. Indeed, resilience is linked to a community's ability to 'use local networks and resources to support actions required during an emergency and to support recovery efforts' [4] (p. 10). As such, this article supports the earlier assertion that animal attachment could be used to increase disaster resilience and survival across the general population [3]. However, animals are arguably more important to people for whom the challenges associated with disaster resilience are compounded by vulnerabilities.

2. Method

Before considering the relationship between animals and disaster resilience, it is necessary to provide a note on the material that supports this paper. The authors searched English language academic literature from October 2013 to December 2013 with a focus on the seven vulnerable groups: Indigenous Australians, culturally and linguistically diverse communities (CALD), children and youth, the elderly, people with disabilities, the homeless and people with mental health issues. Given the paucity of available literature on the topic of improving the resilience of specific vulnerable communities using animal attachment, and given the diversity of the groups, there was no systematic procedure followed, and no time limit on academic literature. However, by synthesizing literature on what makes these groups vulnerable, the challenges to building their disaster resilience and how animals figure in their lives, it was possible to develop some literature-informed propositions.

Notwithstanding the fact that general emergency management for all seven groups is under-researched, this article is the first to synthesize information on vulnerability, disaster resilience and pet ownership across the groups to concurrently consider the topic of animals, disasters and vulnerability. Whilst the majority of research has been focussed on domestic pets such as cats and dogs, this article is interested in animals broadly (pets, companion animals, livestock, wildlife).

3. What Do Animals Have to Do with Disaster Resilience?

Humans form close interpersonal relationships that are commonly referred to as 'attachments.' Within psychology, Attachment Theory is associated with John Bowlby [8] and Mary Ainsworth's [9] research on affectional ties between a primary caregiver and infant. It has since been extended to describe the close bonds formed between humans and non-human animals [10–12]. The essential premise of Attachment Theory is that individuals exercise attachment strategies, with the goal of establishing and maintaining proximity to an attachment figure' [8]. To act as a source of psychological security, attachment figures should provide:

(1) Proximity maintenance—they are sought out and available in times of need;
(2) Safe haven—they offer protection and support to relieve distress;
(3) Secure base—they act as a reliable presence that facilitates and permits risk-taking and exploration; and
(4) Separation distress—prompted by separation from or actual loss of the figure [13].

The threat of actual or symbolic danger to the relationship triggers attachment strategies that employ these criteria seen, for example, in the seeking of proximity to the figure (or the reluctance to abandon an animal).

Research suggests that companion animals—particularly dogs—satisfy the above criteria, with proximity maintenance [14], as well as safe haven and secure base [15] the most salient features. According to Ainsworth, this overall perception of felt security and comfort is a fundamental characteristic of the attachment-type affectional bond to a unique figure that '… is never wholly interchangeable with, or replaceable by another …' [16] (p. 711). Many guardians would agree that their animal charges are unique and irreplaceable. Attachment Theory then represents a valuable tool for understanding why people risk their lives to save animals during natural disasters. However, the willingness of people to save animals such as wildlife with whom they do not demonstrate a 'textbook' attachment relationship suggests that other explanations may be required to explain the willingness of humans to save animal lives; that this behavior is driven by other motivations besides attachment (such as obligation and morality); or that attachment could manifest in more spontaneous and transient forms, such as hope symbolism [17]. Whatever the motivation, such actions are open to public interpretation and re-interpretation, mostly according to the outcome of animal rescue attempts [18].

Regardless of the terminology (for a discussion of 'animal as extended self' [19,20] as an alternative theory to explain human risk-taking behavior to save animals, see Thompson [3], there is clear evidence that the safety of humans and animals is intertwined during disasters [1,2,21]. The literature on animals and disasters is limited, yet diverse. It spans the impact of pet ownership on evacuation failure [1,2], the anthropogenic causes of mass animal deaths during natural disasters—especially in relation to intense animal farming or production [21], emergency accommodation for animals, public health implications of abandoned pets and pets in shelters, implications for responders and emergency services personnel [22,23], implications for animal rights advocates [24], the planning, management and administration of animals during disasters [21,25,26], the emotional impact of pet loss following disasters [23,27], risk factors for pet evacuation failure [1], and risk factors for losing a pet during a disaster [28]. Together, this body of research characterizes animal ownership as a risk factor for disaster survival.

Indeed, over 8% of flood-related fatalities in Australia from 1788 to September 1996 resulted from people's attempts to save 'stock, property or pets'—even when the animal or pet was not their own [29] (p. 406), such as when 'good Samaritans' attempted animal rescue. Further afield, Heath, Kass and others found that Californian animal owners were less likely to evacuate than non-owners [2]. Their study on flood evacuation behavior found ownership of pets the greatest reason for failure to evacuate in houses without children, with the risk of failing to evacuate increasing twofold for every additional companion cat or dog in the household [2]. Howlett and Turnbull cite a USA study finding that more than 80% of animal owners would risk their lives to save their animal [30] (p. 3). Heath, Voeks *et al.* identified that when animal owners do evacuate, they are likely to return to try to rescue their animals [1]. When people risk their lives to save or return to animals, they also endanger the lives of others [24] such as family, friends, neighbors, rescue and relief personnel.

However, given that more than half the population own pets, there is arguably more risk in **not** helping people to safely accommodate animals in their emergency plans. There are high levels of pet ownership in developed societies, such as 63% in Australia and the US [26,31]. That leaves another large percentage of the population with animals in their lives, through co-location or their social relations with pet owners. In fact, pet ownership and animal interactions are an important part of everyday life in Australia, with 91% of Australian pet owners reporting feeling 'very close' to their pet [32] (p. 73). Shifting focus from the risk of animal ownership to the risk of not helping animal owners/guardians to save themselves and their animals might just save more lives. That is, the idea of animal attachment as risk factor could be reconfigured to one of protective factor [3]. By motivating people to develop and activate their emergency preparedness and response [26], animal attachment could improve the survival rates of animal owners, guardians and others who may risk their lives to rescue animals such as the 'good Samaritans' mentioned above in relation to flood-related deaths.

Animals are no less significant in the recovery and rebuilding phases of a disaster, due to the psychological impact of animal loss [33,34]. Whilst the emotional impact of the loss of human life is widely acknowledged, the loss of animals can also result in significant grief and psychological trauma [27]. When animal loss occurs alongside a traumatic event such as a disaster, the impact can be overwhelming [28]. In the case of a natural disaster, humans often experience 'post-disaster distress' [27], especially following 'enforced abandonment' [35] of animals or feelings of blame for not having made the necessary precautions for the life of their animal. They may also experience guilt because their grief of losing an animal is socio-culturally less valued than the grief of losing a human. This trauma is not specific to close relations with domestic companion animals. Farmers can also experience psychological trauma from the loss of livestock and substantial financial losses [23]. For example, the biological disaster of an outbreak of foot and mouth disease in the UK in 2001 which involved the slaughter of more than four million cows, pigs and sheep also resulted in more than 80 suicides by farmers and other affected people [21] (pp. 14–15). Therefore, helping people to save animals is relevant not only to disaster planning and survival but to recovery and rebuilding in the days, weeks, months and years after a disaster.

In the same way that animal attachment could be reconfigured from risk factor to protective factor for natural disaster survival, so too could vulnerability be converted into resilience. The term resilience is widely used across many disciplines, for example ecology, engineering, and psychology; each conveying their own nuance. However, '...all definitions are linked to the ability of a system, entity, community or person to withstand shocks while still maintaining its essential functions' [36] (p. 2). Of particular relevance to this article, is community resilience. Community resilience can be complex, as 'it involves the interaction of individuals, families, groups and the environment' [37] (p. 9) and it 'is dependent on social interaction and collective action based on networks of relationships, reciprocity, trust, and social norms' [37] (p. 11). A resilient community is one whose members are connected to one another and work together, and which can adapt to changes in the physical, social or economic environment. The role that animals can play in community connectedness is revealed in research on pets and social capital [38]. That is, pets provide social capital through which people can interact with others, build social networks and feel good about their local neighborhood [39]. In this way, they can counter social isolation that has been linked with vulnerability.

The Victorian Vulnerable People in Emergencies Policy defines a vulnerable person as 'someone living in the community who is: frail, and/or physically or cognitively impaired; and unable to comprehend warnings and directions and/or respond in an emergency situation' [40] (p.3). For inclusion on the state Vulnerable Persons Register, a person needs to additionally be unable to 'identify personal or community support networks to help them in an emergency' [40] (p. 3). Despite the accepted view that pets provide social capital [39], that social capital is important to resilience [41], and that animals provide psychological, emotional, health, wellbeing and practical benefits to vulnerable people [42], there has been no systematic investigation of the impact of animals on the resilience of vulnerable groups. This article is the first to consider the ways in which animals could be used to increase the disaster resilience of vulnerable groups. They are discussed below, according to their characteristics and prevalence, challenges to their disaster resilience, the role of animals in their lives and the impact of animals on their resilience. Once these aspects are outlined, we hypothesize the potential value of using animal attachment to improve the resilience of these vulnerable groups.

4. Vulnerable Groups and the Roles of Animals in Their Lives

To determine the extent to which animal attachment could be used to increase the disaster resilience of vulnerable groups in the community, it is important to first understand who those groups are, what makes them vulnerable to disasters, and how animals play a role in their lives. Seven vulnerable groups are discussed below, in no particular order.

4.1. Indigenous Australians Living in Remote Communities

The term 'Indigenous Australian' refers to those who identify as being of Aboriginal or Torres Strait Islander origin, and who are accepted as such by the community with which the persons associate [43]. There is a growing movement of Indigenous Australians away from major centers to outstations and homeland communities. This has led to the establishment of small Indigenous settlements in often extremely remote locations [44,45]. The development of remote communities has been identified as a particular challenge for disaster resilience [4] (p. 12) because they are typically located in areas that are susceptible to natural hazards such as cyclones, flooding and bushfire. These communities can be difficult to relocate during natural disasters for reasons of tradition, culture and cost. Communities are often forced to seek shelter or refuge in inappropriate buildings, or forced to evacuate by air due to damage caused to access roads.

Animals feature heavily in the lives of Indigenous lifestyle and spirituality [46]. Dogs are the most common companion animals found in Indigenous communities as they are considered an intrinsic part of the community. Unfortunately, pet ownership numbers are not reported for Indigenous peoples. However, it is not uncommon for domestic dogs to outnumber people in Indigenous communities [47,48]. Indigenous Australians have an enduring relationship with dogs that first began with dingoes [49]. The relationship between dogs and humans is intricately linked, and this relationship has changed over time incorporating new perspectives and dog keeping practices. Both dingoes, and now dogs, are considered sacred animals and deeply incorporated into Aboriginal society. For example, they are formally included in family units, (*i.e.*, they are afforded traditional or kinship names) and incorporated into creation and dreaming knowledge [50]. Indigenous people in contemporary society own dogs for a number of reasons, including companionship, as a physical and spiritual protector, to assist in hunting, and as a source of warmth [51].

There are three categories of dogs found in Indigenous communities; (1) the traditionally valued hunting dogs, (2) the community or free-living community dogs, and (3) the pet dogs. Hunting dogs are named and incorporated into the local kinship system. They are highly valued, play an important role in protecting and feeding the community and are often purchased and/or brought in from outside the community. Community dogs are typically unnamed and loosely attached to households, but not directly owned by anyone. These dogs usually fend for themselves and obtain food through eating disregarded remains or fighting favored dogs (hunting dogs, or those that are owned and directly cared for). Another is the pet dog. These are given names, collars, allowed in the house, and generally well fed and cared for [47].

Regardless of a lack of formal ownership and direct care, community dogs are still highly meaningful and useful to the community [46]. For example, around households the dogs combine with the other dogs to create a body of animals protecting a household from both human and spirit intruders [47]. On a community level, larger dog populations are perceived as having special intuitive powers. It is believed that dogs sense human deaths and usually alert the community of a death by howling [47]. Although many of the dogs in communities appear neglected to outsiders [46], this is not entirely reflective of care and ownership, but more a lack of knowledge and/or access to veterinary care.

In relation to disaster response, if evacuation is essential, it is important to note that there may be some individual dogs that are more likely to influence decision to evacuate. For example, companions and prized hunting dogs are likely to be prioritized for evacuation with people, as they will play an important functional role in the aftermath of a disaster for protection and hunting for food. However, this is not to downplay the important social, cultural and practical function of all dogs in remote Indigenous Communities and other animals. Many Indigenous people also share a special relationship with some natural species, or a particular member of that species (e.g., a totem animal such as a kangaroo, eagle *etc.* [50]). Some may choose to stay to protect or care for these animals instead of evacuating.

Evacuations from remote areas are often conducted by air and residents of the community temporarily relocated, so the evacuation of companion animals is problematic. In one published case study, the entire remote community of Kiwirrkurra, Western Australia (170 people) was evacuated to a military base in 2001 due to flooding. This represented a severe disruption to the social fabric of the community, and members commented that their separation contributed to social difficulties. During interviews, residents spoke specifically about how devastated they were to leave their dogs behind. To them, dogs were (and remain) an important cultural element of the community [52]. This suggests that domestic dogs are likely to be an important factor in successful recovery in remote Indigenous communities.

4.2. Culturally and Linguistically Diverse Communities

Like many countries, Australia's population is culturally and linguistically diverse (CALD). CALD people may be migrants, refugees, asylum seekers, international students or second or third generation Australians. 30.2% of Australia's population was born overseas, and of the 69.8% of the population who were born in Australia, 34.3% had both parents born overseas and 11.9% had one parent born overseas [53]. CALD people bring with them a rich array of cultures and languages. A language other than English is spoken at home by almost one quarter (23.2%) of all Australians. Indeed, CALD people may speak one of some 50 languages other than English as recorded by the Australian Bureau of Statistics, including Mandarin (1.6%), Cantonese (1.2%) and Greek (1.2%) [53].

CALD people are more vulnerable to disasters because they may have limited access to information in a relevant language. Following hurricanes and flooding in the US, numerous studies found that ethnic minorities, particularly those with limited English language skills, were hit hardest [54–57]. Following Hurricane Katrina for example, many CALD residents did not evacuate 'because the government failed to issue warnings, evacuation instructions, or hazard and safety precautions in a language they could understand' [58]. Although translation of these materials is typically offered as a solution, low education attainment can create further challenges for CALD people that are not always resolved by good translation. For example, it is possible that some refugees from South Sudanese may be illiterate in their own language [59]. Moreover, information cannot simply be translated, but needs to be culturally appropriate. Important messages can be lost in literal or cultural translation [58,60,61]. Although CALD people are considered to be vulnerable to hazards and risks associated with disasters [58], those from refugee backgrounds in particular are likely to draw on their experience and skill in surviving adversity [62].

The limited literature on pet ownership amongst CALD communities is largely US-based. For instance, studies have found that 'white' people are more likely to own pets than Hispanics, African Americans or Asians [63–65]. However, the term 'white' is not defined and does not take into consideration the cultural and linguistic diversity that 'white' may encompass. Hood's [66] research on pet ownership amongst Asians in Australia makes a similar point; it is equally important to recognize 'cultural, religious and ethnic differences' in pet ownership amongst Asian communities as it is to avoid the mistake of applying 'unhelpful generalizations and stereotyping' [66].

There are some aspects of pet ownership that are unique and specific to particular CALD cultural and religious groups. Dogs might be seen as unclean by some followers of Islam (in accordance with the Qur'an), and are unlikely to be kept as pets in homes [67]. Consequently, in an emergency shelter scenario, some individuals may not appreciate a dog being present [66]. Walker, Robinson and others [68] found that members of CALD communities were less concerned with the 'fate of pets' than non-CALD (cited in [69]). However, only three of the CALD participants in that particular study had responsibility for pets. Whilst CALD pet ownership levels appear low, they may increase across generations. Any benefits of using animal attachment to increase disaster resilience amongst vulnerable communities should thus not be precluded from CALD communities on the assumption of low ownership levels alone.

4.3. Children and Youth

UNESCO identifies children as those under 18 years of age, and youth as those aged between 15 and 24 years [70]. Children and youth equate to 33% of Australia's population [71]. There is a wealth of literature referring to the psychological effects of disaster on children and youth [72–77]. The degree of psychological symptom development is proportionate to the extent of close-exposure of the disaster experienced by the child [78]. Despite young people being referred to as one of the groups most vulnerable to natural disasters [79], school-age children have been found to lack the emergency management training that could assist them and their families to be more resilient [80]. Indeed, Mitchell *et al.* argue that too much emphasis has been placed by researchers (citing [81,82]) on children's vulnerability as 'passive victims with no role to play in communicating risk and participating in decision-making processes' [83]. Instead, they argue that because of the high toll of child deaths in disasters, children should be involved in disaster planning.

According to Chaseling [84], pet ownership is highest amongst families with children. Dogs and cats are the most popular pets, whilst there are also high numbers of pet birds and fish [84]. Research has found that having a pet improves children's health outcomes [85,86]. Animals improve the lives of children with disabilities, for instance Assistance Dogs Australia supporting children with autism [87–89]. Pets are also understood to 'aid childhood development especially nurturing and social skills' [90]. They can be particularly important in helping children who are experiencing stress [91]. Indeed, studies have found benefits of animals including a decrease in stress including anxiety and fear in hospitalized children when receiving Animal-Assisted Therapy [92]. Of particular importance to the role that animals can play in assisting children to cope with and recover from a disasters, pets 'improve feelings of safety and help create social bridges in our communities' [90]. According to Ross *et al.* [93], children may 'view their pet as they would a human sibling' or as a best friend, confidante, 'source of comfort and protection' [93] (p. 81).

In a study of the extent of evacuation during a flooding disaster in the US, families with children were more likely to evacuate than those without children. The study also found that 'pet ownership is associated with household evacuation failure' [2]. The concern is that a family's likelihood of evacuating decreases with pet ownership. Indeed, in an earlier study, Heath *et al.* [94] found that families with children were most likely to re-enter an evacuated area to rescue their pets. However, the risk to children here is not so much in pet ownership, as it is in failing to ensure that children and pets remain safely together during a disaster event. According to Travis [95], pets have a huge impact on the disaster resilience of children, because of the stability pets provide during a traumatic and disruptive event. Research has found that the death of a pet can have a profound effect on a person's emotional health [96,97]. Indeed, the forced separation of a pet during an evacuation can produce the same grief reaction as would the death of a family member or close friend [98]. The most renowned example of a forced separation was witnessed by people around the world as footage of the Hurricane Katrina evacuations recorded a dog named Snowball being torn from the arms of a distraught young boy who was not allowed to bring his pet on a bus [99].

4.4. Older People

Most developed world countries have accepted the chronological ages of either 60 or 65 years as a definition of an older person, which in many cases aligns with the age at which a person becomes eligible for statutory and occupational retirement pensions [100]. As many disaster researchers have highlighted (for example, [101]), it is not advancing age alone that makes older people vulnerable. Rather, age is accompanied by certain characteristics that may decrease resilience:

> *In addition to chronic health conditions, older adults may have impaired physical mobility or cognitive ability, diminished sensory awareness, and social and economic limitations. For example, declining vision or hearing can make it difficult for an older adult to communicate. Older adults with cognitive problems may become agitated during a crisis or feel overwhelmed by the crowding, noise, and lack of privacy in a shelter. They may need assistance to ensure that they have their medications, adequate nutrition and water, and assistive devices* [102] (p. 2).

Older people are sometimes considered to be a challenge with respect to disaster planning due to their perceived reluctance to prepare and evacuate [103–105]. Following disasters, older people often suffer financial hardship and social isolation, exacerbation of existing health conditions and exposure to new health conditions (linked to loss of social support and assistive aids and to impaired access to health services) [106].

As with other vulnerable groups, the current level of animal ownership amongst older Australians is not well understood. In 1994, 32.3% of lone persons aged 60 years or over had a pet [107]. This level is not necessarily indicative of the significance of pets and other animals to older people, and some older people may actively choose to not have pets. Chur-Hansen *et al.* [108] identified emotional and pragmatic explanations. Emotional reasons included good support networks (*i.e.*, no need to share their lives with an animal), not wanting another 'child', and not wanting to go through the grieving process when the pet dies. Pragmatic reasons included living arrangements (e.g., retirement village which might not allow pets), the desire to travel (and not worry about the care of a pet), health concerns (such as falls, cleanliness of the pet), the expense of keeping a pet, and worries about what would happen to the pet if the older person was no longer able to care for it. This is despite the development of some support programs to help older people keep pets in their lives. One established program is the Royal Society for the Prevention of Cruelty to Animals (RSPCA) *Pets for Older Persons* program, which helps older people by looking after pets during times of personal crisis, such as a medical emergency or requirement of the older person for respite care [83]. The program also can assist with veterinary treatment and pet grooming.

Pets can play a role in the resilience of older people due to their recognized positive effects including companionship, a feeling of purpose and self-identity, and a motivation to engage in daily social activity [109,110]. However, research on the benefits of pet ownership for older people is scant, often anecdotal or methodologically weak, and shows mixed results [108,111]. There may be negative effects relating to pets as trip hazards that increase the likelihood of falls in the older person [112,113].

There is scant evidence in the literature of animal attachment impacting on the behavior of older people during disasters specifically. One US study found that 'pet ownership was not a significant risk factor for evacuation failure of households with seniors' [2] (p. 661). They also recognize the other possible evacuation impediments related to old age in general, as noted above.

4.5. People with Disabilities

A disability is a long-term physical, mental, intellectual or sensory impairment which intersects with social, political and economic barriers to hinder a person's full and equal participation in society [114]. Disabilities and activity limitations include: conditions which interfere with mobility (e.g., arthritis, chronic fatigue syndrome), respiratory conditions (e.g., asthma), cognitive difficulties (e.g., dementia), vision loss and hearing loss [115]. In 2009, four million Australians (18.5% of the population) reported having a disability [116].

People with a disability suffer higher rates of mortality and injury in disasters [117]. In relation to preparedness, research has found that whilst people with a disability may have located a shelter or prepared medical supplies, they were overall inadequately prepared for disasters [118–120]. There is also a lack of preparedness at an institutional level. For example, Kendall-Tackett & Mona [121] found that the majority of emergency personnel are not trained in responding to people with a disability. Rooney and White [122] note that people with a disability have been left behind in emergency situations because they were not assisted or accommodated within building and emergency plans. In relation to accessing information, current emergency communication networks do not take into account people with a hearing disability and those with vision impairment [123]. In relation to evacuation, most evacuation plans require people to be able to walk, drive, see, or hear and thus are not accessible by people with disabilities [124], which means many cannot evacuate under current systems. There are also specific evacuation shelter needs to take into consideration. Takahashi *et al.* [125] found that people with an intellectual disability were rejected and segregated by their neighbors in refuges due to social discomfort, which created extreme distress for the people with disabilities. Finally, in relation to recovery, loss of supports and aids such as vehicles, medical equipment and accessible housing severely limits independence post-disaster [117].

The existing research on animals as disability aids highlights additional benefits to social, emotional and psychological wellbeing. Lane, Nicholas and Collis [126] surveyed 57 people with a disability assistance dog. They reported an increased sense of social integration and enhancement to self-perceived health. Hart, Zasloff & Benfatto [127] surveyed 38 people with hearing assistance dogs and found that, as well as providing assistance by alerting them to sounds, hearing dogs also increased the owner's sense of safety, decreased feelings of loneliness especially through changing their interactions within their family and with the hearing community, and also reduced stress. Whitmarsh [128] surveyed 800 visually impaired people. Their respondents cited the benefits of guide dog ownership as: independence, confidence, companionship, increased and changed social interaction and increased mobility. Guest *et al.* [129] undertook a longitudinal study of 51 people with a hearing impairment which measured psychological health and wellbeing prior to receiving a disability assistance dog and up to 18 months after they received their dog. They found that after receiving a dog there were significant reductions in hearing-related problems, as well as in tension, anxiety and depression, and improvements in social involvement and independence. These findings are supported by Valentine *et al.* [42]. There is also research demonstrating the strong bond between people with a disability and their assistance animals [126], and intense grief when the dog dies [130].

4.6. The Homeless

There were 105,237 homeless people in Australia in 2011, representing 0.5% of the population [131]. There is scant Australian research on homelessness and disaster preparedness and response [132]. From the existing research, there are four risk factors which increase homeless people's propensity to death, injury and loss during a disaster and to poor recovery post disaster: (1) lack of resources, (2) lack of access to services, (3) limited social inclusion, and (4) pre-existing physical, mental and emotional stressors [133]. These factors have significant implications for preparedness, communication, transportation, evacuation, sheltering, health and recovery [134]. In particular, people experiencing homelessness have limited or no access to the media through which disaster warnings and information are commonly communicated such as television, radio, and internet. As homeless people have not been included in disaster planning in Australia, they are less likely to be warned, found and evacuated, or provided with adequate support post-disaster [133,135]. Pre-existing trauma heightens the experience of disaster and may mean that homeless people are more vulnerable to post-traumatic stress disorder [134]. In terms of recovery from a disaster, people experiencing homelessness will also be more vulnerable because of the disruption to safe places, sleeping places and income (e.g., Big Issue, recycling, the underground economy) [134]. Moreover, their homelessness may make them ineligible for post-disaster assistance programs, such as housing support [136].

There are no publicly available statistics on the rate of pet or animal ownership amongst people experiencing homelessness in Australia. Rates are likely to be similar to those in the US, where between five and ten percent of people experiencing homelessness also have a pet [137].

Existing research on the relationship between people experiencing homelessness and their pets is primarily qualitative and is US-based. Brewbaker [138] found that dogs were a source of comfort amidst the hardships of homelessness, improving emotional, physical and social wellbeing. Irvine [139] found that dogs helped reduce the social isolation of homeless people by facilitating contact with others. They also provided a 'moral identity' both for the person and for others. This is important, given that people experiencing homelessness often internalize many of the dominant negative discourses that they are lazy, unacceptable and irresponsible. Caring for and being responsible for a pet helps homeless people change these internalized stories about themselves. Being seen with a dog also tends to discourage passers-by from yelling abuse [140,141]. Rew [142] interviewed 42 homeless young people, all of whom reported deep feelings of loneliness. Thirteen of the young people reported that in coping with this loneliness, their pets provided unconditional love, reduced loneliness, and improved their health. They also provided companionship and friendship [141]. In fact, Taylor *et al.* [143] found that the attachment bond was stronger between homeless people and their pets than for those who have secure housing [144].

When the bond between person and pet is severed, people experiencing homelessness report significant grief. In an Australian study, Slatter *et al.* [141] interviewed 26 homeless people living in Australia's Gold Coast about their experiences of pet ownership. Many spoke of grief, loneliness and declining mental health on losing an animal when they became homeless, not being able to keep their pets in shelters, or through not being able to meet council regulations. Being separated from their pets through loss or death is a time of significant grief [141]. In particular, the loss of a pet is one of the most significant stressors for children who are experiencing homelessness [145,146].

This research on the bonds between homeless people and their pets, and the role of pets in reducing isolation and improving mental and physical wellbeing are supported by anecdotal evidence. For example, Munro [147] presents the story of Chris Curran, who felt that people stopped to chat and smile at him more when he was with his dog Princess, rather than 'looking down on' him. Many people with whom Munro spoke chose to stay with their pets on the streets rather than enter shelters where their pets were not allowed.

As noted above, research on homeless people and disasters is meager, and research on the role that animals might play is non-existent. However, as with other groups, it is expected that homeless people will be reluctant to leave their animals behind as part of a disaster evacuation. They may also struggle to find evacuation shelters that will accommodate them and their animals, due to a lack of animal vaccination records and other documentation.

4.7. People with Mental Health Issues

Mental illness is a general term that encompasses 'a health problem that significantly affects how a person feels, thinks, behaves and interacts with other people' [148]. Disorders include affective and anxiety disorders, substance abuse, and psychotic disorders (schizophrenia and bipolar disorder). In 2007, 45% of the Australian population (7.3 million) had experienced an anxiety or affective disorder (e.g., PTSD, depression, bipolar), or a substance abuse disorder at some stage of their lives, and 20% (3.2 million) had experienced them in the previous 12 months [149]. As with people experiencing homelessness, there are four risk factors which increase the vulnerability to death, injury and loss during a disaster and to poor recovery post disaster for person's experiencing a mental illness: (1) lack of resources, (2) lack of access to services, (3) limited social inclusion, and (4) pre-existing physical, mental and emotional stressors [133].

There are a wide variety of symptoms, treatments, effects and levels of severity of mental illness. People with a panic disorder may struggle to leave the house whereas people with a psychotic disorder may lose touch with reality. The severity can range from mild to severe. Despite this, mental health consumers are no less likely than others to demonstrate heroism, resilience and adaptability to disaster. However, there are some common correlates of mental health issues that may increase their risk in a disaster. These vulnerabilities arise from a lack of resources, services and inclusion that affects their preparedness, communication, transportation and evacuation, sheltering and recovery. For example, people experiencing mental health issues may have fewer social networks. More limited access to the mainstream methods of communicating emergency information can render them unaware of an emergency. They may also be unfamiliar with emergency language and personnel and more likely to react negatively to seeing people in safety clothing, interacting with unknown people, and responding to demands [150]. Post-disaster services may not be appropriate for people with a mental illness [151] and volunteers usually lack appropriate mental health training [150]. There are also particular vulnerabilities relating to pre-existing health conditions. People with a mental illness are more vulnerable to rapid and unplanned changes [151]. A disaster or emergency may trigger the onset of new or recurrent symptoms, or a relapse of substance abuse [152].

There are no comprehensive statistics on pet ownership levels amongst those experiencing a mental health issue in Australia or elsewhere. One study reports that 18.6% of clients of a community mental health service in the US owned a pet, and 63% would like to live with a pet [153]. Other studies examine how pet ownership affects the wellbeing of people with a mental illness. Wisdom *et al.* [154] interviewed 177 adults with a serious mental illness and found that animals assisted recovery through providing empathy and connections which increased social networks, serving as family when these are absent, supporting self-efficacy and a sense of empowerment. In a study of women who had been recently widowed, those who owned pets reported lower drug use and fewer psychiatric symptoms than those who did not own pets [155].

There is also research on the relationship between pet ownership and mental wellbeing more generally [156]. One study of the impact of animal assisted therapy (AAT) on psychiatric patients showed significant decreases in anxiety [157]. AAT decreased violent behavior, and increased language and social skills in children with ADHD [158]. However, responsibility for pet care can exacerbate mental health issues [154].

Further, and relevant for consideration in disaster response, is that higher attachment may be adverse in terms of the effects of the loss of a pet or animal, or the desire/ability to leave them behind [159]. If people with mental health issues do evacuate, they may struggle to find evacuation shelters that will accommodate them due to the stigma attached to their illness, combined with their desire to accommodate their animals.

5. Results and Discussion

5.1. How do Animals Impact the Disaster Resilience of Vulnerable Groups?

Despite the different causes for vulnerability discussed above, and the different ways in which animals are incorporated into the lives and belief systems of the seven vulnerable groups, it is clear that animals contribute positively to the health and wellbeing of vulnerable people. They provide companionship, security, practical assistance and the social capital that counters loneliness and social isolation.

It is therefore hardly surprising that the ways in which vulnerable people perceive and react to natural disasters is influenced by their interactions and relations with pets and other animals. For vulnerable people, animals can influence:

- Perception and recognition of disasters. For example, assistance animals can help in alerting older people to sirens or other emergency warnings.
- Evacuation decisions. For example, homeless people may refuse shelters if they cannot be accompanied by their animals.
- Evacuation behavior. For example, separation from animals can immobilize owners with disability.
- Evacuation experience. For example, separation from animals can exacerbate the social anxiety of those with mental health issues, whilst the presence of animals in shelters may induce anxiety in some CALD people.
- Recovery from disaster. For example, without hunting dogs, Indigenous Australians' ability to hunt for food may be compromised. The loss of pets can increase risk of stress disorders in children and social isolation in older people.

With all of these animal-related impacts on disaster behavior in mind, and to preserve the everyday benefits of pets and other animals to vulnerable groups, animals should be accommodated in disaster management and emergency planning at all jurisdictions and across the community-responder divide.

5.2. What Role Could Animal Attachment Play in Building the Disaster Resilience of Vulnerable People?

Despite different mechanisms and manifestations of vulnerability amongst the seven groups discussed above, the overarching challenges to building their resilience are the four interrelated areas of access, communication, motivation to act, and recovery. To increase their natural disaster resilience, vulnerable people need information that encourages them to make informed decisions leading to action. However, vulnerable people are often socially isolated and thereby difficult to contact for the purposes of successfully delivering information. They may not have the requisite skills or abilities to fully utilize existing initiatives that are mostly in written form and in the English language. They may also face emergencies on an everyday basis that attune them to their short-term needs, and therefore be less engaged with resilience building initiatives for unpredictable events like disasters. Pets, animals and animal-attachment could be used to overcome these challenges in the following ways.

Animals could facilitate better access to vulnerable people. Information about preparing animals and pets for disaster survival should be standard in general disaster resilience initiatives. But how do we make sure that that information reaches vulnerable people with animals? Disaster resilience building information could be distributed to vulnerable people who have pets by utilizing existing animal-related activities and networks. For people with disabilities, this could be Assistance Dogs Australia. For the homeless, it could be through the RSPCA program *Living Ruff*, the New South Wales program *Pets in the Park*, and the Queensland program *Pawprints*, which provide pet health clinics and free veterinary services, as well as food and emergency shelter for animals.

One means of attracting homeless people into animal-related networks could be via encouraging them to microchip and vaccinate their pet. To create new animal-related networks, these services could be provided free of charge to those who could not otherwise afford them. Microchipping and vaccination could increase acceptance of homeless people and their pets in emergency shelters. Using animals as a conduit for disaster resilience initiatives could have the added benefit of building social capital whilst reducing perceived threat from communicators. This is particularly relevant for those vulnerable groups who experience social isolation and those who may be suspicious or feel threatened by strangers.

Animals could facilitate better communication with vulnerable people. In a study of emergency response for the Sudanese community, Glasgow [160] identifies several engagement strategies that can be entirely independent from written material, such as visual resources, face to face demonstrations, settlement support services, ethnic community groups and ethnic radio stations. Similarly, information in animal-related networks and activities (such as pet care seminars, or free animal health checks) could be used to communicate disaster resilience information. As communication should also be accessible to people with different abilities (especially those with hearing and sight impairment), determining how animal attachment can exactly be used to increase disaster resilience could drive innovation in oral or visual media communication.

Animals could facilitate better motivation for vulnerable people to prepare and act. As described in the introduction in relation to the general population, a desire to protect their pets and animals could motivate vulnerable people who would not otherwise take resilience building actions (be that staying and defending, evacuating with pet or evacuating without pet).

Animals could facilitate better recovery for vulnerable people. Vulnerable people often face additional challenges during recovery from a disaster, due to issues with social and cultural isolation, mental health, developmental stresses (in the case of children) and age-related conditions. As pets and other animals provide assistance for these challenges in daily life, recovery without pets can lead to their exacerbation in life after a disaster. During disasters, owners and responders may be faced with the sight of distressed or dying animals, and sometimes the task of euthanizing them. This adds another layer of emotional distress to recovery (see, for example [23]). Avoiding these disturbing experiences, and maximizing the value of pets and other animals in improving the recovery of vulnerable people after disasters is a compelling rationale for ensuring that all measures are taken to ensure that pets as well as people survive natural disasters. As animal lives are so frequently dependent on humans for survival, sometimes animals are reliant on the actions made by (or available to) vulnerable people. The benefits of animals to vulnerable people during disaster recovery and rebuilding are not confined to animal guardians alone. Animal assisted therapy and simple animal-assisted interactions can facilitate and improve interpersonal interactions.

5.3. Recommendations for Further Research

Further empirical research is required to further substantiate the literature and theory based proposition made in this article that animal attachment, activities and networks can be used as conduits for building disaster resilience amongst vulnerable people. The following avenues for research would be valuable:

(1) Systematic collection of data on pet and animal ownership (by the Australian Bureau of Statistics (ABS) or Australian Companion Animal Council (ACAC)) that can indicate or provide:

   a. The vulnerability of respondents.
   b. Incidence and prevalence of pet and animal owners.

c. The numbers and types of pets and animals owned.
d. Language spoken at home.

(2) Forecasting of pet and animal ownership trends, especially for CALD groups.
(3) An understanding of the impact of non-domestic/non-household animals (*i.e.*, birds, horses, donkeys, alpacas) on vulnerable people
(4) A social network analysis to comprehensively understand animal-related social networks, including their reach and media and communication channels
(5) A study of the most effective ways of using animal attachment and animal-related activities and networks to promote disaster resilience (media communication, *etc.*)
(6) A study of the most effective ways for vulnerable people to evacuate with their animals (e.g., interactions with responders)
(7) Practical translation of plans for vulnerable people to evacuate with their animals for the purposes of identifying barriers to best practice and areas requiring further information and assistance (such as walkthroughs)
(8) An understanding of the role of pets and animals in rebuilding lives and communities after a disaster, with a focus on vulnerable groups or a consideration of vulnerability as it applies to all those who have survived disasters
(9) Other vulnerable groups, such as:

a. People who live alone or without 'personal or community support networks to help them in an emergency' (who are likely to meet the criteria for Vulnerable Persons Registers) [40] (pp. 4–5).
b. Indigenous Australians living in non-remote communities.
c. Non-indigenous Australians living in remote communities.
d. People who have previously survived a disaster.
e. Animals (and how humans impact their disaster resilience, building on Irvine's [21] research).

The research proposed above could (a) support further evaluation for the case for using animal attachment to increase the disaster resilience of vulnerable people and (b), identify the best means of doing so (what works best for whom and under what circumstances).

6. Conclusion

This article critically evaluated the proposition that animal attachment could be used to build disaster resilience [3] even for vulnerable groups. It identified the importance of pets and other animals in the lives of vulnerable people as well as their potential contribution to disaster resilience. In particular, animal attachment and animal related activities and networks could be useful conduits for successfully accessing vulnerable people, communicating resilience building information, engaging pet and animal owners and guardians in resilience building behaviors and facilitating recovery. Of course, not all vulnerable people own animals. However, ownership is high in developed countries and those who do not own animals still have animals in their lives or in their social networks. Moreover, this animal-related 'piggybacking' proposition may have analogies to other situations where people (more or less vulnerable) experience Attachment or what Belk [19] refers to as a relationship of 'extended self' such as houses [161]. Animal attachment and animal-related activities and social networks may provide novel and innovative means to improve disaster preparedness and responsiveness, but the success of the kinds of initiatives suggested throughout this paper may be impeded by pragmatic limitations. For example, it has been incredibly difficult to educate non-vulnerable populations in the US about animal friendly shelters during evacuations [162]. Notwithstanding the challenges to any public health initiative such as funding and government support, there is a clear need to identify who is most at risk of natural disasters and determine how best to access and engage them. However, protection is rarely if ever absolute. We are all vulnerable people and we are all non-human animals. Research and planning should therefore aspire to enable and motivate maximum disaster resilience for all members of the community—humans and nonhuman animals alike; pets and their people.

Acknowledgments

The research on which this article is based was commissioned by the World Society for the Protection of Animals for the Australia-New Zealand Emergency Management Committee in line with the direction of the Standing Council on Police and Emergency Management forward work plan and the National Strategy for Disaster Resilience. Special thanks to Jacqueline Mills, Senior Advisor, Corporate Engagement, Asia Pacific, World Society for the Protection of Animals for her trust, support and expert advice.

Author Contributions

Kirrilly Thomson led this research project. She edited contributions and synthesized them as the current article. She researched and wrote Sections 1, 2, 3, 5 and 6. Danielle Every researched and wrote Sections 4.5, 4.6 and 4.7. Sophia Rainbird researched and wrote Sections 4.2 and 4.3. Victoria Cornell researched and wrote Section 4.4, as well as the discussion of resilience in Section 3. Bradley Smith led the research and writing of Section 4.1. Joshua Trigg researched and wrote the discussion of animal attachment in Section 3. All authors contributed to the drafting of the overall article.

Conflicts of Interest

The authors declare no conflict of interest.

References

1. Heath, S.E.; Voeks, S.K.; Glickman, L.T. Epidemiologic features of pet evacuation failure in a rapid-onset disaster. *J. Am. Vet. Med. Assoc.* **2001**, *218*, 1898–1904.
2. Heath, S.E.; Kass, P.H.; Beck, A.M.; Glickman, L.T. Human and Pet-related Risk Factors for Household Evacuation Failure During a Natural Disaster. *Am. J. Epidemiol.* **2001**, *153*, 659–665.
3. Thompson, K. Save me, save my dog: Increasing natural disaster preparedness and survival by addressing human-animal relationships. *Austr. J. Commun.* **2013**, *40*, 123–136.
4. *National Strategy for Disaster Resilience: Building Our Nation's Resilience to Disasters*; Council of Australian Governments: Canberra, Australia, 2011.

5. *Comnmunique 4–5 July 2013*; Standing Council on Police and Emergency Management: Darwin, Northern Territory, Australia, 2013.
6. Higgins, J.W.; Temple, V.; Murray, H.; Kumm, E.; Rhodes, R. Walking Sole Mates: Dogs Motivating, Enabling and Supporting Guardians' Physical Activity. *Anthrozoos* **2013**, *26*, 237–252.
7. Health and Human Services Emergency Management. *Vulnerable Persons Regisgers (VPRs): Getting Started*; Department of Health Services, State Government of Victoria: Melbourne, Australia, 2012.
8. Bowlby, J. *Attachment: Attachment and Loss*, 2nd ed.; Basic Books: New York, NY, USA, 1999.
9. Ainsworth, M.D.S. Attachments and other affectional bonds across the life cycle. In *Attachment Across the Life Cycle*; Parkes, C.M., Stevenson-Hinde, J., Marris, P., Eds.; Routledge: London, UK, 1991; pp. 33–51.
10. Archer, J. Why do people love their pets? *Evol. Human Behav.* **1997**, *18*, 237–259.
11. Archer, J.; Ireland, J.L. The Development and Factor Structure of a Questionnaire Measure of the Strength of Attachment to Pet Dogs. *Anthrozoos* **2011**, *24*, 249–261.
12. Beck, L.; Madresh, E.A. Romantic Partners and Four-Legged Friends: An Extension of Attachment Theory to Relationships with Pets. *Anthrozoos* **2008**, *21*, 43–56.
13. Mikulincer, M.; Shaver, P.R. The attachment behavioral system: Basic concepts and principles. In *Attachment in Adulthood: Structure, Dynamics, and Change*; The Guilford Press: New York, NY, USA, 2007; pp. 3–28.
14. Kurdek, L.A. Pet dogs as attachment figures. *J. Soc. Person. Relat.* **2008**, *25*, 247–266.
15. Kurdek, L.A. Young adults' attachment to pet dogs: Findings from open-ended methods. *Anthrozoos* **2009**, *22*, 359–369.
16. Ainsworth, M.D.S. Attachments beyond infancy. *Am. Psychol.* **1989**, *44*, 709–716.
17. Due, C.; Thompson, K.; Every, D. 'An image of hope in a week of despair': Representations of 'Sam the Koala' in the Australian mainstream news media. *Media Int. Austr.* **2014**, in press.
18. Every, D.; Due, C.; Thompson, K.; Ryan, J. "I know it sounds silly, but my pets mean the world to me": Conflicting perspectives on animal rescues in natural disasters. *Soc. Anim.* **2014**, in press.
19. Belk, R.W. Possessions and the Extended Self. *J. Consum. Res.* **1988**, *15*, 139–168.
20. Belk, R.W. Metaphoric Relationships with Pets. *Soc. Anim.* **1996**, *4*, 121–145.
21. Irvine, L. *Filling the Ark: Animal Welfare in Disasters*; Temple University Press: Philadelphia, PA, USA, 2009.
22. Schaffer, C.B. Human-Animal Bond Considerations During Disasters. 8 April 2011. Available online: http://www.integratedtrainingsummit.org/presentations/2009/main_training_summit/47_-_human-animal_bond_considerations_during_disasters_-_schaffer_caroline.pdf (accessed on 22 April 2014).
23. Hall, M.J.; Ng, A.; Ursano, R.J.; Holloway, H.; Fullerton, C.; Casper, J. Psychological Impact of the Animal-Human Bond in Disaster Preparedness and Response. *J. Psychiat. Pract.* **2004**, *10*, 368–374.
24. Irvine, L. Animals in Disasters: Issues for Animal Liberation Activism and Policy. *Anim. Liber. Phil. Policy J.* **2006**, *4*, 1–16.

25. Irvine, L. *Animals in Disasters: Responsibility and Action (Policy Paper)*; Animals and Society Institute: Boston, MA, USA, 2007.
26. Leonard, H.A.; Scammon, D.L. No Pet Left Behind: Accommodating Pets in Emergency Planning. *J. Publ. Policy Market.* **2007**, *26*, 49–53.
27. Lowe, S.R.; Rhodes, J.E.; Zwiebach, L.; Chan, C.S. The impact of pet loss on the perceived social support and psychological distress of hurricane survivors. *J. Traum. Stress* **2009**, *22*, 244–247.
28. Zottarelli, L.K. Broken Bond: An Exploration of Human Factors Associated with Companion Animal Loss During Hurricane Katrina1. *Sociol. Forum* **2010**, *25*, 110–122.
29. Coates, L. Flood Fatalities in Australia, 1788–1996. *Austr. Geographer.* **1999**, *30*, 391–408.
30. Howlett, M.; Turnbull, C. *Large Animal Emergency Rescue Training*; AgriFoods Skills Australia International Specialised Skills Institute: Carlton, Australia, 2009.
31. ACAC. *Contribution of the Pet Care Industry to the Australian Economy*, 6th ed.; BIS Shrapnel: Sydney, Australia, 2006.
32. ACAC. *Contribution of the Pet Care Industry to the Australian Economy*, 7th ed.; BIS Shrapnel: Sydney, Australia, 2010.
33. Gerwolls, M.K.; Labott, S.M. Adjustment to the Death of a Companion Animal. *Anthrozoos* **1994**, *7*, 172–187.
34. Planchon, L.A.; Templer, D.I. The Correlates of Grief after Death of Pet. *Anthrozoos* **1996**, *9*, 107–113.
35. Hunt, M.; Al-Awadi, H.; Johnson, M. Psychological Sequelae of Pet Loss Following Hurricane Katrina. *Anthrozoos* **2008**, *21*, 109–121.
36. Rockefeller Foundation. Rebound: Building a More Resilient World; Rockefeller Foundation: New York, NY, USA, 2012.
37. McAslan, A. *Community Resilience: Understanding the Concept and it Application*; Torrens Resilience Institute: Adelaide, Australia, 2010.
38. Putnam, R.D. Bowling alone: America's declining social capital. *J. Democr.* **1995**, *6*, 65–78.
39. Wood, L.; Giles-Corti, B.; Bulsara, M. The pet connection: Pets as a conduit for social capital? *Soc. Sci. Med.* **2005**, *61*, 1159–1173.
40. Health and Human Services Emergency Management. *Vulnerable Peple in Emergencies Policy*; Department of Health and Human Services, State Government of Victoria: Melbourne, Australia, 2012.
41. Kirmayer, L.J.; Whitley, R.; Dandeneau, S.F.; Isaac, C. Community Resilience: Models, Metaphors and Measures. *Int. J. Indigenous Health* **2009**, *5*, 62–117.
42. Valentine, D.; Kiddoo, M.; LaFleur, B. Psychosocial Implications of Service Dog Ownership for People Who Have Mobility or Hearing Impairments. *Soc. Work Health Care* **1993**, *19*, 109–125.
43. *Information Paper: Perspectives on Aboriginal and Torres Strait Islander Identification in Selected Data Collection Contexts, 2012*; Australian Bureau of Statistics (ABS): Belconnen, Australia, 2013.

44. Council of Australian Governments (COAG). *Improving Emergency Management Outcomes for Remote Indigenous Communites in Northern Australia*; COAG Review of Natural Disaster Relief and Mitigation Arrangements; Department of Transport and Regional Services: Canberra, Australia, 2002.
45. Ellemor, H. Reconsidering emergency management and indigenous communities in Australia. *Environ. Hazards* **2005**, *6*, 1–7.
46. Constable, S.; Dixon, R.; Dixon, R. For the Love of Dog: The Human & Dog Bond in Rural and Remote Australian Indigenous Communities. *Anthrozoos* **2010**, *23*, 337–349.
47. Senior, K.; Chenhall, R.; McRae-Williams, E.; Daniels, D.; Rogers, K. Dogs and people in Aboriginal communities: Exploring the relationship within the context of the social determinants of health. *Environ. Health* **2006**, *6*, 39–46.
48. White, I. Hunting dogs at Yalata. *Mankind* **1972**, *8*, 201–205.
49. Smith, B.P.; Litchfield, C.A. A Review of the Relationship between Indigenous Australians, Dingoes (*Canis dingo*) and Domestic Dogs (*Canis familiaris*). *Anthrozoos* **2009**, *22*, 111–128.
50. Rose, D.B. *Dingo Makes Us Human: Life and Land in an Australian Aboriginal Culture*; Cambridge University Press: Cambridge, UK, 2000.
51. Phelan, S. *Conducting Dog Health Programs in Indigenous Communities: A Veterinary Guide*; Report Commissioned by Animal Management in Rural and Remote Indigenous Communities (AMRRIC) and International Fund for Animal Welfare (IFAW); AMRRIC: Darwin, Australia, 2007.
52. Brinkley, C. Kiwirrkurra: The flood in the desert. *Austr. J. Emerg. Manag.* **2009**, *24*, 67–70.
53. 2011 Census QuickStats. People. Cultural & Language Diversity. Australian Bureau of Statistics (ABS), 2011. Available online: http://www.censusdata.abs.gov.au/census_services/getproduct/census/2011/quickstat/0 (accessed on 22 April 2014).
54. Elder, K.; Xirasagar, S.; Miller, N.; Bowen, S.A.; Glover, S.; Piper, C. African Americans' decisions not to evacuate New Orleans before Hurricane Katrina: A qualitative study. *Am. J. Publ. Health* **2007**, *97*(Suppl. 1), S124–S129.
55. Ghosh, T.S.; Patnaik, J.L.; Vogt, R.L. Rapid needs assessment among Hurricane Katrina evacuees in metro-Denver. *J. Health Care Poor Underserved* **2007**, *18*, 362–368.
56. Mathew, A.B.; Kelly, K. *Disaster Preparedness in Urban Immigrant Communities: Lessons Learned from Recent Catastrophic Events and Their Relevance to Latino and Asian Communities in Southern California*; Tomás Rivera Policy Institute, University of Southern California: Los Angeles, CA, USA, 2008.
57. Hurworth, R. *CALD Communities and Emergency Management: A Literature Synthesis*; Centre for Program Evaluation, The University of Melbourne: Melbourne, Australia, 2009.
58. Blazer, J.; Murphy, B. Addressing the Needs of Immigrants and Limited English Communities in Disaster Planning and Relief. Lessons for Government, Disaster Relief Agencies, and Community-Based Organizations. *Immigrants' Rights Update* **2008**, *22*, 1–11.
59. Ziaian, T.; de Anstiss, H.; Antoniou, G.; Baghurst, P.; Sawyer, M. Emotional and behavioural problems among refugee children and adolescents living in South Australia. *Austr. Psychol.* **2011**, *48*, 139–148.

60. Dean, B. Emergency Planning for Culturally and Linguistically Diverse (Cald) Communities. In Proceedings of Policing Partnerships in a Multicultural Australia: Achievements and Challenges Conference, Brisbane, Australia, 25–26 October 2001.
61. *CAMS Submission to the Queensland Floods Commission of Inquiry Queensland*; Ethnic Communities Council of Queensland: West End, Australia, 2011.
62. *Guidelines for Emergency Management in Culturally and Linguistically Diverse Communities*; Emergency Management Australia, Commonwealth of Australia: Dickson, Australia, 2007.
63. Elmore, R.G. Reasons for the lack of racial diversity in veterinary medicine. *J. Vet. Med. Educ.* **2004**, *31*, 414–416.
64. Gardyn, R. Animal magnetism. *Am. Demogr.* **2002**, *24*, 31–37.
65. *1999–2000 APPMA National Pet Owners Survey*; American Pet Products Manufacturing Association (APPMA): Greenwich, CT, USA, 2000.
66. Hood, J. Pet Ownership and Asian Multiculturalism. In Proceedings of the Urban Animal Management Conferences in Australia, Perth, Australia, 7–9 October 1998.
67. Raja, M.A. *Muslim Modernity: Poetics, Politics, and Metaphysics. Muslim Societies and the Challenge of Secularization: An Interdisciplinary Approach*; Springer: Dordrecht, The Netherlands, 2010; pp. 99–111.
68. Walker, R.; Robinson, P.; Tebbutt, J.; Lin, V.; Bisset, P.; Burns, R.; Schauble, J. *Emergency Management Risk Communication Project*; Final Report to Department of Human Services (Victoria); School of Publica Health, La Trobe University: Melbourne, Australia, 2006.
69. Farrow, D.; Rutter, A.; Hurworth, R. *Evaluation of the Inclusive Emergency Management with Culturally and Linguistically Diverse (CALD) Communities Program, July 2006–June 2010*; Centre for Program Evaluation, The University of Melbourne: Melbourne, Australia, 2009.
70. *Understanding Policy Development and Implementation for Children and Young People*; UNESCO, Children and Youth Programme: Galway, Ireland, 2012.
71. 2011 Census of Population and Housing: Basic Community Profile—Australia. Available online: http://www.censusdata.abs.gov.au/census_services/getproduct/census/2011/communityprofile/0 (accessed on 22 April 2014).
72. Green, B.L.; Korol, M.; Grace, M.C.; Vary, M.G.; Leonard, A.C.; Gleser, G.C.; Smitson-Cohen, S. Children and disaster: Age, gender, and parental effects on PTSD symptoms. *J. Am. Acad. Child Adolescent Psychiat.* **1991**, *30*, 945–951.
73. Shannon, M.P.; Lonigan, C.J.; Finch, A.; Taylor, C.M. Children exposed to disaster: I. Epidemiology of post-traumatic symptoms and symptom profiles. *J. Am. Acad. Child Adolescent Psychiat.* **1994**, *33*, 80–93.
74. Thienkrua, W.; Cardozo, B.L.; Chakkraband, M.S.; Guadamuz, T.E.; Pengjuntr, W.; Tantipiwatanaskul, P.; Sakornsatian, S.; Ekassawin, S.; Panyayong, B.; Varangrat, A.; *et al.* Symptoms of posttraumatic stress disorder and depression among children in tsunami-affected areas in southern Thailand. *JAMA* **2006**, *296*, 549–559.
75. Udwin, O.; Boyle, S.; Yule, W.; Bolton, D.; O'Ryan, D. Risk Factors for Long-term Psychological Effects of a Disaster Experienced in Adolescence: Predictors of Post Traumatic Stress Disorder. *J. Child Psychol. Psychiat.* **2000**, *41*, 969–979.

76. Vernberg, E.M.; La Greca, A.M.; Silverman, W.K.; Prinstein, M.J. Prediction of posttraumatic stress symptoms in children after Hurricane Andrew. *J. Abnormal Psychol.* **1996**, *105*, 237–248.
77. Wooding, S.; Raphael, B. Psychological impact of disasters and terrorism on children and adolescents: experiences from Australia. *Prehospital Disaster Med.* **2004**, *19*, 10–20.
78. Gurwitch, R.H.; Kees, M.; Becker, S.M.; Schreiber, M.; Pfefferbaum, B.; Diamond, D. When disaster strikes: Responding to the needs of children. *Prehospital Disaster Med.* **2004**, *19*, 21–28.
79. Ronan, K.; Johnston, D. *Promoting Community Resilience in Disasters: The Role for Schools, Youth, and Families*; Springer, New York, NY, USA, 2005.
80. Foster, H.; Towers, B.; Whittaker, J.; Handmer, J.; Lowe, T. *Peri-Urban Melbourne in 2021: Changes and Implications for the Victorian Emergency Management Sector*; Bushfire and Natural Hazards CRC: Melbourne, Australia, 2012; Volume 28.
81. Ansell, N. *Children, Youth and Development*; Routledge: London, UK, 2004.
82. Anderson, W.A. Bringing children into focus on the social science disaster research agenda. *Int. J. Mass Emerg. Disasters* **2005**, *23*, 159–175.
83. Mitchell, T.; Haynes, K.; Wei, C.; Oven, K. The Roles of Children and Youth in Communicating Disaster Risk. *Child. Youth Environ.* **2008**, *18*, 254–279.
84. Chaseling, S. Pet populations in Australia. Dogs increasing and cats decreasing—Why is it so? In Proceedings of the 10th Urban Animal Management Conference in Australia, Melbourne, Australia, 2001.
85. Kaminski, M.; Pellino, T.; Wish, J. Play and pets: The physical and emotional impact of child-life and pet therapy on hospitalized children. *Child. Health Care* **2002**, *31*, 321–335.
86. Timperio, A.; Salmon, J.; Chu, B.; Andrianopoulos, N. Is dog ownership or dog walking associated with weight status in children and their parents? *Health Promot. J. Austr.* **2008**, *19*, 60–63.
87. Assistance Dogs Australia. 2013. Available online: http://www.assistancedogs.org.au/pages/paws-program.html (accessed on 22 April 2014).
88. Smart Pup. Autism Assist Dogs 2013. Available online: http://www.smartpups.org.au/ (accessed on 2 December 2013).
89. Dogs for Kids with Disabilities (DKD). 2013. Available online: http://www.dogsforkidswithdisabilities.com/default.html (accessed on 2 December 2013).
90. *The Power of Pets: The Benefits of Companion Animal Ownership*; Australian Companion Animal Council Inc.: St Leonards, Australia, 2009.
91. Nagengast, S.; Baun, M.; Megel, M.; Liebowitz, J. The effects of the presence of a companion animal of physiological arousal and behavioral distress in children. *J. Pediat. Nurs.* **1997**, *12*, 323–330.
92. Tsai, C.-C.; Friedmann, E.; Thomas, S.A. The effect of animal-assisted therapy on stress responses in hospitalized children. *Anthrozoos* **2010**, *23*, 245–258.
93. Ross, C.B.; Baron-Sorensen, J. *Pet Loss and Human Emotion*; Taylor & Francis: New York, NY, USA, 2007.
94. Heath, S.E.; Voeks, S.K.; Glickman, L.T. A study of pet rescue in two disasters. *Int. J. Mass Emerg. Disasters* **2000**, *18*, 361–381.

95. Travis, H.J. Children and the Human-Animal Bond: Minimizing Pet Loss During Disasters. In *Teaching Compassion: Humane Education in Early Childhood*; Springer: Dordrecht, The Netherlands, 2014; Volume 8, pp. 133–145.
96. Zottarelli, L.K. Broken Bond: An Exploration of Human Factors Associated with Companion Animal Loss During Hurricane Katrina. *Sociol. Forum* **2010**, *25*, 110–122.
97. Sharkin, B.S.; Knox, D. Pet loss: Issues and implications for the psychologist. *Prof. Psychol. Res. Pract.* **2003**, *34*, 414–421.
98. Chur-Hansen, A. Grief and bereavement issues and the loss of a companion animal: People living with a companion animal, owners of livestock, and animal support workers. *Clin. Psychol.* **2010**, *14*, 14–21.
99. *Organizing Pet-Friendly Evacuation Shelters: Best Practices for Florida—Training Guide*; University of Florida: Gainesville, FL, USA, 2008.
100. World Health Organization. Definition of an older or elderly person. 30 November 2013. Available online: http://www.who.int/healthinfo/survey/ageingdefnolder/en/index.html (accessed one 22 April 2014).
101. Fernandez, L.S.; Byard, D.; Lin, C.-C.; Benson, S.; Barbera, J.A. Frail Elderly as Disaster Victims: Emergency Management Strategies. *Prehospital Disaster Med.* **2002**, *17*, 67–74.
102. Aldrich, N.; Benson, W. Disaster preparedness and the chronic disease needs of vulnerable older adults. *Prev. Chron. Dis.* **2008**, *5*. Available online: http://www.cdc.gov/pcd/issues/2008/jan/07_0135.htm (accessed one 22 April 2014).
103. Paek, H.-J.; Hilyard, K.; Freimuth, V.; Barge, J.K.; Mindlin, M. Theory-based approaches to understanding public emergency preparedness: Implications for effective health and risk communication. *J. Health Commun.* **2010**, *15*, 428–444.
104. Loke, A.Y.; Lai, C.K.Y.; Fung, O.W.M. At-home disaster preparedness of elderly people in Hong Kong. *Geriat. Gerontol. Int.* **2012**, *12*, 524–531.
105. Morrow, B.H. Social vulnerabilities and Hurricane Katrina: An unnatural disaster in New Orleans. *Marine Technol. Soc. J.* **2007**, *40*, 16–26.
106. *Older Persons in Emergencies: An Active Ageing Perspective*; World Health Organization: Geneva, Switerland, 2008.
107. Australian Bureau of Statistics. 4102.0—Australian Social Trends, 1995. Available online: http://www.abs.gov.au/AUSSTATS/abs@.nsf/2f762f95845417aeca25706c00834efa/5EF8016F420622A3CA2570EC00753524 (accessed one 22 April 2014).
108. Chur-Hansen, A.; Winefield, H.; Beckwith, M. Reasons given by elderly men and women for not owning a pet, and the implications for clinical practice and research. *J. Health Psychol.* **2008**, *13*, 988–995.
109. McNicholas, J.; Gilbey, A.; Rennie, A.; Ahmedzai, S.; Dono, J.-A.; Ormerod, E. Pet ownership and human health: A brief review of evidence and issues. *BMJ* **2005**, *331*, 1252–1254.
110. Enders-Slegers, M. The meaning of companion animals: Qualitative analysis of the life histories of elderly cat and dog owners. In *Companions Animals and Us: Exploring the Relationships Between People and Pets*; Podberscek, A., Paul, E., Serpell, J., Eds.; Cambridge University Press: Cambridge, UK, 2000; pp. 237–256.

111. Winefield, H.R.; Black, A.; Chur-Hansen, A. Health effects of ownership of and attachment to companion animals in an older population. *Int. J. Behav. Med.* **2008**, *15*, 303–310.
112. Kurrle, S.E.; Day, R.; Cameron, I.D. The perils of pet ownership: A new fall-injury risk factor. *BMJ* **2004**, *181*, 682–683.
113. Pluijm, S.M.; Smit, J.H.; Tromp, E.A.; Stel, V.S.; Deeg, D.J.; Bouter, L.M.; Lips, P. A risk profile for identifying community-dwelling elderly with a high risk of recurrent falls: Results of a 3-year prospective study. *Osteoporosis Int.* **2006**, *17*, 417–425.
114. Convention on the Rights of Persons with Disabilities 2006. Available online: http://www2.ohchr.org/english/law/disabilities-convention.htm (accessed on 15 December 2013).
115. Kailes, J. Disaster services and "special needs": Term of art or meaningless term? Nobody Left Behind 2005. Available online: http://www2.ku.edu/~rrtcpbs/findings/pdfs/SpecialsNeeds.pdf (accessed on 15 November 2013).
116. *Disability, Australia 2009*; Australian Bureau of Statistics: Canberra, Australia, 2011.
117. White, G.; Fox, M.; Rooney, C.; Cahill, A. Assessing the impact of Hurricane Katrina on persons with disabilities. 2007. Available online: http://www.rtcil.org/products/NIDRR_Executive SummaryKatrinaReport.pdf (accessed on 22 April 2014).
118. Uscher-Pines, L.; Hausman, A.; Powell, S.; DeMara, P.; Heake, G.; Hagen, M. Disaster preparedness of households with special needs in southeastern Pennsylvania. *Am. J. Prev. Med.* **2009**, *37*, 227–230.
119. Bethel, J.; Foreman, A.; Burke, S. Disaster preparedness among medically vulnerable populations. *Am. J. Prev. Med.* **2011**, *40*, 139–143.
120. Hogaboom, N.; Oyster, M.; Riggins, M.; Boninger, M. Evacuation preparedness in full-time wheelchair users with spinal cord injury. *J. Spinal Cord Med.* **2013**, *36*, 290–295.
121. Kendall-Tackett, K.; Mona, L. The impact on 9/11 of people with disabilities: Committee on Disability Issues in Psychology. In Proceedings of the American Psychological Association Conference, Washington, DC, USA, 18–21 August 2005.
122. Rooney, C.; White, G. Narrative analysis of a disaster preparedness and emergency response survey from persons with mobility impairments. *J. Disabil. Policy Stud.* **2007**, *17*, 206–215.
123. Sullivan, H.; Hakkinen, M.; Kawamura, H. Preparedness and warning systems for populations with special needs: Ensuring everyone gets the message (and knows what to do). In Proceedings of the International Conference on Energy, Environment and Disasters, Charlotte, NC, USA, 24–30 July 2005.
124. Njelesani, J.; Cleaver, S.; Tataryn, M.; Nixon, S. Using a Human Rights-Based Approach to Disability in Disaster Management Initiatives. 2012. Available oneline: http://www.intechopen.com/books/natural-disasters/using-a-human-rights-based-approach-to-disability-in-disaster-manatement-initiatives (accessed on 10 November 2013).
125. Takahashi, A.; Watanabe, K.; Oshima, M.; Shimada, H.; Ozawa, A. The effect of the disaster cause by the great Hanshin earthquake on people with intellectual disability. *J. Intell. Disabil. Res.* **1997**, *41*, 193–196.
126. Lane, D.; Nicholas, J.; Collis, G. Dogs for the disabled: Benefits for the recipients and welfare of the dogs. *Appl. Anim. Behav. Sci.* **1998**, *5*, 49–60.

127. Hart, L.; Zasloff, R.; Benfatto, A. The socialising role of hearing dogs. *Appl. Anim. Behav. Sci.* **1996**, *47*, 7–15.
128. Whitmarsh, L. The benefits of guide dog ownership. *Vis. Impair. Res.* **2005**, *7*, 27–42.
129. Guest, C.; Collis, G.; McNicholas, J. Hearing dogs: A longitudinal study of social and psychological effects on deaf and hard-of-hearing recipients. *J. Deaf Stud. Deaf Educ.* **2005**, *11*, 252–261.
130. Kwong, M.; Bartholomew, K. "Not just a dog": An attachment perspective on relationships with assistance dogs. *Attach. Human Dev.* **2011**, *13*, 421–436.
131. *Census of Population and Housing: Estimating Homelessness 2011*; Australian Bureau of Statistics: Canberra, Australia, 2012.
132. Every, D.; Thompson, K. Disaster Resilience: Can the Homeless Afford It? *Aust. J. Emerg. Manag.* **2014**, in press.
133. Wisner, B. Marginality and vulnerability: Why the homeless of Tokyo don't 'count' in disaster preparations. *Appl. Geogr.* **1998**, *18*, 25–33.
134. Edgington, S. *Disaster Planning for People Experiencing Homelessness*; National Health Care for the Homeless Council, Inc.: Nashville, TN, USA, 2009.
135. Uitto, J.I. The geography of disaster vulnerability in megacities: A theoretical framework. *Appl. Geogr.* **1998**, *18*, 7–16.
136. Greene, M. *Housing Recovery and Reconstruction: Lessons from Recent Urban Earthquakes*; Bay Area Regional Earthquake Preparedness Project; Governor's Office of Emergency Services: Oakland, CA, USA, 1992.
137. Pets of the Homeless 2012. Available online: http://www.petsofthehomeless.org/ (accessed on 5 December 2013).
138. Brewbaker, E. The experience of homelessness and the human-animal bond: A qualitative study. M.Sc. Thesis, Smith College of Social Work, Massachusetts, MA, USA, 2012.
139. Irvine, L. *My Dog Always Eats First: Homeless People and Their Aniamls*; Lynne Rienner Publishers: Boulder, CO, USA, 2013.
140. Irvine, L. Animals as Lifechangers and Lifesavers: Pets in the Redemption Narratives of Homeless People. *J. Contemp. Ethnogr.* **2013**, *42*, 3–30.
141. Slatter, J.; Lloyd, C.; King, R. Homelessness and companion animals: More than just a pet?. *Brit. J. Occup. Ther.* **2012**, *75*, 377–383.
142. Rew, L. Friends and pets as companions: Strategies for coping with loneliness among homeless youth. *J. Child Adolescent Psychiat. Nurs.* **2000**, *13*, 125–132.
143. Taylor, H.; Williams, P.; Gray, D. Homelessness and dog ownership: An investigation into animal empathy, attachment, crime, drug use, health and public opinion. *Anthrozoos* **2004**, *17*, 353–368.
144. Kidd, A.; Kidd, R. Benefits and liabilities of pets for the homeless. *Psychol. Rep.* **1994**, *74*, 715–722.
145. Lee, S. *Homeless—Non English Speaking Background Women and Children Who are Victims of Domestic Violence: Discussion Paper*; Immigrant Women's Speakout Association: Sydney, Australia, 2008.

146. Keys, D. *Children and Homelessness: Literature Review*; Salvation Army, Melbourne City Mission, Research and Social Policy Unit: Melbourne, Australia, 2009.
147. Munro, P. Man's Best Friend. *Sydney Morning Herald* 25 October 2013.
148. *What is Mental Illness?*; Department of Health and Ageing: Canberra, Australia, 2012.
149. *National Survey of Mental Health and Wellbeing 2007*; Australian Bureau of Statistics: Canberra, Australia, 2008.
150. Substance Abuse and Mental Health Services Administration. *Building Bridges: Mental Health Consumers and Representatives of the Disaster Response Community in Dialogue*; HHS Publication No. 4250; Center for Mental Health Services: Rockville, MD, USA, 2007.
151. Speier, T. Introduction to crisis counselling programs and services to persons with serious and persistent mental illness. In *Responding to the Needs of People with Serious and Persistent Mental Illness in Times of Disaster*. Available from: http://cretscmhd.psych.ucla.edu/nola/Video/MHR/Governmentreports/1-Responding_to_Needs_Serious_Mental_Illness.pdf (accessed on 1 December 2013).
152. Fornili, K. Disasters and substance use disorders: Response and responsibility. *J. Addict. Nurs.* **2006**, *17*, 71–77.
153. Zimolag, U.; Krupa, T. Pet ownership as a meaningful community occupation for people with a serious mental illness. *Am. J. Occup. Ther.* **2009**, *63*, 126–137.
154. Wisdom, J.; Saedi, G.; Green, C. Another breed of "service animals": STARS study findings about pet ownership and recovery from serious mental illness. *Am. J. Orthopsychiat.* **2009**, *79*, 430–436.
155. Akiyama, H.; Holtzman, J.; Britz, W. Pet ownership and health status during bereavement. *J. Death Dying* **1986**, *17*, 187–193.
156. Smith, B.B. The 'pet effect'—Health related aspects of companion animal ownership. *Austr. Family Phys.* **2012**, *41*, 439–442.
157. Barker, S.; Dawson, K. The Effects of Animal-Assisted Therapy on Anxiety Ratings of Hospitalized Psychiatric Patients. *Psychiat. Serv.* **1998**, *49*, 797–801.
158. Nagengast, S.; Baun, M.; Megel, M.; Leibowitz, J. The effects of the presence of a companion animal on physiological arousal and behavioral distress in children during a physical examination. *J. Pediat Nurs.* **1997**, *12*, 323–330.
159. Peacock, J.; Chur-Hansen, A.; Winefield, H. Mental Health Implications of Human Attachment to Companion Animals. *J. Clin. Psychol.* **2012**, *68*, 292–303.
160. Glasgow, K. *The Sudanese Refugees and Fire Hazard Study*; Bushfire CRC: East Melbourne, Australia, 2006.
161. Lollar, K. The Liminal Experience: Loss of Extended Self After the Fire. *Qual. Inq.* **2010**, *16*, 262–270.
162. Hunt, M.G.; Bogue, K.; Rohrbaugh, N. Pet Ownership and Evacuation Prior to Hurricane Irene. *Animals* **2012**, *2*, 529–539.

Characteristics of Loads of Cattle Stopping for Feed, Water and Rest during Long-Distance Transport in Canada

Hannah E. Flint [1], Karen S. Schwartzkopf-Genswein [2], Ken G. Bateman [1] and Derek B. Haley [1,*]

[1] Department of Population Medicine, Ontario Veterinary College, University of Guelph, 50 Stone Rd E., Guelph, ON, N1G 2W1, Canada; E-Mails: flinth@uoguelph.ca (H.E.F.); kbateman@uoguelph.ca (K.G.B.)

[2] Agriculture and Agri-Food Canada, Lethbridge, AB, T1J 4B1, Canada; E-Mail: karen.genswein@agr.gc.ca

* Author to whom correspondence should be addressed; E-Mail: dhaley@uoguelph.ca.

Simple Summary: This study was designed to benchmark the characteristics of loads of cattle stopping for feed, water and rest during long distance transport in Canada. Another objective of this study was to determine how well these loads were following current Canadian regulations for the length of time animals can spend in transit, and how long they must be rested for. The majority of loads stopping for feed water and rest were transporting cattle to feedlots rather than processing plants. All loads were under the 48 hour maximum allowable time in transit defined under the Canadian transport regulations and all loads exceeded the minimum duration of 5 hours required for feed, water and rest.

Abstract: This study is the first comprehensive examination of long-haul cattle being transported across Canada and off-loaded for feed, water and rest. A total of 129 truckloads were observed at one of two commercial rest stations near Thunder Bay, Ontario. Data collected included information regarding the truck driver, the trailer, the trip, the animals and animal handling. The majority of the loads stopping were feeder calves (60.94%) while 21.09% were weaned calves, and the remaining 14.84% were market weight cattle. The truck loads surveyed were in transit for, on average, 28.2 ± 5.0 hours before stopping and cattle were rested for an average of 11.2 ± 2.8 hours. These data suggest that loads stopping at the rest station were adhering to the regulations stated in the Health of Animals Act, which outline a maximum of 48 hours in transit before a mandatory stop of at least

5 hours for feed, water and rest. There was a large amount of variability around how well recommendations, such as stocking density were followed. Further research is required to assess how well cattle are coping with long-distance transport under current regulations and industry practices.

Keywords: long-distance transport; transportation; cattle; welfare; rest

---

1. Introduction

A census conducted by the Ontario Ministry of Agriculture and Food (OMAF) in 2012 found that over 600,000 cattle were slaughtered at federally and provincially inspected processing plants within the province, this despite a provincial beef herd population of only 321,000 cows [1]. Thus, large proportion of the beef cattle finished for slaughter in Ontario come from out of province, and most come from western Canada, arriving by road transport.

The transportation of livestock within Canada is federally regulated by the Health of Animals Act, which is the enabling Statute of the Health of Animals Regulations [2]. These regulations cover, among other items, definitions for animals that are unfit for transport, facility requirements for loading and unloading, specifications for the vehicle/container, and requirements for the provision of feed and water en route. These regulations state that weaned cattle cannot be confined on the truck for more than 48 hours without being unloaded for a minimum of 5 hours for feed, water and rest somewhere along their journey. The time in transit can be extended to 52 hours if the cattle are expected to reach their final destination within that time. [2].

Several aspects of long distance transport can impact the well-being of the animals. The experience and skill of the truck driver can have a large impact on cattle welfare both through their handling of the cattle at loading (and unloading) and via their actual driving [3]. As loading and unloading have been suggested to be the most stressful portion of transportation [4], good handling practices are important. Transport of longer duration has also been shown to result in animals suffering more injuries and greater weight loss, or shrink, and time in transit can also affect morbidity once the cattle reach their destination [5–7]. Stocking density is another factor that can impact welfare during transport. High stocking densities have been shown to limit the animals' ability to position themselves in their preferred orientation of either parallel or perpendicular to the direction of travel, and this can lead to more animals losing their balance and struggling to maintain footing [8]. This may contribute to the increase in injuries, such as bruises, in cattle transported at high stocking densities [8].

The number and variety of potential welfare concerns arising from long-distance transport inevitably raise the question about the well-being of cattle being transported long distances in Canada, given current industry practices. As a first step to answering this question, the present project was initiated to benchmark the characteristics of loads of cattle stopping for rest as part of their long-distance journey and to also document the practice of providing opportunity for rest.

2. Experimental Section

2.1. Information Gathered

All methods used in this study were approved by the Animal Care Committee (#12R038) and Research Ethics Board (#12SE009) at University of Guelph. A survey was administered on a voluntary basis and in an interview format to 104 truck drivers who had stopped at a commercial cattle rest station near Thunder Bay, Ontario between April 23, 2012 and June 13, 2012 (spring), and between September 27, 2012 and December 13, 2012 (fall). To collect information on truckloads arriving during the summer months, between June and September, surveys were left available at the rest station for completion by willing drivers, providing information about an additional 25 loads for a total of 129 completed surveys.

When administered in person, the survey was completed immediately after the cattle had been unloaded. The survey was a modified version of the survey used by González *et al.* [9], with questions added to describe the characteristics of the cattle being transported. The survey was designed to collect information regarding five general aspects of cattle transport: the driver, the trailer, the trip, the animals, and the animal handling (Table 1).

Table 1. Information that was collected through administering a survey to truck drivers and observing the unloading and reloading of cattle from trucks stopped for feed, water and rest near Thunder Bay, ON (TB).

Driver	Trailer	Trip	Animal	Animal Handling
Sex	No. axles	Origin type	Space allowance	Time to unload
Years of experience	No. compartments	Destination type	No. animals on load	Time to load
CLT [1] training (Y/N)	Bedding condition	Distance travelled to TB	Type	Slips unload
	Weather boards	Total distance travelled	Weight class	Falls unload
		Time in transit to TB	Sex	Slips load
		Time at rest station	No. compromised	Falls load
		Weather at unloading	No. down	Carry cattle prod (Y/N)
		Weather during trip	No. dead	
			Lying down in truck	

[1] Canadian Livestock Transport certification program.

2.1.1. Driver Characteristics

Information collected regarding driver skill included the number of years' experience hauling cattle and whether they had taken Canadian Livestock Transport (CLT) certification program, a voluntary course that teaches truck drivers proper livestock handling, loading, and biosecurity practices. In order to match the study conducted by González *et al.* [9] on truckloads of cattle leaving Alberta, drivers' years of experience was split into categories according to the following criteria: <2, 2 to 5, 5 to 10 or >10 years of experience hauling cattle.

2.1.2. Trailer Characteristics

Information about the trailer was gathered to assess the environment in which the cattle were transported. Drivers were asked what the make and year of their trailer was, as well as the number of trailer axles, the number of compartments being used in the trailer for the present load, and the percentage of the trailer that was covered by weather boards. The condition of the bedding at the time of unloading was scored as no bedding, dry, wet, or soupy where wet bedding was defined as the bedding being moist and clumping together, and soupy was defined as the bedding being saturated and dripping liquid. Dry bedding was defined as the bedding being loose and neither wet nor soupy. Weather boards are plastic or wood panels that can be attached to the side of the livestock trailer in order to reduce air flow into the trailer during cold weather. The use of weather boards was scored as the number of vertical strips of boarding attached to one side of the trailer.

2.1.3. Trip Characteristics

Trip information gathered related to the point of origin, and the date and time of departure. The date and time of arrival at, and departure from, the rest station were also recorded. We were interested in how well trucks were meeting the requirements for maximum allowable times for animals in transit and the duration of rest outlined by Canadian federal legislation. To do this, distances travelled both to the rest station and to the final destination and time in transit were estimated and, and time spent at the rest station was calculated. Distance travelled (km), to the rest station was estimated using Google Maps [10] and the city, town or village nearest to the point of departure. The total distance to be travelled was also estimated by finding the distance between the place of origin and the city, town or village nearest to the driver's reported final destination. The time spent in transit was estimated as the difference between the date and time of the start of the trip reported by the driver and the date and time that the truck arrived at the rest station, accounting for time zone differences. The time spent at the rest station was calculated as the difference between the dates and times of arrival at and departure from the rest station.

We recorded the type of property where the cattle were loaded as being from a ranch/farm, a feedlot or an auction market. Farms and feedlot were ultimately combined in the dataset as the truck drivers were not always able to distinguish between the two types. Lastly, weather at unloading was recorded using the temperature from a thermometer at the rest station and by scoring the weather as clear, cloudy, foggy, raining, snowing or windy. Information about the route taken was provided by the truck driver and combined with historical weather data available at Weather.org [11] to estimate the maximum and minimum temperatures during the trip. The sum of the maximum and minimum temperatures along the route was divided by two in order to obtain an estimated midpoint temperature for the trip to the rest station.

2.1.4. Animal Characteristics

Information regarding the total number of animals that were on the truck as well as the number of animals in each compartment was collected. The type of animal was also recorded as beef or dairy. The estimated average weight of the animals on the truck, as reported by the driver, was recorded. As precise animal weight measures were not available for every load, approximate average animal weight was used to categorize the animals into weight classes. Weaned calves were defined as animals weighing under 300 kg, feeder calves were animals between 300 and 550 kg and market weight cattle were animals over 550 kg. Animals were also defined as cull cattle when they were over 550 kg and identified by the driver as such. The sex of the animals on a load was recorded as steers, heifers, bulls, cows, or mixed for loads containing more than one sex category.

We were interested in how well space allowances on the truck matched those outlined in the Canadian Code of Practice for the transportation of farm animals [12]. To determine this, space allowances (m^2/animal) were calculated for each compartment of the truck by dividing the area of the compartment [13] by the number of animals in that compartment. This was then used to find the percentage deviation from the recommended stocking density for animals of that body weight [13] as defined by the Code [12]. The allometric coefficient (space allowance/[body weight]$^{2/3}$) was also calculated for each compartment of the truck as this measure allowed for comparison between animals of different body weights [13].

The number of animals that were compromised, down or dead was recorded. Compromised is defined by the Canadian Food Inspection Agency's (CFIA) transportation of animals program as an animal with reduced capacity to withstand the stress of transportation, due to injury, fatigue, infirmity, poor health, distress, very young or old age, impending birth or any other cause [14]. Down or non-ambulatory animals are defined in the Health of Animals Act as animals that are unable to stand without assistance or to move without being dragged or carried [2]. Truck drivers were also asked whether or not they had observed any of their animals lying down in the truck at any point in the journey.

2.1.5. Animal Handling Characteristics

Information was collected on animal handling practices through video recordings and live observations during the unloading and reloading of the animals at the rest station. We recorded the time at which these processes started and ended, scored the number of slips and falls, and recorded whether the driver carried an electric cattle prod during handling. Unloading started when the first foot of the first animal stepped off the truck and ended when the last foot of the last animal stepped off the truck. Reloading started when the first foot of the first animal stepped onto the truck and ended when the last foot of the last animal stepped fully onto the truck. Time taken to unload and reload was calculated as the difference between their respective start and end times. Time taken to unload and reload was also calculated as the number of seconds per animal by dividing the time taken to unload and reload by the number of animals on the trailer.

Video recordings of both unloading and reloading were reviewed to count the number of slips and falls of animals both on the ramp to the truck and in the holding pen at the base of the ramp. Slips were counted when an animal lost its balance and had one or more of its feet slide, but still maintained an upright position and no part of the body other than the limbs came in contact with the ground. A fall was counted when an animal experienced a loss of balance such that they were no longer upright and some part of its body other than the limbs (e.g., flank) came into contact with the ground. The proportion of animals that slipped or fell was documented to compare any loads with different numbers of animals. Proportion was calculated by dividing the number of times animals slipped or fell by the number of animals in that load. This was then used to determine if the load was over or under the 1.0% level used by the American Meat Institute (AMI) transportation audit to differentiate acceptable handling [15].

Whether drivers carried an electric cattle prod was scored on a yes/no basis, with all drivers who were seen handling animals with a prod in their hand at any point during handling scoring a "yes". It was not possible to determine whether or not the cattle prod was actually used or activated on the animals during handling. The drivers were not observed while they were on the truck and it was not clear whether the prod was on when it made contact with the animals.

2.2. Statistical Analysis

Descriptive statistics were run on the data using SAS 9.3 in order to find maximum, median, minimum, mean and standard deviations for all continuous variables. Frequencies and proportions were calculated for all categorical variables. Further statistics were run to provide descriptive statistics for continuous split up by weight class of animals. Variables relating to space allowance were analyzed by compartment and animal weight class.

3. Results and Discussion

All the results for the continuous variables that were recorded are summarized in Table 2 and results for categorical variables are summarized in Table 3. Table 4 shows results for continuous animal and animal handling characteristics that are separated by the weight class of cattle.

Table 2. Continuous variables collected for loads of cattle stopping for feed, water and rest near Thunder Bay, ON (TB).

Variable	Min.	Median	Max.	Mean	SD	N
Years of experience	0.00	20.00	48.00	18.68	13.97	66
Distance travelled to TB (km)	823.00	1639.00	2167.00	1566.40	306.30	129
Total distance travelled (km)	2262.00	3111.00	3833.00	3069.30	333.06	126
Time in transit to TB (h:mm:ss)	11:00:00	28:41:00	44:00:00	28:11:52	4:56:35	102
Time spent at rest station (h:mm:ss)	5:00:00	11:18:30	21:55:00	11:13:43	2:45:13	96
Temperature at unloading (°C)	−12.00	10.50	28.00	10.53	9.89	122
No. animals on truck	39.00	62.00	118.00	68.95	21.59	129
Time taken to unload (h:min:s)	0:06:12	0:14:50	0:37:41	0:16:26	0:05:48	89
Time taken to load (h:min:s)	0:07:19	0:14:45	0:37:50	0:15:42	0:05:27	99
Time to unload per animal (s)	6.31	13.61	41.50	14.29	5.54	89
Time to load per animal (s)	6.76	12.54	30.71	13.45	4.46	99
Slips unload (slips/animal/load)	0	0	0.088	0.0095	0.016	89
Slips load	0	0.016	0.22	0.023	0.034	96
Falls unload (falls/animal/load)	0	0	0.035	0.0021	0.0061	89
Falls load	0	0	0.051	0.0054	0.011	96

Table 3. Categorical variables collected for loads of cattle stopping for feed, water and rest near Thunder Bay, ON.

Variable	N	Category	Frequency	Proportion
Driver sex	66	Male	64	0.97
		Female	2	0.030
Driver experience	66	<2	7	0.11
		2–5	10	0.15
		6–10	7	0.11
		>10	42	0.64
CLT [1] training	66	Yes	16	0.24
		No	50	0.76
Trailer axles	128	Tri	122	0.95
		Tandem	6	0.047
No. compartments	128	4	25	0.20
		5	57	0.45
		6	46	0.36
Weather boards (strips)	121	0	109	0.90
		1	2	0.017
		5	7	0.058
		6	3	0.025
Bedding condition	116	Dry	56	0.48
		Wet	59	0.51
		Soupy	1	0.0086
Origin province	128	Alberta	42	0.33
		Saskatchewan	73	0.57
		Manitoba	13	0.10
Destination province	128	Ontario	113	0.88
		Quebec	15	0.12
Origin type	99	Farm	75	0.76
		Salesbarn	24	0.24
Destination type	103	Farm	75	0.73
		Slaughter	20	0.19
		Other	8	0.078

Table 3. *Cont.*

Variable	N	Category	Frequency	Proportion
Weather at unloading	123	Clear	58	0.47
		Cloudy	49	0.40
		Foggy	1	0.0081
		Rain	13	0.11
		Windy	2	0.016
Weight class	128	Weaned	27	0.21
		Feeder	78	0.61
		Slaughter	19	0.15
		Cull	1	0.0078
		Mixed	3	0.023
Animal sex	128	Steer	104	0.81
		Heifer	17	0.13
		Cow	1	0.0078
		Bull	0	0.00
		Mixed	6	0.047
Lying down in truck	125	Yes	105	0.84
		No	20	0.16
Falls unloading	89	Acceptable (≤0.01)	79	0.89
		Unacceptable (>0.01)	10	0.11
Prod carried	102	Yes	95	0.93
		No	7	0.069

[1] Canadian Livestock Transportation certification program.

Table 4. Continuous variables by weight class of loads stopping for feed, water and rest near Thunder Bay, ON.

Weight Class	Variable	Min.	Median	Max.	Mean	SD	N
Weaned	No. animals on load	79.00	98.00	118.00	100.74	10.01	27
	Time taken to unload (h:mm:ss)	0:11:23	0:18:34	0:32:47	0:19:20	0:06:18	21
	Time taken to load (h:mm:ss)	0:12:51	0:17:54	0:30:18	0:18:49	0:05:01	26
	Time to unload per animal (sec)	7.27	10.41	20.25	11.34	3.67	21
	Time to load per animal (sec)	6.76	10.75	18.74	11.25	3.05	26
	Slips unload (slips/animal/load)	0	0	0.046	0.0089	0.013	21
	Slips load	0	0.014	0.15	0.020	0.031	24
	Falls unload (falls/animal/load)	0	0	0.011	0.00094	0.0030	21
	Falls load	0	0	0.032	0.0044	0.0097	24

Table 4. *Cont.*

Weight Class	Variable	Min.	Median	Max.	Mean	SD	N
Feeder	No. animals on load	48.00	61.00	96.00	64.08	11.14	78
	Time taken to unload (h:mm:ss)	0:06:12	0:14:44	0:37:41	0:15:36	0:05:15	57
	Time taken to load (h:mm:ss)	0:07:19	0:13:31	0:37:50	0:14:20	0:05:11	61
	Time to unload per animal (sec)	6.31	13.89	41.50	15.10	6.08	57
	Time to load per animal (sec)	8.19	12.68	28.02	13.57	3.82	61
	Slips unload (slips/animal/load)	0	0	0.088	0.0095	0.017	57
	Slips load	0	0.017	0.22	0.026	0.036	60
	Falls unload (falls/animal/load)	0	0	0.035	0.0021	0.0063	57
	Falls load	0	0	0.051	0.0066	0.012	60
Market	No. animals on load	39.00	39.00	48.00	40.58	2.39	19
	Time taken to unload (h:mm:ss)	0:09:18	0:12:10	0:15:04	0:12:10	0:02:00	7
	Time taken to load (h:mm:ss)	0:08:22	0:14:05	0:21:30	0:14:05	0:05:34	7
	Time to unload per animal (sec)	14.31	17.38	19.93	17.02	2.05	7
	Time to load per animal (sec)	11.67	21.53	30.71	19.66	7.39	7
	Slips unload (slips/animal/load)	0	0	0.063	0.012	0.024	7
	Slips load	0	0	0.10	0.015	0.039	7
	Falls unload (falls/animal/load)	0	0	0.023	0.0063	0.011	7
	Falls load	0	0	0.021	0.0030	0.0079	7

3.1. Driver Characteristics

In this survey there were 66 different truck drivers who stopped at the rest station during the study period. The truck drivers had on average 18.7 ± 14.0 (mean ± SD) years of experience hauling cattle with a median of 20.0 years of experience. A majority of the drivers (63.6%) had > 10 years experience hauling cattle, which González *et al.* categorically defined as "extensive" [9]. The rest of the drivers were split fairly evenly between the experience categories: 10.2% = 5 to 10 years; 15.2% = between 2 and 5 years; 10.6% = <2 years of experience hauling cattle. There is limited research that indicates that driver experience affects the welfare of animals during transportation, however, González *et al.* [9] found that drivers with more experience had animals with less shrink at their final destination. Further, Hemsworth *et al.* [16] have documented the beneficial effects of training in improving the attitudes and behaviour of stockpersons towards dairy cattle.

Roughly one quarter (24.2% or 16) of the drivers surveyed had taken CLT training. This result is close to the 30% of drivers that Thrower [17] found had received some form of training in a study where 666 loads of feeder and yearling cattle arriving at Ontario feedlots and auction markets where surveyed. Warren *et al.* [18] surveyed 1,348 loads of market weight cattle arriving at a processing plant in Ontario in 2009 and reported that a majority of truck drivers had not received CLT training, but instead were trained on the job. Warren *et al.* [18] attributed this result to the fact that a majority of drivers surveyed were from Ontario companies, as were a majority of the drivers in this study. Although CLT training is available nationwide, it was developed and first launched by the Alberta Farm Animal Care Association in Alberta and Saskatchewan in 2007 and likely had the highest participation in those provinces, especially early after the program was launched. González *et al.* [9]

found that the policy of most of the transport companies in Alberta was that all drivers must receive CLT training. According to Temple Grandin, stockperson attitude and training is the most important factor affecting animal welfare [3], however there is minimal research indicating specifically that driver experience and training affects the welfare of animals during transportation.

3.2. Trailer Characteristics

A majority (95.3%) of trailers in this study had three rear axles (tri-axle) with the remaining 4.7% of trailers having two rear axles (tandem). Tandem trailers have shorter back and doghouse compartments and therefore can fit fewer animals in these compartments. The number of compartments that were used ranged from four to six and varied based on the animal weight class and trailer type. All loads of weaned calves used six compartments, in both tandem and tri-axle trailers, as these animals were small enough to be able to split the nose compartment into top and bottom decks. Feeder weight animals in tri-axle trailers had the greatest variation in the number of compartments used with 12.5% of loads using four compartments, 66.7% with five compartments and 20.8% with six compartments. This difference is likely due to the variation in size and weight of these animals and whether they were too tall for the low ceilings in the nose and doghouse compartments. All loads of feeder cattle in tandem trailers had five compartments. Loads of slaughter weight animals were only observed in tri-axle trailers and 57.9% used four compartments while 42.1% used five compartments. The use of the doghouse as a fifth compartment depended on the number of animals that needed to be transported, and whether the animals were short enough to fit into the compartment. A majority of trucks surveyed used no weather boards (90.0%) while the remaining 10.0% of trailers had between 4 and 25% of the vehicle covered. As expected, all the trucks that utilized boards occurred during the months of November and December when the coldest ambient temperatures were recorded.

All of the trucks in this study were bedded with straw, which is in keeping with the Health of Animals Regulations, which state that all vehicles used to transport animals should be "littered with straw, wood shavings, or other bedding material" [2]. This result was also found in a survey of 666 loads of feeder and yearling cattle transported to auction markets and feedlots in Ontario, which found that over 99% of loads were bedded [17]. The present results differ from those found by González *et al.* [9] when they surveyed 6,152 truckloads of cattle leaving Alberta, a majority of which (89.0%) were destined for the United States. That study found only 22.7% of loads used bedding. The difference in bedding use documented by González *et al.* [9] may be due in part to the different weight classes of cattle observed. In their study, González *et al.* [9] reported that a higher proportion of loads carrying feeders and weaned calves were bedded, compared to slaughter weight cattle. They explained this difference as possibly being due to the perception of younger animals being more fragile. That study also documented a higher proportion of slaughter weight cattle than was seen in our study (82.2% *vs.* 14.8%), however all loads of slaughter weight cattle in our study were bedded. As González *et al.* [9] found that bedding was used for 97.5% of loads from companies that provided bedding for free, it is also possible that differences in bedding usage between our studies is due to different company policies on bedding fees. Bedding was reported as being wet 50.9% and dry 48.3% of the time. Only 1 load of cattle (0.86%) had soupy bedding. As expected, a higher proportion of truckloads (83.3%) with wet bedding was seen when the weather at unloading was recorded as being rainy.

Weather conditions were only recorded upon arrival at the rest station and not during the whole of the trip. This means that even loads recorded as 'clear' may have experienced rain at some other point during the trip resulting in wet bedding from spray coming through the vents.

3.3. Trip Characteristics

A majority of loads (57.0%) stopping for feed, water and rest originated in Saskatchewan, followed by Alberta (32.8%) and Manitoba (10.2%). Most of the loads 88.3% were destined for Ontario, with 11.7% destined for Quebec.

We found that 75.8% of cattle came directly from a farm or feedlot, while 24.2% of cattle came from an auction market. However, this differed by season, as a higher proportion of cattle originated from auction markets in the fall months than in the spring (45.5% *vs.* 8.70%, respectively). This may be attributed to the fact that a majority (75.0%) of the weaned calves originated from auction markets and weaned calves were mainly observed being transported in the fall months. Cattle were destined for farms or feedlots for 72.8% of loads, and for slaughter in 19.4% of loads, while the remaining 7.76% were heading to other destinations, such as quarantine or auction markets.

On average, loads observed in this study stopped close to the midway point (distance) between the point of origin and their reported final destination. The average distance travelled to the point of rest was 1,566 ± 306 (mean ± SD) km with a median of 1,639 km. The average total distance trucks would ultimately travel to reach the final destination was 3,069 ± 333 km with a median of 3,833 km. Market weight cattle were transported shorter distances to the rest station (1,156 ± 330 km) compared to either feeder (1,643 ± 222 km) or weaned calves (1,625 ± 266 km). Market weight cattle were also transported shorter distances to their final destination with an average of 2,609 ± 338 km when compared to either feeder (3,166 ± 248 km) or weaned calves (3,110 ± 297 km). One possible explanation for this finding could be that producers are more concerned about the effects of long-distance transportation on shrink and meat quality when cattle are going directly to slaughter. They may believe that cattle heading to feedlots will have adequate time to recover from this stress without unmanageable economic or animal welfare costs. This may cause the producer to choose processing plants closer to the point of origin. Another possible explanation could be that there is a greater proportion of feedlots closer to Thunder Bay, than backgrounding operations or cow-calf farms. This difference could also be due to the small sample size of market weight loads, with a majority of them originating from near one of three towns in Manitoba and Saskatchewan.

The average duration of the trip to the rest station from the point of origin was 28.2 ± 5.0 hours with a maximum of 44.1 and a minimum of 11.0 hours. This indicates that all the trucks surveyed in this study were well below the maximum of 48 hours in transit when they stopped at the rest station [2]. With trucks stopping, on average, around the midway point in their journey, it is expected that none of the trucks that were surveyed would exceed 48 hours for the second half on the journey. The load that came closest to the maximum time allowed originated in Alberta and stopped to pick up cattle at four separate locations. This practice was relatively uncommon as only 7.75% (10 loads) of the observed loads picked up cattle from multiple locations, and a majority of those (8 loads) picked up cattle from only two different locations. The load with the shortest transport time originated in Manitoba and stopped at the rest station in order to make truck repairs. In support of our findings, Warren *et al.* [18]

found that out of 1,348 trucks surveyed at a processing plant in Ontario, only 2 loads (0.15%) had been in transit for over 48 hours. As our study found that slaughter weight cattle were transported shorter distances, the proportion of loads that exceeded the maximum time in transit may be greater in cattle destined for feedlots. This is supported in findings by Thrower [17] who, when looking at feeder cattle arriving at auction markets and feedlots in Ontario, found that 10 of 54 trucks (18.5%) that had been in transit for over 52 hours had not stopped for feed, water and rest. This suggests that there are trucks that do not stop at the rest station, and obviously those loads were not benchmarked as part of this study population.

Every load that stopped for feed, water and rest exceeded the regulated requirement of providing a minimum of 5 hours rest. The average duration of the stay at the rest station was more than double that duration: 11.2 ± 2.8 hours with a minimum of 5.0 and a maximum of 16.8 hours. A single exception was a truck that stayed for 21.9 hours due to a mechanical issue. Previous work by where drivers self-reported the duration of their rest stop found averages of 12 hours in the study by Warren *et al.* [18] and 13 hours in the study by Thrower [17]. These long durations of rest maybe due to the regulated required rest periods for the drivers of transport vehicles, which state that drivers must rest for a minimum of ten hours per day, with at least eight hours being consecutive [19].

3.4. Animal Characteristics

All loads of cattle surveyed in our study were transporting beef cattle. The majority of loads were feeder cattle (60.9%) while 21.1% were weaned calves and 14.8% market weight cattle. A small number of loads 2.34% (3 loads) had both weaned and feeder weight cattle. There was only one load of cull cows surveyed (0.78%) and no loads of bulls were encountered or surveyed. The majority of loads were steers (81.3%) with 13.3% of loads heifers and 4.69% of loads with a mixture of sexes. The number of animals on the truck ranged from 79 to 118 for weaned calves, 48 to 96 for feeder weight cattle, and 39 to 48 for slaughter weight cattle. When asked whether any of their animals laid down during the trip 84.0% of drivers reported yes, that at least some animals had laid down, although this was not further quantified. Drivers were able to observe their animals lying down when they stopped during the trip and checked on their animals.

Due to the small number of loads in tandem trailers surveyed in this study, space allowance was only calculated for tri-axle trailers. Space allowance results are summarized in Table 5 and these varied by cattle weight class and truck compartment as shown in Table 6. Cattle in the nose and doghouse compartments typically had more space than the minimum recommended with the top deck of the nose having on average 59% more space, the bottom deck of the nose 46% more space, and the doghouse 26% more space than the minimum recommended in the Canadian Code of Practice [12]. The back, belly and deck compartments were typically closer to the minimum recommended space allowance with the back compartment having on average 5.4% more space, the belly 7.2% less space and the deck 6.2% less space than the minimum. These results are consistent with those reported by González *et al.* [13]. When we discussed the extra space in the nose and doghouse compartments with truck drivers they explained that due to the smaller size and different shape of these compartments adding another animal would cause them to be too crowded, even if on paper they would be closer to the minimum stocking density. This suggests that recommendations may need to be reassessed to better reflect the usable space in these compartments. These results may be concerning as a majority (80.2%) of the cattle were transported in the back, belly and deck compartments, and were thus more likely to be exposed to overcrowded conditions.

Table 5. Space allowances (m^2/head) for cattle on tri-axle trailers that were unloaded at feed, water and rest stations in Thunder Bay, ON.

Variable	Compartment	Min.	Median	Max.	Mean	SD	N
SA [1] (m^2/head)	Back	0.60	1.06	1.81	1.07	0.28	116
	Belly	0.56	0.93	1.64	1.00	0.27	114
	Deck	0.59	0.94	1.64	1.01	0.26	111
	Nose bottom	0.91	1.36	2.72	1.58	0.53	112
	Nose top	0.91	1.36	1.63	1.30	0.25	40
	Doghouse	0.69	1.08	2.42	1.26	0.50	94
DRSA [2]	Back	−0.45	0.021	0.19	0.0012	0.11	113
	Belly	−0.20	0.086	0.23	0.075	0.066	111
	Deck	−0.20	0.079	0.21	0.065	0.068	108
	Nose bottom	−1.13	−0.44	0.043	−0.47	0.26	109
	Nose top	−1.39	−0.611	−0.14	−0.60	0.23	38
	Doghouse	−1.16	−0.18	0.16	−0.23	0.26	90
AC [3]	Back	0.015	0.019	0.027	0.019	0.0021	113
	Belly	0.014	0.018	0.022	0.018	0.0014	111
	Deck	0.015	0.018	0.022	0.018	0.0014	108
	Nose bottom	0.018	0.027	0.040	0.028	0.0050	109
	Nose top	0.021	0.030	0.044	0.030	0.0044	38
	Doghouse	0.016	0.022	0.042	0.023	0.0053	90

[1] Space allowance (m^2/head); [2] Deviation from recommended space allowance ((recommended-observed)/recommended); [3] Allometric coefficient (space allowance/(body weight)$^{2/3}$).

Table 6. Space allowances (m^2/head) for cattle on tri-axle trailers that were unloaded at feed, water and rest stations near Thunder Bay, ON by weight class.

Variable	Weight Class	Compartment	Min.	Median	Max.	Mean	SD	N
SA [1]	Weaned	Back	0.60	0.74	0.97	0.75	0.090	29
		Belly	0.56	0.70	0.82	0.69	0.069	27
		Deck	0.59	0.70	0.83	0.70	0.066	26
		Nose bottom	0.91	1.17	1.63	1.15	0.19	27
		Nose top	0.91	1.17	1.63	1.20	0.22	27
		Doghouse	0.69	0.81	1.08	0.80	0.10	27
	Feeder	Back	0.79	1.06	1.41	1.08	0.15	67
		Belly	0.73	1.04	1.23	0.99	0.13	67
		Deck	0.76	1.04	1.23	1.00	0.12	65
		Nose bottom	0.91	1.63	2.04	1.50	0.29	64
		Nose top	1.02	1.63	1.63	1.51	0.20	12
		Doghouse	0.81	1.38	2.42	1.35	0.38	58

Table 6. *Cont.*

Variable	Weight Class	Compartment	Min.	Median	Max.	Mean	SD	N
	Market	Back	1.27	1.58	1.81	1.53	0.15	19
		Belly	1.31	1.41	1.64	1.46	0.11	19
		Deck	1.31	1.41	1.64	1.46	0.96	19
		Nose bottom	1.63	2.72	2.72	2.52	0.36	19
		Nose top	-	-	-	-	-	-
		Doghouse	1.94	2.43	2.43	2.24	0.25	8
DRSA [2]	Weaned	Back	−0.33	0.057	0.19	0.019	0.12	29
		Belly	−0.020	0.099	0.23	0.085	0.081	27
		Deck	−0.20	0.089	0.16	0.067	0.090	26
		Nose bottom	−1.00	−0.45	−0.14	−0.52	0.20	28
		Nose top	−1.39	−0.53	−0.14	−0.58	0.26	26
		Doghouse	−0.58	0.0014	0.10	−0.049	0.15	27
	Feeder	Back	−0.45	0.014	0.15	−0.0068	0.10	65
		Belly	−0.051	0.084	0.21	0.080	0.057	65
		Deck	−0.072	0.073	0.21	0.070	0.057	63
		Nose bottom	−1.13	−0.36	0.043	−0.40	0.27	62
		Nose top	−0.79	−0.75	−0.20	−0.66	0.18	12
		Doghouse	−1.16	−0.22	0.16	−0.28	0.26	55
	Market	Back	−0.24	0.0045	0.11	0.0016	0.097	19
		Belly	−0.037	0.039	0.17	0.044	0.066	19
		Deck	−0.079	0.080	0.12	0.044	0.66	19
		Nose bottom	−0.91	−0.73	−0.25	−0.64	0.18	19
		Nose top	-	-	-	-	-	-
		Doghouse	−0.86	−0.52	−0.29	−0.50	0.19	8
AC [3]	Weaned	Back	0.015	0.018	0.024	0.018	0.0022	29
		Belly	0.014	0.017	0.022	0.017	0.0015	27
		Deck	0.016	0.017	0.022	0.017	0.0016	26
		Nose bottom	0.021	0.027	0.037	0.028	0.0037	28
		Nose top	0.021	0.028	0.044	0.029	0.0047	26
		Doghouse	0.017	0.019	0.029	0.019	0.0027	27
	Feeder	Back	0.016	0.019	0.027	0.019	0.0019	65
		Belly	0.015	0.018	0.020	0.018	0.0011	65
		Deck	0.015	0.018	0.020	0.018	0.0011	63
		Nose bottom	0.018	0.026	0.040	0.027	0.0051	62
		Nose top	0.022	0.033	0.034	0.031	0.0034	12
		Doghouse	0.016	0.023	0.042	0.025	0.0050	55

Table 6. *Cont.*

Variable	Weight Class	Compartment	Min.	Median	Max.	Mean	SD	N
	Market	Back	0.017	0.020	0.025	0.020	0.0019	19
		Belly	0.017	0.019	0.021	0.019	0.0013	19
		Deck	0.018	0.018	0.021	0.019	0.0013	19
		Nose bottom	0.024	0.034	0.038	0.033	0.0037	19
		Nose top	-	-	-	-	-	-
		Doghouse	0.026	0.030	0.036	0.030	0.0036	8

[1] Space allowance (m^2/head); [2] Deviation from recommended space allowance; [3] Allometric coefficient (space allowance/(body weight)$^{2/3}$).

Market weight cattle had the highest values for space allowance compared to weaned and feeder cattle, as shown by the larger allometric coefficient for these animals across compartments. These results are consistent with those reported by González *et al.* [13]. This was explained by González *et al.* [13] as being the result of limitations on the amount of weight allowable per axle by Ministry of Transportation regulations. With larger animals there is more weight per square metre and with slaughter weight cattle, the number of animals that can be loaded is more often limited by weight regulations than by stocking density. Therefore, market weight cattle are often loaded with a higher space allowance (less crowded) than smaller cattle.

Transporting cattle at stocking densities exceeding the values recommended in the Canadian Code of Practice [12] has been shown to result in significantly increased levels of bruising and muscle damage [8], which is both an issue for the well-being of cattle and the person marketing them. It was suggested by Tarrant *et al.* [8] that more animals fall down at higher stocking densities and also that animals that fall or lie down during the journey at high stocking densities may not be able to stand-up easily and may be trampled, resulting in increased bruising.

Results for the number of compromised, down or dead cattle on each load are summarized in Table 7. No cattle were dead on arrival at the rest station for any loads surveyed in this study. Just one load (0.96% of all loads) contained an animal recorded as down, and 2.88% of loads had an animal that was deemed to be compromised (3 loads). Overall, there were three animals (0.040%) that were lame at unloading and one animal (0.013%) that was down on the trailer, for a total of four (0.053%) compromised animals. Compromised animals observed in this study were unloaded and kept in a separate pen for the duration of their stay at the rest station. When it was time to reload they were assessed for fitness for transport and in all cases those animals were left at the rest station and later euthanized. Having animals on the truck that are compromised, down or dead is an obvious welfare issue and perhaps a likely an indicator of poor transportation practices. The AMI transportation audit program developed by Temple Grandin assesses the welfare of animals, including cattle, arriving at processing plants in the United States. This audit uses a level of 1.9% of cattle on the truck being compromised or down as acceptable [15]. Every load in our study was within the acceptable limits outlined by the AMI transportation audit [15]. All of the cases of compromised animals in this survey were due to lameness. The proportion of compromised animals seen in this study were either similar to, or lower than, those seen in other studies. The percentage of lame animals was similar to the 0.022% reported by González *et al.* [9] and the 0.065% reported by Thrower [17]. Warren *et al.* [18]

reported higher percent of lame animals at 0.16%. One possible reason for this higher proportion of lameness could be that the researchers used a more sensitive definition for lameness. However, lameness was not operationally defined in their paper and so this could not be verified as the cause. Another explanation could be that lameness is more prevalent among market weight cattle arriving at processing plants than in the feeder and weaned calves that were predominant in our study. The percentage of animals that were down, or needed assistance was similar in our study (0.013%) to the 0.002%–0.025% reported by the others [9,17,18]. No dead animals were seen in this study, but this may be due to the present sample size of 8,894 animals when compared to the other studies that have looked at this variable, which have found 0.008%–0.015% of animals dead had sample sizes of 19,977–290,362 animals [9,17,18].

Table 7. Number of compromised, down, and dead cattle observed for loads stopping for feed, water and rest in Thunder Bay, ON, based on their production classes. No load contained more than one compromised, down, or dead animal.

Weight Class	Compromised [1]	Down [2]	Dead	Loads [3]	Animals [4]
Weaned	1	1	0	27	4,154
Feeder	2	0	0	65	2,720
Market	0	0	0	7	300
Other	0	0	0	5	405
All	3	1	0	104	7,579

[1] Defined as an animal with reduced capacity to withstand the stress of transportation, due to injury, fatigue, infirmity, poor health, distress, very young or old age, impending birth or any other cause; [2] Defined as an animal that is unable to stand without assistance or to move without being dragged or carried; [3] Number of truckloads of animals observed; [4] Number of individual animals observed.

When the characteristics of loads with compromised or down animals were examined we found that all of the affected loads arrived at the rest station during the month of October. This might indicate that season plays a role in the probability of an animal becoming compromised or down during transport and could be an area for future research. The single load with an animal down in the trailer had mixed steers and heifers within the belly compartment, where the animal was down. This may have caused problems due to differences in size between steers and heifers, although we did not quantify this directly. The mixing of sexes may have caused increased activity within the compartment leading to one of the animals getting injured. However, Yeh *et al.* [20] did not find any increase in bruising when mixing sexes of cattle on a transport truck. It was noted by both the researcher (Hannah Flint) and the rest station manager that the compartment had a couple of animals, including the one that was down, that were noticeably smaller than the rest. Variability in the size of animals within compartments was not measured in this study, but could be a contributing factor in incidence of compromised or down animals. One of the loads with a compromised animal due to lameness had the longest time in transit (44 hours). As studies have shown that injuries increase with journeys of longer duration [6,21] it is possible that the long time in transit was a contributing factor to the lameness seen in that particular load. Other loads with compromised animals had no measured unique characteristics that in any way seemed to set them apart from other loads.

3.5. Animal Handling Characteristics

In this study, it took on average 16.4 ± 5.81 (mean ± SD) minutes to unload and 15.7 ± 5.45 minutes to load cattle. The time taken to unload in our study was less than the 30 minutes reported by González *et al.* [9]. One reason for this difference could be due to differences in facility design. González *et al.* had unloading times from various facilities. This difference in time could also be due to variation in handling techniques, or differences in speed in market weight animals observed in their study, compared to predominantly feeder weight animals observed in our study. This last possibility is supported by the fact that we saw longer unloading times in market weight animals when the number of animals on the truck was accounted for. The time taken to unload was greater than the 8.4 minutes taken to unload cattle in Europe reported by Villarroel *et al.* [22]. The reason for this difference could be due to the fact that the average number of animals on the trucks in Europe was much lower (16 *vs.* 69) than the present study, and the majority of the trucks in the study from Europe were small, two-axle, vehicles designed to carry eight animals and had fewer compartments than the trailers we observed [22]. When time taken to unload per animal was calculated the time of 14.29 seconds per animal seen in our study was roughly half of the 31.50 seconds calculated from the study conducted by Villarroel *et al.* [22]. The unloading time per animal seen in our study was also much less than the 72.0 seconds reported by Maria *et al.* [23], which like the study conducted by Villarroel *et al.* [22] was conducted in Europe. Differences in trucks and handling techniques in Europe may result in longer unloading times. The time to load in our study was similar to the 20.0 minutes reported by González *et al.* [9] and 16.8 minutes reported by Villarroel *et al.* [22]. However, when the time to load per animal was calculated the 13.45 seconds per animal seen in our study was considerably less than the 63.00 seconds found by Villarroel *et al.* [22] and 86.0 seconds found by Maria *et al.* [23]. This could be due to differences in the amount time needed to open and close dividers in European trucks compared to those used in North America. Loading and unloading can be the most stressful period during transportation [4]. Thus, it could be argued that a faster loading and unloading time is beneficial to the animals as it reduces the time spent being handled. This is supported by the fact that Maria *et al.* [23] found trucks that experienced shorter unloading times (under 1 minute) had animals with lower levels of cortisol, creatine kinase and lactate at slaughter when they also had fewer slips, falls and balks. Conversely, it could indicate that the cattle are rushing off of, or onto, the truck in order to escape a negative environment or handling stimuli, which we attempted to control for/quantify by counting the number of slips and falls. The data collected here does not suggest the truck is a negative environment for the cattle as the time to load was less than the time to unload, indicating that the cattle are returning to the trailer easily. However there is the possibility that cattle may be moving quickly to escape negative handling stimuli when being loaded, despite potentially finding the truck environment aversive. One limitation to using the gross duration of unloading and reloading as a measure of handing is that it included time the driver spent opening and closing compartments, moving bedding, counting animals (in some cases recounting animals), *etc*. This means the actual ‘hands-on’ animal handling time is likely less than what we recorded.

In this study, an average of 0.74% of cattle slipped in each load during unloading and 0.16% fell with a maximum of 8.77% and 3.51% respectively. More cattle slipped and fell during reloading with an average of 2.26% of cattle in each load slipping during reloading and 0.44% falling, with maximums of 22.0% and 5.08% respectively. Under the AMI transportation audit program the number of cattle that fall during unloading must be less than 1% in order to be deemed acceptable [15]. When the AMI cut off of 1% is applied to the loads surveyed here, 89.0% of all loads would be deemed acceptable. Slips and falls during unloading and reloading can be an indicator of improper facilities or handling techniques as cattle may be rushing to avoid a negative stimulus or may not have proper footing [3]. In order to further assess the behaviour and welfare of cattle during unloading and reloading the speed of cattle movement, or number of balks could additionally be recorded.

Truck drivers were seen holding a cattle prod during either unloading or reloading in 93.1% of loads, but it was not possible to record whether the prod was being activated by the handlers as it some do touch the cattle with the prod as they count them, without applying any shock. Huertas *et al.* [6] found that the use of devices that force cattle to move, such as a cattle prod, during loading or unloading en route to processing plants increased the level of bruising seen in the carcasses. Even if the prod was not used here, it has been suggested when an electric prod is not the primary driving tool worker attitude improves and handlers are less likely to yell at or hit the animals [3]. Some drivers stated they felt the need to carry a cattle prod during loading to ensure their personal safety, which may suggest that there is a need for more training on other, more welfare-friendly, driving tools.

A major limitation of the present sample is that only trucks that stopped for feed, water and rest at the studied rest station were surveyed and thus, the results are limited to drivers and companies that are actually operating under compliance with the regulations. This study did not include loads that chose to stop at the other commercial rest station near Thunder Bay, which may have a different demographic of clientele. There may be loads that legally should be stopping for rest, but that disobey the laws and regulation. To further assess how well all cattle being transported long-distances in Canada are coping, further studies that include loads from the other rest station near Thunder Bay, as well as loads that do not stop for feed, water and rest should be examined.

4. Conclusions

This study is the first comprehensive examination of loads of commercial cattle being transported long distances within Canada. Results confirmed that a majority of the loads stopping for feed, water and rest were calves destined for further feeding (82.0%). Loads were being rested after 28.2 ± 5.0 hours on the road, well under 48 hours, which is the maximum allowed by law. Additionally the loads observed offered, on average, 11.2 ± 2.8 hours of rest, which is more than double the minimum of 5 hours legislated. These results indicate the loads observed were following the regulations stated by Canada's Health of Animals Act. However, there is variability around how closely recommendations, such as stocking density, were being followed. The results relating to stocking density indicate that it may be beneficial to update the recommendations to provide stocking densities for different compartments to reflect differences in usable space. In order to assess how well cattle themselves are coping under the current transportation regulations and practices, further research into how these factors affect the cattle needs to be undertaken. Further research should also be conducted to determine how many loads fail to stop for feed, water and rest and how this transgression of the regulations might be affecting the health and welfare of cattle transported under those conditions.

Acknowledgments

We would like to acknowledge the owner and manager of the rest station observed in this study, for his help and cooperation in conducting this study and livestock truck drivers for their participation. This study was funded by OMAF.

Author Contributions

H.E. Flint was a Master of Science graduate student responsible for the fieldwork, collation of the data, and leading the writing of the manuscript. K.S. Schwartzkopf-Genswein and K.G. Bateman were project collaborators. D.B. Haley initiated the project and was the Principle Investigator and funding holder for the work. All co-authors contributed to the preparation of the final manuscript.

Conflicts of Interest

The authors declare no conflict of interest.

References and Notes

1. Cattle Statistics. In *Statistics Canada Catalogue*; Statistics Canada: Ottawa, Canada, 2012.
2. *Health of Animals Act*; c. 296; Department of Justice: Ottawa, Canada, 1990; pp. 138, 143, 148.
3. *Livestock Handling and Transport*, 3rd ed.; Grandin, T., Ed.; CABI: Cambridge, UK, 2007.
4. Pettiford, S.G.; Ferguson, D.M.; Lea, J.M.; Lee, C.; Paull, D.R.; Reed, M.T.; Hinch, G.N.; Fisher, A.D. Effect of loading practices and 6-hour road transport on the physiological responses of yearling cattle. *Austr. J. Exper. Agr.* **2008**, *48*, 1028–1033.
5. Cernicchiaro, N.; White, B.J.; Renter, D.G.; Babcock, A.H.; Kelly, L.; Slattery, R. Associations between the distance traveled from sale barns to U.S. commercial feedlots and overall performance, risk of respiratory disease and cumulative mortality in feeder cattle during 1997 to 2009. *J. Anim. Sci.* **2012**, *90*, 1929–1939.
6. Huertas, S.M.; Gil, A.D.; Piaggio, J.M.; Van Eerdenburg, F.J.C.M. Transportation of beef cattle to slaughterhouses and how this relates to animal welfare and carcase bruising in an extensive production system. *Anim. Welf.* **2010**, *19*, 281–285.
7. Jarvis, A.M.; Harrington, D.W.J.; Cockram, M.S. Effect of source and lairage on some behavioural and biochemical measurements of feed restriction and dehydration in cattle at a slaughterhouse. *Appl. Anim. Behav. Sci.* **1996**, *50*, 83–94.
8. Tarrant, P.V; Kenny, F.J.; Harrington, D.W.J.; Murphy, M.R. Long distance transportation of steers to slaughter: Effect of stocking density on physiology, behaviour and carcass quality. *Livestock Prod. Sci.* **1992**, *30*, 223–238.
9. González, L.A.; Schwartzkopf-Genswein, K.S.; Bryan, M.; Silasi, R.; Brown, F. Benchmarking study of industry practices during commercial long haul transport of cattle in Alberta, Canada. *J. Anim. Sci.* **2012**, *90*, 3606–3617.
10. Google Maps. Available online: http://maps.google.ca (accessed on 23 April 2012).
11. Weather.org. Available online: http://www.weather.org/weatherorg_records_and_averages.htm (accessed on 23 April 2012).

12. Canadian Agri-Food Research Council (CARC). *Recommended Code of Practice for the Care and Handling of Farm Animals—ansportation*; 2001. Available online: http://www.nfacc.ca/codes-of-practice/transport (accessed on 18 March 2013).
13. González, L.A.; Schwartzkopf-Genswein, K.S.; Bryan, M.; Silasi, R.; Brown, F. Space allowance during commercial long distance transport of cattle in North America. *J. Anim. Sci.* **2012**, *90*, 3618–3629.
14. Canadian Food Inspection Agency. Transportation of animals program. Compromised animals policy. Available online: http://www.inspection.gc.ca/animals/terrestrial-animals/humane-transport/compromised-animals-policy/eng/1360016317589/1360016435110 (accessed on 3 June 2013).
15. Grandin, T.; American Meat Institute. *Recommended Animal Handling Guideline and Audit Guide: A Systematic Approach to Animal Welfare*; American Meat Institute: Washington, DC, USA, 2010.
16. Hemsworth, P.H.; Coleman, G.J.; Barnett, J.L.; Borg, S.; Dowling, S. The effects of cognitive behavioral intervention on the attitude and behavior of stockspersons and the behavior and productivity of commercial dairy cows. *J. Anim. Sci.* **2002**, *80*, 68–78.
17. Thrower, M.J.C. Transporation conditions for feeder and yearling cattle transported by road to Ontario sales barns or feedlots. M.S. Thesis, University of Guelph, Guelph, Canada, 2009.
18. Warren, L.A.; Mandell, I.B.; Bateman, K.G. An audit of transport conditions and arrival status of slaughter cattle shipped by road at an Ontario processor. *Can. J. Anim. Sci.* **2010**, *90*, 159–167.
19. *Commercial Vehicle Drivers Hours of Service Regulations*; S.O.R./2005-313; Department of Justice: Ottawa, Canada, 1985; p. 14.
20. Yeh, E.; Anderson, B.; Jones, P.; Shaw, F. Bruising in cattle transported over long distances. *Vet. Record* **1978**, *103*, 117–119.
21. Minka, N.S.; Ayo, J.O. Effects of loading behaviour and road transport stress on traumatic injuries in cattle transported by road during the hot-dry season. *Livestock Sci.* **2007**, *107*, 91–95.
22. Villarroel, M.; María, G.A.; Sierra, I.; Sañudo, C.; Garćia-Belenguer, S.; Gebresenbet, G. Critical points in the transport of cattle to slaughter in Spain that may compromise the animals' welfare. *Vet. Record* **2001**, *149*, 173–176.
23. Maria, G.A.; Villarroel, M.; Chacon, G.; Gebresenbet, G. Scoring system for evaluating the stress to cattle of commercial loading and unloading. *Vet. Record* **2004**, *154*, 818–821.

4

Establishing Bedding Requirements during Transport and Monitoring Skin Temperature during Cold and Mild Seasons after Transport for Finishing Pigs

John McGlone [1,*], Anna Johnson [2], Avi Sapkota [1], Rebecca Kephart [2]

[1] Department of Animal and Food Sciences, Texas Tech University, Lubbock, TX 79409, USA; E-Mail: asapkota@purdue.edu

[2] Department of Animal Science, Iowa State University, Ames, IA 50011, USA; E-Mails: johnsona@iastate.edu (A.J.); rkdavis@iastate.edu (R.K.)

* Author to whom correspondence should be addressed; E-Mail: john.mcglone@ttu.edu.

Simple Summary: Typically, bedding is used to improve pig comfort and welfare during transport. This study assesses the level of bedding required during transport of finishing pigs in semi-truck trailers. The present study shows that adding more than six bales/trailer of bedding in cold weather and more than three bales/trailer of bedding in mild weather provides no benefit to the pigs. Economic forces would not favor increased bedding with no benefit. Use of infrared thermography may provide a useful tool to indicate when cooling interventions are needed during warm weather.

Abstract: The broad aim of this study was to determine whether bedding level in the transport trailer influenced pig performance and welfare. Specifically, the objective was to define the bedding requirements of pigs during transportation in commercial settings during cold and mild weather. Animals (n = 112,078 pigs on 572 trailers) used were raised in commercial finishing sites and transported in trailers to commercial processing plants. Dead on arrival (DOA), non-ambulatory (NA), and total dead and down (D&D) data were collected and skin surface temperatures of the pigs were measured by infrared thermography. Data were collected during winter (Experiment 1) and fall/spring (Experiment 2). Total D&D percent showed no interaction between bedding level and outside air temperature in any experiments. Average skin surface temperature during unloading increased with outside air temperature linearly in both experiments ($P < 0.01$). In conclusion, over-use of bedding may be economically inefficient. Pig skin surface temperature could be a useful measure of pig welfare during or after transport.

Keywords: bedding; microenvironment; pigs; skin surface temperature; transportation; welfare

---

1. Introduction

More than 100 million pigs are transported to processing plants yearly in the U. S. [1]. Losses from dead and down (D&D) pigs arriving at the processing plants represent a significant financial loss [2] and suggest an animal welfare concern. Losses have been defined as any mortality or non-ambulatory pigs occurring during transportation from finishing sites to the processing plant. These losses include:

- Dead on arrival (DOA) defined as pigs that die during transit; and
- Non-ambulatory (NA), which are pigs unable to move or keep up with other unloaded pigs and have to be killed in suspect of disease. The NA category can be delineated into two further sub-categories:
    - Non-ambulatory, non-injured (NANI) defined as pigs that cannot move or walk, but do not have any obvious signs of injury, trauma, or disease; and
    - Non-ambulatory, injured (NAI), pigs that cannot move or walk due to injury during any stage of transportation and show clear signs of injury, trauma, or disease [2].

Factors that may influence losses during transit include: micro-environment inside the trailer, stocking density, animal health, transit time, wait time both at the farm (from loading to leaving) and plant (prior to unloading) [2,3], and handling of the pigs throughout the entire process [4]. Temperature, humidity, air speed, air pressure, level of gases (ammonia, carbon dioxide), and the amount and condition of any bedding have been identified as major microenvironment components that may affect transport losses [5,6]. The level of bedding material may be a crucial component in controlling the microenvironment and thereby improve swine welfare during transport.

The National Pork Board introduced a training program for swine transporters, producers, and handlers, now known as the Transport Quality Assurance (TQA) program, in 2002. As new research is done in swine transport, the National Pork Board updates the TQA, with the most recent edition published in 2008 [7]. This program outlines recommendations to help those in the pork industry understand handling and transport of pigs. The TQA Handbook gives the following guidelines regarding bedding: at temperatures lower than −12 °C, pigs should be provided with four bags of bedding (heavy); at temperatures of −12 °C to 3.8 °C, pigs should be provided with three bags of bedding (medium); and at temperatures above 3.8 °C, pigs should be provided with two bags of bedding (light). These recommendations were based on professional judgment and experience as opposed to scientific data. Therefore, the present study was designed to determine the level of bedding that might decrease transport losses, thereby improving pig welfare and lowering economic losses.

2. Experimental Section

2.1. General

Institutional Animal Care and Use Committees at Texas Tech- and Iowa State University approved the experimental protocol for this study. This research was conducted using commercial finishing sites, trailers, and processing plants. A total of 112,078 finisher barrows and gilts (mixed commercial genetics) from farms in Iowa and Minnesota were observed during loading and unloading from trailers going to commercial processing plants in Missouri or Iowa. Trailers were primarily pot-belly styles (center portion lower than the top of the tires), though some straight-deck styles (each of 2 decks were level) were also used (1.7% of trailers were straight deck). Trailer dimensions were 14.7 m long × 2.6 m wide or 16.3 m long × 2.6 m wide. Each trailer transported an average of 166.9 ± 0.63 pigs (minimum = 27, maximum = 193). Duration of travel varied due to varying distances between finishing sites and processing plants. The processing plants that cooperated wish to remain anonymous.

2.2. Treatments

This study was divided into 2 experiments: cold and mild weather. Each bale of wood shavings used was 22.7 kg and 0.2 m^3. Bedding levels were assigned randomly to trailers and applied by the 13 transport companies. A single bedding level was assigned to each trailer, with the same amount of bedding applied to each deck. Researchers confirmed the amount of bedding was appropriate. Weather data were available on 70% of transport groups of pigs. Trailers utilized natural ventilation, and boarding was applied to each trailer as specified by McGlone [8].

The first experiment (January to February 2011; −13 °C to 20 °C) consisted of 2 treatment groups. Treatment 1: 6 bales/trailer (n = 103; 17,100 pigs). Treatment 2: 12 bales/trailer (n = 69; 11,403 pigs). Most (74%) observations were at air temperatures <10 °C. Data collection was done at 2 plants (1 in Iowa, 1 in Missouri) and 32 finishing sites.

The second experiment (March and May 2011, −2 °C to 21 °C) consisted of 3 treatment groups. Treatment 1: 3 bales/trailer (n = 105; 17,745 pigs), Treatment 2: 6 bales/trailer (n = 122; 21,080 pigs), and Treatment 3: 12 bales/trailer (n = 38; 6,075 pigs). Most (69%) observations occurred at air temperatures between 5 °C and 20 °C. Data collection occurred at 1 plant located in Iowa and at 37 finishing sites.

2.3. Trailer Characteristics at the Finishing Site and Processing Plant

Bedding levels applied to each trailer, number of loads of pigs (one load is considered a group of pigs loaded and subsequently unloaded from the trailer after transport) that had been previously transported on that bedding, and loading percentage on the trailer was collected at the finishing site and processing plant.

Data on the following aspects of transport was collected both at the finishing site and at the processing plant:

- Bedding level applied to the trailer;
- Number of loads previously transported on the bedding currently in the trailer; and,
- Loading percentage, or percent of intended load that was actually loaded onto the trailer.

2.4. Temperature and Relative Humidity Inside the Trailers

Sensors (Extech model RHT10, Extech Instruments, Nashua, NH and HOBO Model H08-003-02, Onset Computer Corp., Bourne, MA) collected temperature and relative humidity every 5 min during loading, waiting time at the farm, transit, waiting time at the plant, and unloading. Sensors were installed inside the trailers in 4 locations. All sensors were placed approximately 1 m above the trailer floor, which allowed data to be collected near the pigs, but were out of reach of the pigs. Two sensors were placed on each deck of the trailer, 1 in the frontmost compartment and 1 in the rearmost compartment of each deck. Sensors were placed opposite of the other sensor on the same deck. Additionally, sensors were placed opposite of the corresponding sensor on the other deck, e.g., if the sensor on the top deck in the frontmost compartment was placed on the left side, then the sensor on the bottom deck in the frontmost compartment would be placed on the right side [9].

Air temperature and relative humidity (RH) were recorded as a single measure at the processing plant upon arrival of each trailer using the Kestrel sensors (Kestrel 4500 Pocket Weather Tracker and Extech model RHT10, Extech Instruments, Nashua, NH). Air temperature and RH are available for 70% of the trailers.

2.5. Transport Losses over the Two Experiments

Total numbers of DOA, NA, and total D&D (including dead in pen) pigs for each load were recorded by auditors and matched with plant records. The NA counts included both injured and non-injured pigs as plant protocol did not differentiate between NA and NAI.

2.6. Pig Surface Temperature

Skin surface temperatures were taken with a dual laser infrared laser thermometer (Extech model # 42570, Extech Instruments, Nashua, NH, USA) laterally near the midline of randomly selected animals at loading and unloading. As surface temperatures were relatively uniform at farm site (loading), surface temperature data at the plant will be used. Ten pigs were randomly selected from each load, 5 of first 50 unloaded and 5 of last 50 unloaded. Because the trailer was the experimental unit, data from the 10 pigs sampled for surface temperature at the plant were averaged to get a single value per trailer.

2.7. Bedding Moisture

Bedding samples were collected for moisture percentage analysis after pigs had been unloaded. Researchers collected 1 sample of at least 100 g of bedding from the center of each deck, ensuring that the entire thickness of the bedding was represented. Samples were stored in resealable zipper storage bags, which in turn were sealed into larger resealable zipper storage bags, so as to prevent moisture loss. The samples were not frozen until the end of the week due to lack of freezer space at the plant; therefore, the time from collection to freezing varied from 1 to 5 days. Samples were stored at −80 °C until analyzed. Moisture percentage was estimated by drying 3 to 4 g of bedding in an aluminum cup at 100 °C for 24 h and calculating the percentage loss of moisture as shown [10]:

$$\% \, Total \; dry \; matter = \frac{(wt. \, dried \; sample + container) - wt. \, container}{(wt. \, wet \; sample + container) - wt. \, container} \times 100\%$$

$$\% \, total \; moisture = 100 - \% \, total \; dry \; matter$$

Samples were analyzed in duplicate. If the coefficient of variation (CV) between the samples was greater than 10%, samples were analyzed again in duplicate until the CV was less than 10%.

2.8. Statistical Analyses

The statistical model included the effects of bedding level, outside air temperature (in 5 °C bins), and the interaction of bedding level and outside air temperature. The experimental unit was the trailer containing all pigs (average of 166.9 ± 0.63 pigs/trailer) in all studies that examined bedding and air temperature effects. The experimental unit was also the trailer, with a sample of 10 pigs from a given trailer for surface temperature assessment data set. All data were analyzed using SAS 9.2 General Linear Models procedure (SAS, 2010 SAS Inst., Inc., Cary, NC, USA). When the treatment P-values were less than 0.10, a T-test (unprotected if P = 0.10 to 0.05) was performed using the Predicted Difference test within the Least Squares Means procedure of SAS. Regression analyses were calculated to determine linear and quadratic effects for air temperature in relation to DOA, NA, D&D, and pig skin surface temperatures at the plant.

3. Results and Discussion

3.1. Temperature and relative humidity inside the trailers

Averages and ranges of temperatures and RH inside the trailers during transport for all experiments are presented in Table 1.

Table 1. Average and range of temperatures and relative humidity (RH) inside trailers during Experiment 1 (cold) and Experiment 2 (mild) during transportation of finishing pigs.

Experiment	Number of trailers	Temperature [°C] [2]			RH [%] [2]		
		Average	Minimum	Maximum	Average	Minimum	Maximum
1 [1]	172	7.8 ± 0.10	−6.80	26.60	69.2 ± 0.25	23.60	98.80
2 [1]	265	12.1 ± 0.09	−3.70	33.20	60.9 ± 0.25	19.40	100.00

[1] Experiment 1 was conducted in January and February 2011. Experiment 2 was conducted in March and May 2011. [2] Temperature and RH data were collected at 5 minute intervals via sensors placed throughout the trailer.

3.2. Transport Losses over the Three Experiments

3.2.1. Experiment 1—Cold Weather

A total of 166.0 ± 1.98 pigs were transported in trailers with six bales of bedding and 165.36 ± 2.43 pigs in trailers with 12 bales of bedding ($P = 0.81$). There were no observed main effects for bedding level on the trailer, outside air temperature, or the interaction for transport losses in the finishing pig ($P > 0.13$). Table 2 shows the effect of bedding level on transport losses in cold weather.

The percentage of DOA, NA, and D&D pigs in relation to outside temperature bins in cold weather is presented in Figure 1.

Figure 1. Least square means of dead on arrival (DOA), non-ambulatory (NA), and total dead and down (D&D) pigs, respectively, in relation to outside temperature bins in cold weather. Total number of loads for each temperature bin is given in parentheses: −5 °C (14), 0 °C (44), 5 °C (24), 10 °C (15), 15 °C (9), and 20 °C (4). A total of 110 trailers each carrying an average of 164.28 pigs were used for this study.

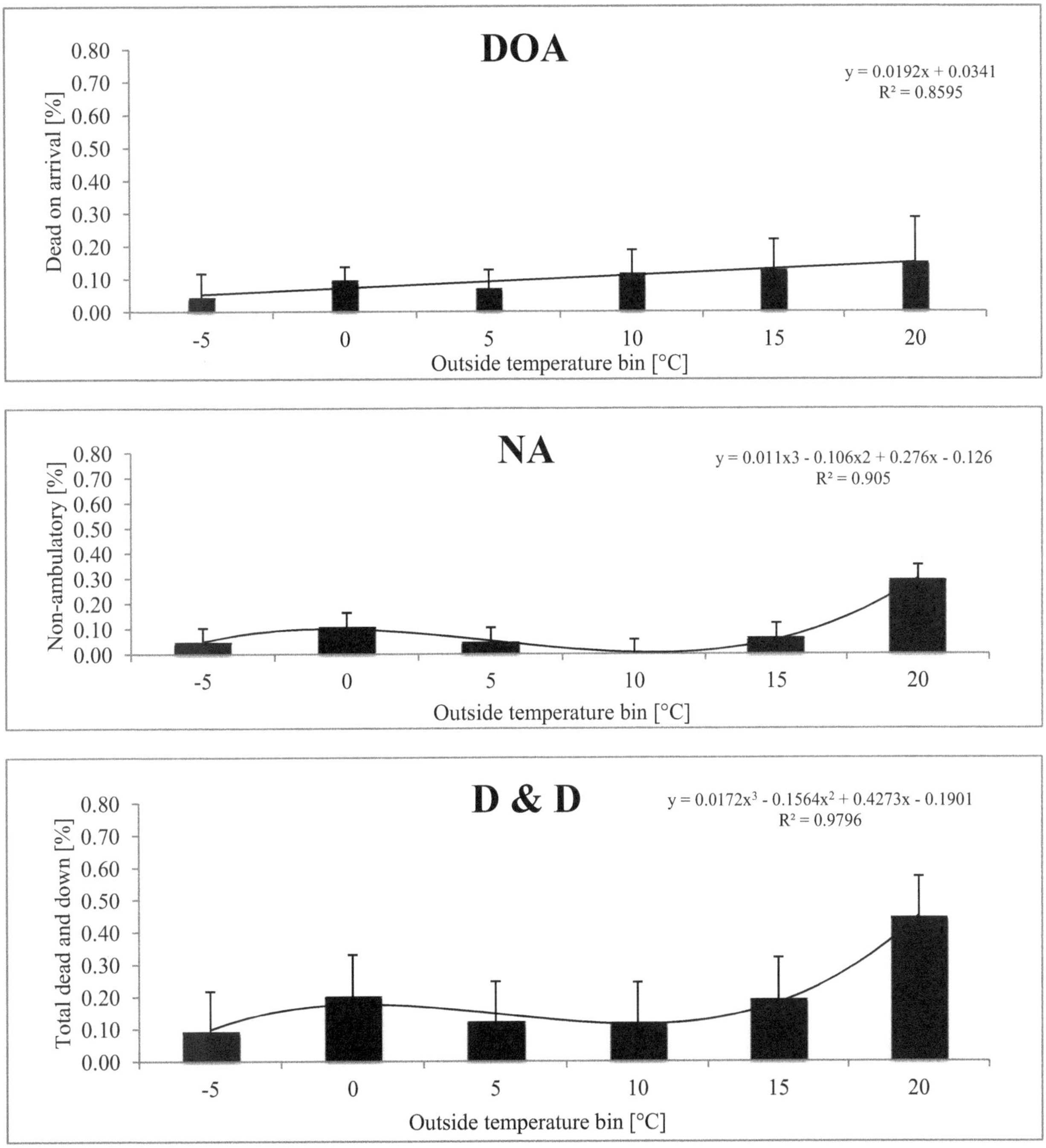

Table 2. Effect of bedding level on the percentage of dead on arrival (DOA), non-ambulatory (NA), and total dead and down (D&D) pigs during Experiment 1 (cold weather, air temperature −13 °C to 20 °C).

Condition upon arrival [%]	Bedding level [bales [1]/trailer]		SEp	*P*-values		
	6	12		Bedding	Temperature	Bedding × Temperature
No. of trailers	103	69				
No. of pigs	17,100	11,403				
DOA	0.06	0.12	0.03	0.13	0.95	0.56
NA	0.05	0.07	0.03	0.73	0.53	0.54
D&D	0.11	0.18	0.04	0.29	0.73	0.47

[1] One bale = 22.7 kg, 0.2 m^3.

3.2.2. Experiment 2—Mild Weather

There was a difference in the number of pigs loaded with three (169.0 ± 1.98 pigs), six (172.8 ± 1.83 pigs), and 12 (159.9 ± 3.29 pigs) bales of bedding ($P < 0.01$). There was no observed main effect for bedding or for the bedding by temperature interaction on transport losses in the finishing pig (Table 3) ($P > 0.05$). There was no temperature effect on DOA (P = 0.86); however temperature did affect NA ($P < 0.01$), and tended to affect D&D ($P = 0.07$). Table 3 shows the effect of bedding level on types of losses in mild weather.

Table 3. Effect of bedding level on percentage of dead on arrival (DOA), non-ambulatory (NA), and total dead and down (D&D) pigs during Experiment 2 (mild weather, air temperature −2 °C to 21 °C).

Condition upon arrival [%]	Bedding level [bales [1]/trailer]			SEp	*P*-values		
	3	6	12		Bedding	Temperature	Bedding × Temperature
No. of trailers	105	122	38				
No. of pigs	17,745	21,080	6,075				
DOA	0.11	0.12	0.03	0.03	0.21	0.86	0.30
NA	0.09	0.10	0.13	0.03	0.84	0.01	0.19
D&D	0.20	0.22	0.09	0.05	0.34	0.07	0.17

[1] One bale = 22.7 kg, 0.2 m^3

Figure 2 represents percentages of DOA, NA, and D&D pigs in relation to outside temperature bins in mild weather.

Figure 2. Least square means of Dead on arrival (%), Non-ambulatory (%), Total dead and down (%), respectively, in relation to outside temperature bins in mild weather. Total number of loads for each temperature bins represented in parenthesis: 0(6), 5(23), 10(29), 15(47), 20(27), 25(2). 134 trailers with 32,962 (average = 171.67) pigs were used for this study.

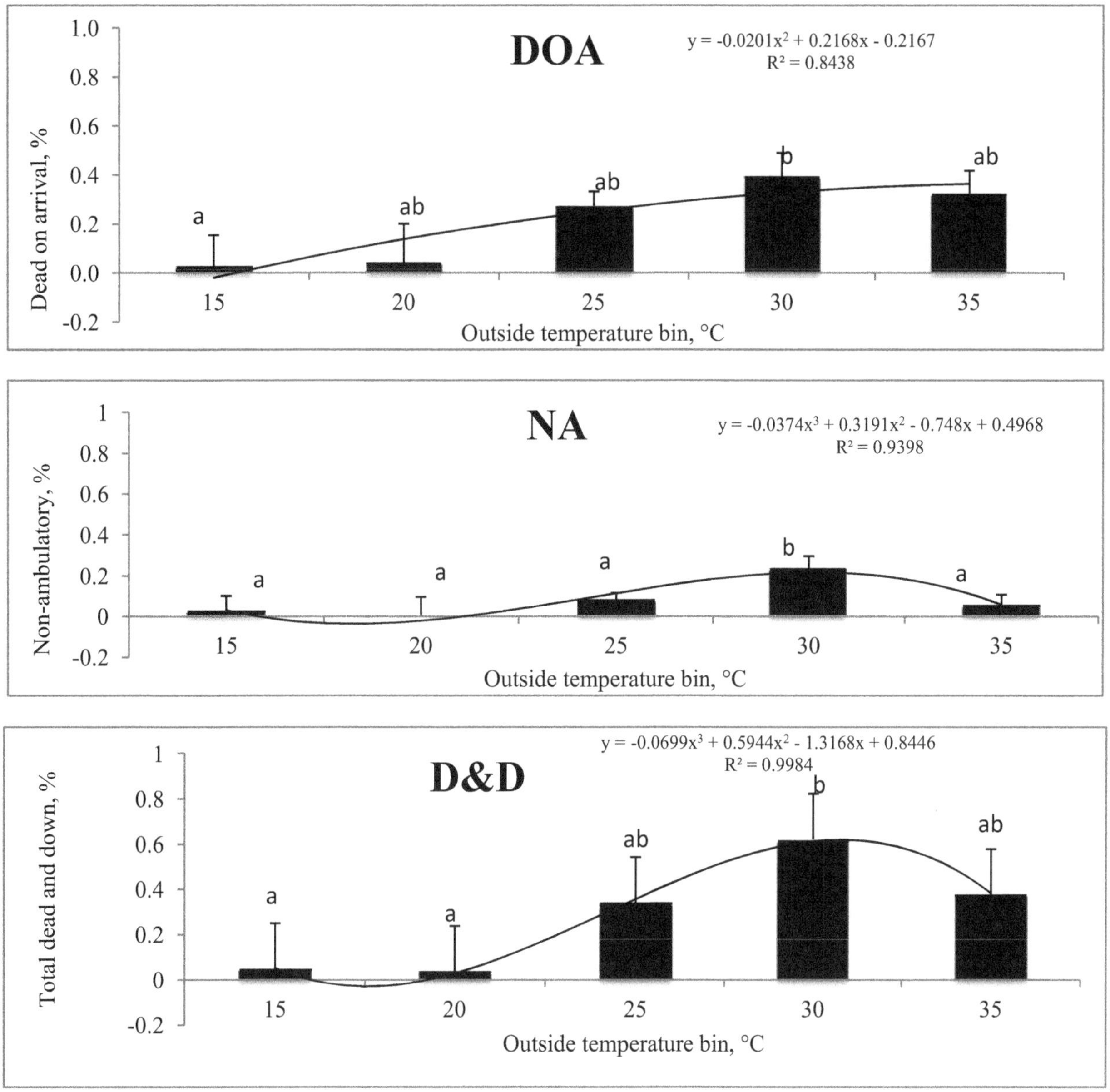

3.3. Pig Surface Temperature at the Plant

In cold weather there was no difference for surface temperatures at the plants for pigs transported with six *vs*. 12 bales (23.8 ± 0.85 °C *vs*. 23.98 ± 0.98 °C) ($P = 0.96$).

In mild weather, skin surface temperature of pigs transported with three or six bales of bedding was not different and skin surface temperature of pigs transported with 12 bales of bedding was lower than that of pigs transported with three or six bales ($P < 0.05$). Surface temperatures differed at the plant (28.9 ± 0.50 °C for three bales, 29.2 ± 0.49 °C for six bales, and 25.9 ± 0.84 °C for 12 bales ($P < 0.01$)) but were not different at the finishing site ($P > 0.05$).

3.4. Overall Effect of Air Temperature

Pig surface temperature at the plant responded to outside air temperature with approximately a 0.37 °C increase per 1.0 °C increase in outside air temperature. The DOA, NA, and D&D percentages increased as outside temperature increased at the plant ($P < 0.01$, 0.05, and < 0.01, respectively). A sharp rise in D&D rates was observed when pig surface temperature exceeded 32 °C.

When skin surface temperature at the plant was plotted against outside air temperatures for all temperature bins (−5 °C to 20 °C, in 5°C bins), skin surface temperature increased linearly with increasing outside air temperature ($P < 0.01$). The regression line linear fit had an r^2 of 0.95, which indicates a strong relationship. In addition, above 30 °C, D&D increased linearly with increasing skin surface temperature after transportation ($r^2 = 0.81$), indicating that skin surface temperature can be used as an indicator of D&D following transportation. This method does not apply to losses occurring on the trailer (DOA, specifically), but may be beneficial in determining if cooling interventions are necessary when pigs arrive at their destination. Figure 3 shows the linear relationship between skin surface temperature and outside air temperature at the processing plant.

Figure 3. Skin surface temperature of pigs in relation to outside air temperature when unloaded at the processing plant. Total number of loads for each temperature bin is given in parentheses: −5 °C (14), 0 °C (14), 5 °C (31) 10 °C (25), 15 °C (70), 20 °C (39), and 25 °C (86). A total of 335 loads with 56,106 pigs were used for this analysis.

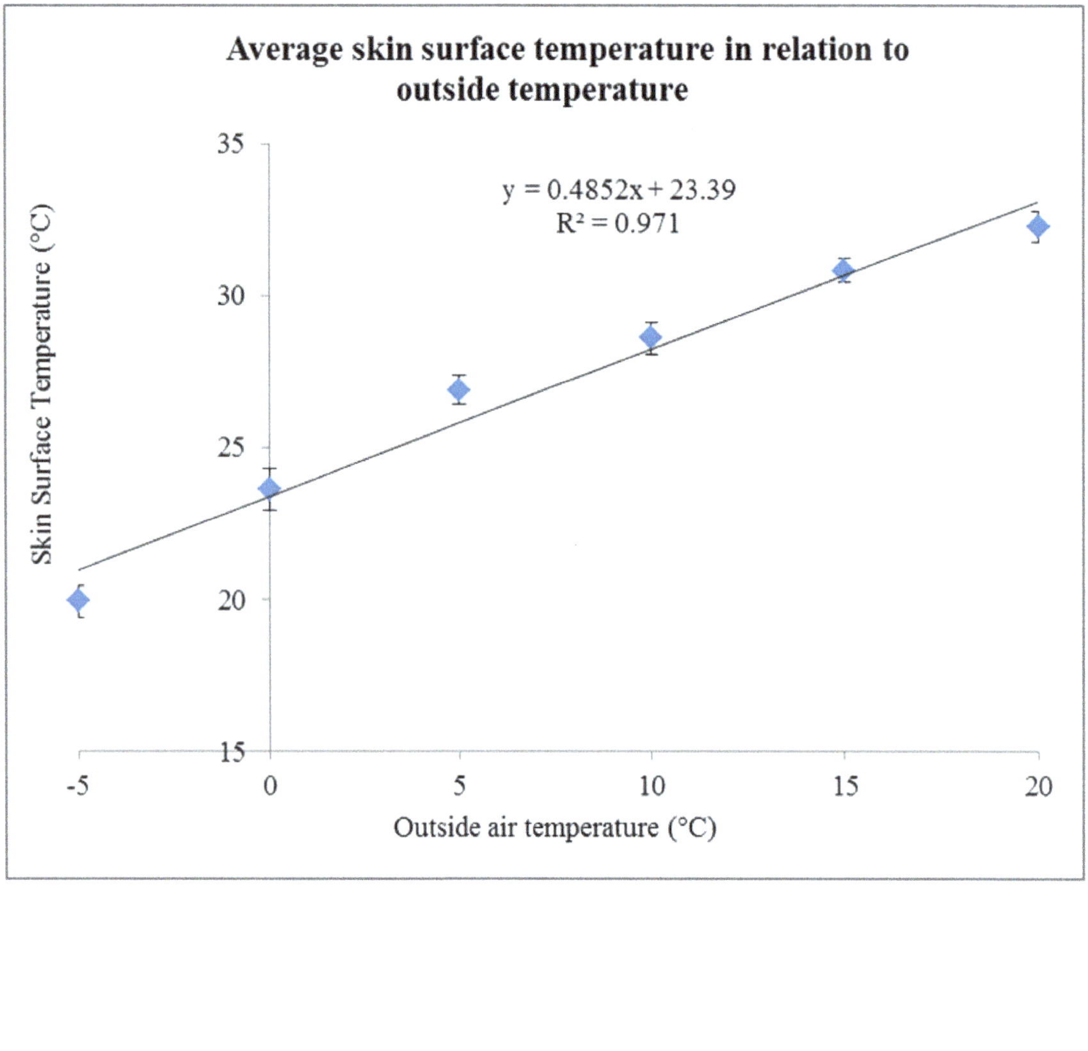

3.5. Bedding Moisture

Bedding samples were not collected in January, and 42 samples were available for moisture analysis in February. Of these samples, average moisture content in the bedding after pigs were unloaded was 60.4 ± 1.86% (minimum 35.8%, maximum 74.4%). Of 213 samples collected and analyzed in March and May, average moisture content in the bedding collected at the plant after unloading was 58.2 ± 1.07% (minimum 25.6%, maximum 80.8%). Moisture content of the bedding did not have a significant effect on losses in cold or mild temperatures.

4. Conclusions

Ethical and economical transport of finishing pigs is an important aspect of swine production and welfare. Annual transportation losses in the U.S. were estimated at approximately $46 million in 2006 [2]. Transportation is a known stressor for swine that has been previously assessed measuring metabolic products such as cortisol, and by determining decreases in carcass yield and the percentage of DOA, NAI, and NANI pigs [6,11,12]. Factors like stocking density, travel distance, total time to transport, feed withdrawal, handling at loading and unloading, season, trailer type, and microenvironment have been identified as factors associated with in-transit losses [13–15].

The results of this study showed that in cold weather, bedding level neither improved nor worsened the percentages of DOA, NA, and D&D. Based on this finding it would be advisable to provide six bales of bedding in cold weather, as there is no proven benefit of providing more. However, there is no data on rates of losses with less than six bales of bedding; therefore, more research is needed on fewer than six bales of bedding to make an accurate recommendation.

There was no effect of bedding level in mild weather. This study showed that there is no advantage of providing more than three bales of bedding. As in cold weather, there is no available data for rates of losses when animals are transported with less than three bales, so more research is needed to provide an accurate recommendation.

The findings of the present study agree with those of Fitzgerald [16], in that the percentage of total losses per trailer was greater during winter compared to mild weather. Also, losses during winter were mainly a result of fatigued pigs, possibly attributed to shivering. Past research correlates in-transit losses with stocking density, season, trailer design, and ventilation [17], but no studies have measured in-transit losses associated with the bedding level used. Results obtained from this study showed that higher levels of bedding did not result in fewer losses in terms of DOA, NA, and D&D during winter as opposed to the bedding levels recommended by the TQA handbook. Similarly, no benefit was observed from using higher levels of bedding during mild weather. The present study showed that skin surface temperature increased linearly by 0.37 °C for every 1.0 °C increase in outside air temperature during unloading at the processing plant. In a preliminary study, skin surface temperature was shown to increase by 0.19 °C for every 1.0°C rise in outside air temperature after being transported for 14 h [18]. Chung *et al.* [19] determined that skin surface temperature could be used to predict rectal temperature after piglets are transported. The results of their study suggested that rectal temperature increases by 0.30 °C for every 1 °C increase in abdominal surface temperature. In addition, D&D rate during the summer increased linearly with skin surface temperature above 30 °C, suggesting that this relationship may be useful as a means of predicting D&D rates during summer transportation.

When bedding samples were assessed for moisture content after transportation, it was found that moisture levels were approximately 2-fold greater after the second load of pigs when compared to the first. Unused bedding contained approximately 5% moisture. After the first load moisture content increased to 26%. After two loads of pigs had been transported on the same bedding, moisture content was nearly 51%. This moisture in the bedding may contribute to transport losses in winter, where the dampness combined with cold air may cause the pigs to shiver more, supporting the knowledge that winter losses are primarily a result of fatigued pigs. Reuse of bedding occurs due to the costs of washing out and applying new bedding to a trailer after each transport. Kephart *et al.* [20] estimates the annual cost of washing out and rebidding to be between 22 and 135 million dollars.

Overall, excessive use of bedding should be avoided. It has no direct benefit to the animals, and may even be harmful. The authors of this paper determined that overuse of bedding results in approximately $4 million in extra expenses annually. This represents a large economic impact to the transport industry. The current study needs to be expanded upon in order to make accurate recommendations for transport during each season and in different climate ranges.

Acknowledgments

We thank National Pork Board for funding this study. The cooperation of graduate and undergraduate farmers, trucking companies, and processing plants during data collection is greatly appreciated. Glenna Pirner helped with the preparation of this manuscript.

Author Contributions

John McGlone conceived the idea for this work and designed the experiments. Anna Johnson contributed to the experimental design. Avi Sapkota carried out the experiments, conducted data analysis, and drafted the article. Rebecca Kephart assisted with carrying out the experiments.

Conflicts of Interest

The authors declare no conflict of interest. This work was supported by the National Pork Board, Texas Tech University, and Iowa State University.

References and Notes

1. United States Department of Agriculture National Agricultural Statistics Service. Available online: http://www.nass.usda.gov/Statistics_by_Subject/result.php?D137063F-E35A-32C3-9919-CB2865784714&sector=ANIMALS%20%26%20PRODUCTS&group=LIVESTOCK&comm=HOGS (accessed on 12 August 2013).
2. Ritter, M.J.; Ellis, M.; Berry, N.L.; Curtis, S.E.; Anil, L.; Berg, E.; Benjamin, M.; Butler, D.; Dewey, C.; Driessen, B.; DuBois, P.; Hill, J.D.; Marchant-Forde, J.N.; Matzat, P.; McGlone, J.; Mormede, P.; Moyer, T.; Pfalzgraf, K.; Salak-Johnson, J.; Siemens, M.; Sterle, J.; Stull, C.; Whiting, T.; Wolter, B.; Niekamp, S.R.; Johnson, A.K. Review: Transport Losses in Market Weight Pigs: I. A Review of Definitions, Incidence, and Economic Impact. *Prof. Anim. Sci.* **2009**, *25*, 404–414.

3. Sutherland, M.A.; McDonald, A.; McGlone, J.J. Effects of variations in the environment, length of journey and type of trailer on the mortality and morbidity of pigs being transported to slaughter. *Vet. Rec.* **2009**, *165*, 13–18.
4. Grandin, T. Assessment of stress during handling and transport. *J. Anim. Sci.* **1997**, *75*, 249–257.
5. Ellis, M.; Wang, X.; Funk, T.; Wolter, B.; Murphy, C.; Lenkaitis, A.; Sun, Y.; Pilcher, C. Development of improved trailer designs and transport management practices that create the optimum environment for market weight pigs during transport and minimize transport losses. Available online: http://www.pork.org/FileLibrary/ResearchDocuments/05-192-Ellis-UofILL.pdf (accessed on 6 August 2012).
6. Warriss, P.D.; Dudley, C.P.; Brown, S.N. Reduction of carcass yield in transported pigs. *J. Sci. Food Agr.* **1983**, *34*, 351–356.
7. National Pork Board. Transport Quality Assurance Handbook. 2008. Available online: http://www.pork.org/filelibrary/TQAAdvisor/TQA4Manual.pdf (accessed on 16 July 2012).
8. McGlone, J.; Sapkota, A.; Johnson, A. Establishing boarding requirements for finishing pigs during transport. *Animals* **2014**, submitted.
9. Kephart, R.K.; Johnson, A.K.; Stalder, K.J.; McGlone, J.J.; Fitzgerald, R.F. Internal temperature and relative humidity of trailers hauling market-weight pigs in the Midwest during warm weather. *Animals* **2014**, submitted.
10. Combs, S.; Hoskins, B.; Jarman, J.; Kovar, J.; Watson, M.; Wolf, A.; Wolf, N. *Recommended Methods of Manure Analysis*; Cooperative Extension Publishing: Madison, WI, USA, 2003; p. 16.
11. Bradshaw, R.H.; Parrott, R.F.; Forsling, M.F.; Goode, J.A.; Lloyd, D.M.; Rodway, R.G.; Broom, D.M. Stress and travel sickness in pigs: Effects of road transport on plasma concentrations of cortisol, beta-endorphin and lysine vasopressin. *Anim. Sci.* **1996**, *63*, 507–516.
12. Minka, N.S.; Ayo, J.O. Physiological responses of food animals to road transportation stress. *Afr. J. Biotechnol.* **2010**, *40*, 6601–6613.
13. Lambooy, E.; Engel, B. Transport of slaughter pigs by truck over a long distance: some aspects of loading density and ventilation. *Livest. Prod. Sci.* **1991**, *28*, 163–174.
14. Lewis, N.J.; Berry, R.J.; Crow, G.; Wamnes, S. Assessment of the effects of the season of transport on the performance of early-weaned piglets. *Can. J. Anim. Sci.* **2005**, *85*, 449–454.
15. Haley, C.; Dewey, C.E.; Widowski, T.; Poljak, Z.; Friendship, R. Association between in-transit loss, internal trailer temperature, and distance traveled by Ontario market hogs. *Can. J. Vet. Res.* **2008**, *72*, 385-389.
16. Fitzgerald, R.F.; Stadler, K.J.; Matthews, J.O.; Schultz-Kaster, C.M.; Johnson, A.K. Factors associated with fatigued, injured, and dead pig frequency during transport and lairage at a commercial abattoir. *J. Anim. Sci.* **2009**, *87*, 1156–1166.
17. Gade, P.B.; Christensen, L. Effect of different stocking densities during transport on welfare and meat quality in Danish slaughter pigs. *Meat Sci.* **1998**, *48*, 237–247.
18. Costa, L.N.; Redaelli, V.; Magnani, D.; Cafazzo, S.; Amadori, M.; Razzuoli, E.; Verga, M.; Luzi, F. Preliminary study on the relationship between skin temperature of piglets measured by infrared thermography and environmental temperature in a vehicle in transit. In *Veterinary Science: Current Aspects in Biology, Animal Pathology, Clinic and Food Hygiene*; Pugliese, A., Gaiti, A., Boiti, C., Eds.; Springer: Berlin, Germany, 2012; pp. 193–197.

19. Chung, T.; Jung, W.; Nam, E.; Kim, J.; Park, S.; Hwang, C.Y. Comparison of rectal infrared thermometry for obtaining body temperature of gnotobiotic piglets in conventional portable germ free facility. *Asian-Austr. J. Anim. Sci.* **2010**, *23*, 1364–1368.
20. Kephart, R.K.; Johnson, A.K.; Stalder, K.J.; Huiatt, T.W.; Sapkota, A.; McGlone, J.J. *Costs of Bedding, Trailer Washout, and Transport Losses in Market Weight Pigs*; Iowa State University Animal Industry Report; AS 660, ASL R2908; Iowa State University: Ames, Iowa, USA, 2014.

5

The Effect of Age, Stocking Density and Flooring during Transport on Welfare of Young Dairy Calves in Australia

Ellen C. Jongman [1,*] and Kym L. Butler [1,2]

[1] Animal Welfare Science Centre, The Melbourne School of Land and Environment, University of Melbourne, Parkville, VIC 3010, Australia

[2] Biometrics Group, Department of Environment and Primary Industries (Victoria), Werribee, VIC 3030, Australia; E-Mail: kym.butler@depi.vic.gov.au

* Author to whom correspondence should be addressed; E-Mail: ejongman@unimelb.edu.au.

Simple Summary: Young calves are vulnerable to the stressful conditions associated with transport. This study examined the effect of age, stocking density and flooring during transport on lying behaviour and some physiological measurements of metabolic state, dehydration and muscle damage in young calves. While physiology and behaviour changed with age, there were no clear effects of transport. More space and straw bedding however was of benefit to calves of all ages, with some indication that straw bedding could ameliorate some of the negative effects of reduced space on lying behaviour.

Abstract: Transport of young ('bobby') calves for slaughter is a contentious welfare issue for some sectors of the Australian community. Factors of age, stocking density and flooring need further research to develop appropriate welfare standards for transport of bobby calves. The objective of this study was to identify the space allowance requirements for transport of bobby calves and to understand factors such as age and flooring that minimise risks to calf welfare during transport. Animals aged 3-, 5- and 10-day old were transported for 12 h in a custom-made cattle truck fitted with 9 pens, with movable mesh divisions. Each pen contained 4 calves, with space allowances of 0.2, 0.3 and 0.5 m^2 per calf and flooring of solid metal, mesh or straw bedding. A total of 432 male dairy calves were transported in 12 trips during the 2-year study. Behavioural measurements included lying during transport, and lying and drinking for 12 h after transport during recovery. Blood samples were taken prior to transport, immediately after transport and 12 h after transport.

Blood samples were analysed for metabolic state (glucose, beta-hydroxy-butyrate (BOHB)), hydration (packed cell volume (PCV)) and exhaustion/bruising (creatine kinase (CK) activity). It was found that several measures were affected by age, which indicates that the physiology and in particular lying behaviour of 3-day old calves is fundamentally different from that of older calves. It is unclear how this affects their ability to cope with the stressors of transport. Space affected the posture changes and CK activity during and after transport and it is concluded that space allowance should be at least 0.3 m^2 per calf for calves of average size, while CK activity suggested that providing more space to 0.5 m^2 per calf may provide even greater benefits. Straw bedding is of clear benefit to calves during transport, to the extent that it may even reduce some of the negative effects of reduced space on lying behaviour.

Keywords: bobby calves; transport; space allowance; flooring; dairy cattle

---

1. Introduction

In Australia, a bobby calf is defined as a calf not accompanied by its dam and under 4 weeks of age [1]. It is usually a dairy breed or cross, often male, and is destined for slaughter. Most bobby calves are slaughtered within the first week of life.

Because of their age and vulnerability the transport of bobby calves is a contentious welfare issue for some sectors of the Australian community. Overcrowding of bobby calves during transport can result in injury and death, and calves that lie down during transport in overcrowded pens can find it difficult to rise and can become trampled. While there is no law regarding the loading density for bobby calves during transport in Australia, for either short or long duration journeys, the Australian Animal Welfare Standards [1] stipulates that during transport all calves should have sufficient space to lie down on their sternum. It also recommends that all calves less than 30 days old that are transported should have bedding. Calves less than 5 days old travelling without mothers to rearing facilities however must be provided with thick bedding and room to lie down and not be transported for longer than 6 h. These standards are based on the premise that, with bobby calves, extra space and bedding will increase lying and improve welfare. However, there is no experimental evidence to support this premise using behavioural and physiology measures.

Given there is sufficient space, young calves prefer to lie down during transport. In several studies calves were found to lie down 50% [2] to more than 70% [3] of the transport time. Smaller calves may be more affected by transport than bigger calves, as they show a greater need to lie down [4].

Mortalities occur during transport and lairage and have been found to increase with transport duration, with truck design being considered a major contributing factor [5]. Although few calves die during transport, Knowles [6] describes an inverse correlation between age at the time of travel and mortality. This effect was particularly noticeable in the weeks after transport, where calves may die due to secondary infections as a consequence of impaired immune function due to transport stress.

Young calves are vulnerable to the stresses of transport and the associated handling during loading and unloading [5,7]. They are particularly hard to handle as a group, as they have not yet developed a herding instinct [8,9]. Even when handled individually, calves become easier to move as their age increases from 3 to 10 days of age [10]. The Welfare Standards for transport for slaughter in Australia [1] states that calves should not be transported for slaughter until they are 5 days old, be fed within 6 h before loading and be transported for no more than 12 h. The guidelines recommend that calves should be of minimum live weight of 23 kg, have hooves that are firm and worn flat and a navel cord that is wrinkled, withered and shriveled. According to the Animal Husbandry Survey 2010, commissioned by Dairy Australia [11], 73% of all farms which sell calves have a permanent record of birth dates and/or a permanent identification tag or collar. However, if calves on farms are not identified by date of birth, it is possible that some calves are transported at an earlier age, as weight and navel cord dryness alone (often used as an indicator of fitness for transport) cannot be used for an indicator of age [12].

Factors of age, stocking density and flooring need further research to develop appropriate welfare standards for the transport of bobby calves. The objective of this study was to identify the space allowance requirements for transport of bobby calves and to understand factors such as age and flooring that minimise risks to welfare during transport of bobby calves. The interactions between these factors may lead to better recommendations on the transport of bobby calves of different ages. The effect of transport conditions on the welfare of calves in this study was measured using variables that may indicate effects on metabolic state (glucose, beta-hydroxy-butyrate (BOHB)), hydration (packed cell volume (PCV)) and assessment of muscle exhaustion/bruising (creatine kinase (CK) activity), as have been used in previous studies on transport of calves [2,4,7,13].

2. Materials and Methods

This experiment was conducted at the Department of Environment and Primary Industries (DEPI), Werribee Centre, Victoria, Australia with the approval from the DEPI-Victoria Agricultural Research and Extension Animal Ethics Committee and in accordance with the Australian Code of Practice for the Care and Use of Animals for Scientific Purposes [14].

2.1. Animals

A total of 432 calves (Friesian and Friesian-cross) were transported from commercial farms in Victoria, Australia, where they were kept under commercial conditions in group housing until transport. Each journey consisted of 36 calves sourced from 1 commercial farm in spring or a combination of 4 different farms within close proximity owned by the same farmer in autumn. Transport dates were determined in consultation with each farmer to coincide with dates when large numbers of calves were expected. They were than instructed to keep 36 calves born on certain dates (with 12 calves on each date) in relation to the date of transport. This ensured that a full consignment within three age groups (3, 5 and 10 days old) could be transported on the allocated transport date. Calves were fed 4 L of colostrum in the morning and were loaded onto the truck via a ramp about 1 h after feeding and blood sampling.

2.2. Transport

Animals were transported for 12 h in a custom-made cattle truck, where they were protected from the elements as per a standard Australian cattle truck (solid front, ventilation from the sides and no roof). The truck was fitted with 9 pens, with movable mesh divisions so stocking densities could be changed according to the allocated location within the truck. The calves were loaded individually via a portable ramp, and careful handling aimed to reduce stress during loading as much as possible. The route consisted of a mix of country roads, main roads and freeways. A total of 6 trips in spring and 6 trips in autumn were conducted over a 2-year period and no climate extremes of hot, cold or very wet weather were encountered, with temperatures within the range of 10 °C to 25 °C and only an occasional brief shower. All pens could be observed with fixed digital cameras (Ness 2.9 mm transit cameras) and data were recorded on a digital recorder (Ness 8-channel mobile MPEG4 DVR) fitted in the cabin of the truck.

2.3. Recovery

After transport, animals were unloaded and housed within one indoor facility in pens in the same groups of 4, with a pen size of 3 m × 3.8 m, where they were observed for another 12 h during recovery. Every pen was observed with fixed digital cameras (b/w CCD infrared cameras fitted with 4.3 mm lenses) and data were recorded on a digital recorder (16-channel I-Watch DVR system) in an adjacent shed. Pen divisions in the shed were made of steel mesh. The animals were provided with straw bedding during recovery from transport. They were not fed during recovery, but did have access to fresh drinking water.

2.4. Treatments

The experimental design was a 3 stocking density × 3 age of calf × 3 flooring type factorial, with treatments combinations allocated to trips, and truck position for each trip (see Table 1). The stocking density treatments consisted of space allowances of 0.2 m^2, 0.3 m^2 or 0.5 m^2 per calf. Movable mesh dividers could be placed at different locations to form pens that were 1m wide and either 0.8 m, 1.2 m or 2 m long. Calves were aged 3, 5 and 10 days old at the day of transport. The truck floor consisted of solid steel. A second floor made out of steel mesh (2.5 cm^2) or a comfortable layer of cereal straw bedding (approximately 10 cm deep) was added on top of the steel floor to the allocated pens so the effect of flooring of either solid steel, steel mesh or straw could be studied. Each pen contained 4 calves, with a total number of 9 pens per trip, with a total of 432 male dairy calves transported over 12 trips during the 2-year study.

Table 1. Diagrammatic representation of the allocation of treatments to trips, and to the truck position for each trip. St denotes straw flooring, So denotes solid flooring and Me denotes mesh flooring. Number of days is the age of calf and the area is the space per calf in a pen of four calves.

	Replicate 1 and 2								
	Trips 1 and 4			*Trips 2 and 6*			*Trips 3 and 5*		
	Left	Mid	Right	Left	Mid	Right	Left	Mid	Right
Front	St/3 day/0.2 m^2	St/5 day/0.3 m^2	St/10 day/0.5 m^2	So/10 day/0.3 m^2	So/3 day/0.5 m^2	So/5 day/0.2 m^2	Me/5 day/0.5 m^2	Me/10 day/0.2 m^2	Me/3 day/0.3 m^2
Centre	Me/10 day/0.3 m^2	Me/3 day/0.5 m^2	Me/5 day/0.2 m^2	St/5 day/0.5 m^2	St/10 day/0.2 m^2	St/3 day/0.3 m^2	So/3 day/0.2 m^2	So/5 day/0.3 m^2	So/10 day/0.5 m^2
Rear	So/5 day/0.5 m^2	So/10 day/0.2 m^2	So/3 day/0.3 m^2	Me/3 day/0.2 m^2	Me/5 day/0.3 m^2	Me/10 day/0.5 m^2	St/10 day/0.3 m^2	St/3 day/0.5 m^2	St/5 day/0.2 m^2
	Replicate 3								
	Trip 7			*Trip 8*			*Trip 9*		
	Left	Mid	Right	Left	Mid	Right	Left	Mid	Right
Front	St/10 day/0.3 m^2	St/5 day/0.5 m^2	St/3 day/0.2 m^2	St/5 day/0.2 m^2	St/3 day/0.3 m^2	St/10 day/0.5 m^2	St/3 day/0.5 m^2	St/10 day/0.2 m^2	St/5 day/0.3 m^2
Centre	Me/5 day/0.2 m^2	Me/3 day/0.3 m^2	Me/10 day/0.5 m^2	Me/3 day/0.5 m^2	Me/10 day/0.2 m^2	Me/5 day/0.3 m^2	So/5 day/0.2 m^2	So/3 day/0.3 m^2	So/10 day/0.5 m^2
Rear	So/3 day/0.5 m^2	So/10 day/0.2 m^2	So/5 day/0.3 m^2	So/10 day/0.3 m^2	So/5 day/0.5 m^2	So/3 day/0.2 m^2	Me/10 day/0.3 m^2	Me/5 day/0.5 m^2	Me/3 day/0.2 m^2
	Replicate 4								
	Trip 10			*Trip 11*			*Trip 12*		
	Left	Mid	Right	Left	Mid	Right	Left	Mid	Right
Front	Me/5 day/0.3 m^2	Me/10 day/0.2 m^2	Me/3 day/0.5 m^2	Me/3 day/0.2 m^2	Me/5 day/0.5 m^2	Me/10 day/0.3 m^2	St/5 day/0.3 m^2	St/10 day/0.2 m^2	St/3 day/0.5 m^2
Centre	St/3 day/0.2 m^2	St/5 day/0.5 m^2	St/10 day/0.3 m^2	St/10 day/0.5 m^2	St/3 day/0.3 m^2	St/5 day/0.2 m^2	So/3 day/0.2 m^2	So/5 day/0.5 m^2	So/10 day/0.3 m^2
Rear	So/10 day/0.5 m^2	So/3 day/0.3 m^2	So/5 day/0.2 m^2	So/5 day/0.3 m^2	So/10 day/0.2 m^2	So/3 day/0.5 m^2	Me/10 day/0.5 m^2	Me/3 day/0.3 m^2	Me/5 day/0.2 m^2

The design had the feature that each calf age and each space allowance were represented once in each left to right position of each trip and represented once in each front to rear position in each trip, so that the main effects of calf age and space could be efficiently estimated. Another feature was that the flooring treatment was represented in all 3 pens of one front to rear position of each trip, so that the flooring main effect was efficiently estimated using between front to rear variation within trips. Other features of the design were that each combination of calf age and space, each combination of calf age and flooring and each combination of space and flooring occurred in one pen in each trip, and each combination of calf age, space and flooring occurred in one pen in each replicate of 3 trips. The randomisation used in creating the design plan for replicates 1, 3 and 4 can be symbolically represented as: Replicate/((Trip/Front to rear position within trips)*(Left to right position across trips)). The symbols '/' and '*' represent nesting and crossing, respectively [15].

Apart from a change trip order, the design of replicate 2 is a duplicate of the design of replicate 1.

2.5. Measurements

The neck area of the calves was clipped the night prior to transport to expose the jugular vein for ease of blood sampling. At the same time, calves were weighed on portable scales in their home pen. Animals were randomly allocated to transport pens. However, due to concerns for the welfare of the animals, if more than 2 very large calves (45 kg or more) were initially allocated to the smallest pens, then one of those large calves was substituted by a smaller calf. This did affect the kg/pen during the study, with a slightly lower weight in the smaller pens (see Results section).

Animals were individually identified within each pen by symbols applied with spray marker on their back. In addition, they were fitted with a nylon animal collar around their neck, fastened with Velcro and marked with the same symbols. Each pen was identified with a number, visible on the video recordings.

Calves were observed by video during transport and in the shed for 12 h after transport. Behavioural measurements included lying during transport, and lying and drinking after transport during recovery. Behaviour was observed through continuous sampling, with each transition from standing to lying and vice versa recorded for each calf. While drinking was difficult to observe, when a calf was observed with the head above the drinking bucket it was recorded as 'drinking'.

Prior to transport and approximately 1 h after feeding in the morning, blood samples were taken via jugular venepuncture, after which the animals were loaded on to the truck and transported for 12 h. Further blood samples were taken immediately after transport and 12 h after transport. Blood samples were analysed for metabolic state (glucose, beta-hydroxy-butyrate (BOHB)), hydration (packed cell volume (PCV)) and assessment of muscle exhaustion/bruising (creatine kinase (CK) activity) by a commercial laboratory (IDEXX Laboratories, Melbourne). Three samples were collected at each blood sampling point: 4-mL serum separator tubes were used to collect blood for analysis for CK activity and BOHB; 2.0-mL fluoride oxalate tubes were used to collect blood for glucose determination; and 4-mL EDTA tubes were used to collect blood for PCV measurement. The whole blood samples were stored at −4 °C before transportation on ice to the laboratory.

2.6. Statistical Analysis

With the exceptions of replicates 1 and 2, the unit of analysis was the average of all calves in a pen in a given trip. Corresponding pens (those with the same treatment combination) in trips 1 and 4, trips 2 and 6, and trips 3 and 5 were averaged to form single units of analysis because, other than a randomisation of trip order, the treatments were inadvertently not re-randomised between replicates 1 and 2. Each measurement was analysed using REML mixed model analyses, that in addition to factorial treatment effects, had a fixed effect for replicates and random effects for trip within replicate, left to right position within replicate (but not trip), front to rear position within each trip, and interaction of trip within replicate and front to back within replicate. These particular random effects were included to be in accord with the randomisation used in the experimental design. In accord with standard experimental design principles, when a variance component was estimated to be less than zero, its estimated value was allowed to stand. Some models did not numerically converge, and in these cases some random effect terms were set to be 0 so as to allow numerical convergence. Prior to REML analyses, some measurements were transformed (see Results section) so that the residual variation did not substantially change with the fitted mean and to reduce skewness of the residuals.

For each variable, factorial treatment effects were tested using Wald F tests. Preliminary analyses indicated that there was only weak evidence between age of calves and the space and flooring treatments, and thus P values for the following effects are presented;

(1) Interaction of calf age with space or flooring treatments (*i.e.*, a combined effect of calf age by space, calf age by flooring and calf age by space by flooring interactions) by comparing a model including all treatment combinations with a model including main effects of calf age, space and flooring, and the two-factor interaction of space and flooring,
(2) Effect of calf age by comparing a model including main effects of calf age, space and flooring, and the two-factor interaction of space and flooring with a model including main effects of space and flooring, and the two-factor interaction of space and flooring,
(3) Interaction of space and flooring treatments by comparing a model including main effects of calf age, space and flooring, and the two-factor interaction of space and flooring with a model including main effects of calf age, space and flooring,
(4) Effect of space treatment by comparing a model including main effects of calf age, space and flooring with a model including main effects of calf age and flooring,
(5) Effect of flooring treatment by comparing a model including main effects of calf age, space and flooring with a model including main effects of calf age and space.

In a few cases the denominator degrees of freedom for the Wald F test was not obtainable, and in these cases a Wald chi-squared test was used as a replacement for the Wald F test. Results are presented as predicted means for each calf age and for each combination of space and flooring measurement. The predicted means for calf age are adjusted for combinations of space and flooring treatments and the predicted means for combinations of space flooring treatments are adjusted for the effects of age. Accordingly all the presented predicted means were obtained using a model with fixed effects for replicate, calf age, space, flooring and the interaction of space and flooring, together with the random effects that were used in all models. Back transformed predicted means are calculated for measurements that were transformed prior to REML analysis by performing the inverse of the transformation (e.g., the inverse of square root is squaring, the inverse of log_{10} is the power of 10). Back transformed predicted means are mostly easily interpreted as a predicted median of a pen, but calculated parametrically. All analyses were carried out using the REML mixed models facilities in the GenStat 16 statistical package [15].

3. Results

The results indicate that there were effects of calf age on both lying behaviour and several of the metabolic parameters (Table 2). In particular, 3-day-old calves lie down more during transport, as well as during the recovery period. They were also lying down more at the time of arrival of the truck at its destination. Three-day-old calves also showed less interest in drinking water during recovery compared with older calves, although this did not affect their hydration. Physiological measures showed that 3-day-old calves were different from older calves, even before transport. However, there were no interactions between age and space/flooring, so restrictions of space and flooring on lying behaviour affected calves of all ages equally.

Table 2. Effect of age on behaviour and physiology before, during and after transport, and after 12 h of recovery. The interaction *P* value is the *P* value for testing for any interaction between calf age and the space or flooring treatments. Approximate least significant differences can be calculated as the sed multiplied by 2.

Measurement	3 days	5 days	10 days	sed	*P* value	Interaction *P* value
Lying (% of time)	59	48	42	3.1	**0.000**	0.87
√σLying (% of time)	3.7	3.7	3.8	0.26	0.80	0.40
-Back transformed	13	14	15			
√# ofposture changes	3.7	3.9	3.7	0.17	0.60	0.55
-Back transformed	14.0	14.9	13.6			
Lying at arrival (% of animals)	59	37	36	6.3	**0.000** *	0.095 [a]
Log_{10}(CK)						
-Before transport	2.21	1.97	2.08	0.045	**0.000**	**0.002** *
--Backtransformed (iu/L)	160	90	120			
-Immediately after transport	2.51	2.27	2.37	0.054	**0.001**	0.29 [b]
--Backtransformed (iu/L)	320	190	230			
-After recovery	2.29	2.11	2.24	0.051	**0.004**	0.86
--Backtransformed (iu/L)	190	130	170			
Glucose						
-Before transport (mmol/L)	6.9	6.1	6.2	0.30	**0.018**	0.49
-Immediately after transport (mmol/L)	6.1	5.8	5.8	0.18	0.058	0.061
-After recovery (mmol/L)	4.5	4.2	4.2	0.16	0.086	0.19

Table 2. *Cont.*

Measurement	3 days	5 days	10 days	sed	*P* value	Interaction *P* value
√(BOHB)						
-Before transport	0.38	0.37	0.40	0.014	0.058	0.54
--Backtransformed (mmol/L)	0.15	0.13	0.16			
-Immediately after transport	0.36	0.37	0.40	0.016	**0.032**	0.063
--Backtransformed (mmol/L)	0.13	0.14	0.16			
-After recovery	0.42	0.46	0.49	0.021	**0.006**	0.083
--Backtransformed (mmol/L)	0.18	0.21	0.24			
PCV						
-Before transport (%)	0.42	0.43	0.43	0.009	0.90	**0.013**
-Immediately after transport (%)	0.42	0.41	0.41	0.011	0.59	**0.001**
-After recovery (%)	0.43	0.42	0.42	0.010	0.41	**0.042**
Lying (% of time) during recovery	85	85	81	1.4–1.5	**0.006**	0.59
√# of Lying bouts during recovery	3.1	3.1	3.1	0.09	0.94	0.93
--Backtransformed	9.6	9.5	9.4			
√# of Drinking bouts during recovery	1.0	1.3	1.9	0.15	**0.000**	0.44 [a]
--Backtransformed	0.9	1.8	3.4			
Weight	37.6	36.6	39.8	0.80	**0.001**	0.39

* Used Wald chi-squared test as calculations for denominator degrees of freedom for the Wald F test did not numerically converge; [a] To achieve numerical convergence of models used in calculating test, the Trip within replicate random component was taken to be 0; [b] To achieve numerical convergence of models used in calculating test, the Trip within replicate and Front to rear position within trips random components were taken to be 0.

The only measurements with a statistically significant interaction ($P < 0.05$) between calf age and the space and flooring treatments were the logarithm of CK activity before transport and PCV before and immediately after transport and after recovery. The statistically significant result for the logarithm of CK activity before transport must be a chance result because they are sampled prior to transport and prior to animals being randomly allocated to treatment. The PCV results are also likely to be by chance, because the result prior to transport must be by chance, and the subsequent results simply follow the pattern of the first result.

Space did not affect the mean time spent lying, however there was a reduction of the number of posture changes (from lying to standing and vice versa) in truck pens with the lowest space allowance (Table 3). This was also reflected in the significant difference in the standard deviation (sd) in the % of time animals spent lying. In addition, the time spent lying during recovery increased with reduced space allowance during transport. Activity of CK was increased in calves transported at 0.2 m^2, compared with both 0.3 m^2 and 0.5 m^2, with more than double the activity of CK recorded in animals transported at 0.2 m^2 compared with the other stocking densities. Calves transported at 0.3 m^2 compared with 0.5 m^2 also showed some elevated activity of CK.

Table 3. Effect of space allowance and flooring on behaviour and physiology before, during and after transport, and after 12 h of recovery. The standard error of difference between means (sed) differs somewhat depending on which pair of predicted means is being compared, and thus the smallest (min) and largest (max) sed are presented for each measurement. The interaction *P* value is the *P* value for testing for any interaction between flooring and the space treatments. Approximate least significant differences can be calculated as the sed multiplied by 2.

Measurement	**Solid**			**Mesh**			**Straw**			**sed**		***P* value**		
	0.2	**0.3**	**0.5**	**0.2**	**0.3**	**0.5**	**0.2**	**0.3**	**0.5**	**min**	**max**	**Flooring**	**Space**	**Interaction**
Lying (% of time)	43	38	42	54	38	42	58	59	71	5.3	5.9	**0.000**	0.069	**0.035**
√σLying (% of time)	4.6	2.9	3.6	5.0	4.2	3.0	3.7	3.5	3.3	0.38	0.42	0.071	**0.001**	**0.011**
-Backtransformed	21	9	13	25	17	9	14	12	11					
√# of posture changes	3.4	4.0	4.0	3.1	4.1	4.4	3.2	4.0	3.8	0.24	0.27	0.43	**0.000**	0.18
-Back transformed	11	16	16	9	17	19	10	16	14					
Lying at arrival (% of animals)	54	24	46	38	29	32	48	64	59	12.1	13.4	**0.016**	0.37	0.14 *
Log_{10}(CK)														
-Before transport	2.14	2.02	2.12	2.03	2.03	2.10	2.12	2.00	2.21	0.077	0.079	0.47	**0.030**	0.54 *
--Backtransformed (iu/l)	140	110	130	110	110	120	130	100	160					
-Immediately after transport	2.69	2.33	2.13	2.85	2.40	2.29	2.53	2.16	2.07	0.083	0.091	**0.004**	**0.000**	0.68
--Backtransformed (iu/L)	490	210	140	710	250	190	340	140	120					
-After recovery	2.45	2.19	2.04	2.60	2.26	2.09	2.22	2.04	2.04	0.069	0.080	**0.002**	**0.000**	**0.012**
--Backtransformed (iu/L)	280	150	110	400	180	120	170	110	110					
Glucose														
-Before transport (mmol/L)	6.1	6.8	6.7	6.4	6.0	6.3	6.2	6.4	6.6	0.45	0.50	0.32	0.58	0.63
-Immediately after transport (mmol/L)	5.8	6.1	6.1	5.8	5.6	5.9	6.1	5.8	5.7	0.23	0.28	0.25	0.93	0.33
-After recovery (mmol/L)	4.2	4.9	4.4	4.3	4.1	4.2	4.5	4.2	4.2	0.20	0.25	**0.028**	0.87	0.58

Table 3. *Cont.*

Measurement	Solid			Mesh			Straw			sed		*P* value		
	0.2	**0.3**	**0.5**	**0.2**	**0.3**	**0.5**	**0.2**	**0.3**	**0.5**	**min**	**max**	**Flooring**	**Space**	**Interaction**
√(BOHB)														
-Before transport	0.40	0.40	0.36	0.38	0.38	0.41	0.40	0.36	0.36	0.026	0.027	0.65	0.67	0.23
--Backtransformed (mmol/L)	0.16	0.16	0.13	0.14	0.14	0.17	0.16	0.13	0.13					
-Immediately after transport	0.43	0.38	0.40	0.35	0.41	0.37	0.34	0.36	0.35	0.024	0.027	**0.009**	0.74	**0.032**
--Backtransformed (mmol/L)	0.19	0.15	0.16	0.12	0.17	0.14	0.11	0.13	0.12					
-After recovery	0.46	0.43	0.44	0.41	0.46	0.48	0.46	0.49	0.47	0.030	0.033	0.31	0.67	0.13
--Backtransformed (mmol/L)	0.21	0.19	0.19	0.17	0.21	0.23	0.21	0.24	0.22					
PCV														
-Before transport (%)	0.43	0.43	0.43	0.43	0.43	0.42	0.42	0.41	0.43	0.015	0.018	0.18	0.77	0.86
-Immediately after transport (%)	0.43	0.42	0.42	0.42	0.42	0.41	0.40	0.40	0.41	0.017	0.020	**0.015**	0.91	0.96
-After recovery(%)	0.43	0.43	0.42	0.43	0.42	0.42	0.41	0.40	0.41	0.016	0.019	**0.022**	0.84	0.97
Lying (% of time) during recovery	87	85	84	85	83	82	84	83	80	1.4	1.5	0.052	**0.049**	0.93
√# of Lying bouts during recovery	3.0	3.3	3.1	2.9	3.0	3.0	3.2	3.1	3.2	0.14	0.16	0.057	0.39	0.56
--Backtransformed	8.7	10.8	9.4	8.6	9.1	9.1	10.1	9.9	10.1					
√# of Drinking bouts during recovery	1.0	1.6	1.5	1.2	1.3	1.2	1.5	1.5	1.5	0.26	0.29	0.41	0.29	0.50
--Backtransformed	1.1	2.7	2.1	1.5	1.8	1.5	2.4	2.3	2.2					
Weight	35.5	38.2	40.6	37.0	38.0	38.6	37.0	38.8	38.3	1.12	1.23	0.93	**0.007**	0.16

* Used Wald chi-squared test as calculations for denominator degrees of freedom for the Wald F test did not numerically converge; [a] Left to right position within replicate variance component set to be 0 to allow numerical convergence of model (except for tests of main effects of space and flooring).

Straw bedding had a large effect on lying behaviour, with calves on straw spending more time lying, both as a percentage during transport and at arrival (Table 3). Straw bedding also resulted in lower levels of CK activity and PCV There were some mixed effects of flooring on glucose, with the lowest concentrations of glucose found after recovery in calves transported on mesh floors.

Interestingly, there were several interactions found of space and flooring. In general they indicated that the effect of space was less pronounced when straw bedding was provided, particularly regarding lying behaviour as well as CK activity at 12 h after transport and BOHB immediately after transport.

4. Discussion

The results indicate a clear difference in measurements depending on age. However, these effects are apparent even before transport, which indicates that the physiology and particularly lying behaviour of 3-day old calves is fundamentally different from older calves.

Little research has been conducted on the physiological changes in calves during their first week of life. However, a few studies have included physiological data of young calves, and they show clear effects of age within the first 7 days of life on physiological parameters such as creatin, glucose, NEFA, bilirubin, IGF-I, thyroxine and insulin [16]. In another study similar effects were seen on cortisol, glucose and lymphocyte:neutrophil ratio, which the authors interpreted as immune suppression due to higher levels of cortisol early in life [17]. Indeed, Knowles [6] reported a negative correlation between age at the time of travel and mortality in the weeks after travel in calves less than 4 weeks old, possibly due to impaired immune function as a consequence of transport stress.

It is unclear if physiological differences across ages affected how well calves coped with the stressors of transport in this study. Since there were no interactions between age and space/flooring, it appears that restrictions of space and flooring affected behaviour and physiology of calves of all ages equally. However, 3-day old calves did lie down more than older calves, which indicates that a comfortable area to lie down is particularly important for these animals. Even though the Australian Animal Welfare Standards and Guidelines for Land Transport of Livestock [1] state that calves should not be transported for slaughter until they are 5 days of age, there is no specific requirement for calves to be identified on farm by their date of birth. While fitness for transport is generally assessed to be represented by a minimum live weight of 23 kg and a dry and shriveled umbilical cord at the junction with the skin, all 3-day-old calves in this experiment had dry, withered navel cords and were over 23 kg live weight. Indeed, anecdotal observations suggest that some calves are transported for slaughter as young as 3 days of age, and greater enforcement of documentation of age on farm may prevent the transportation of calves as young as 3 days of age and may contribute to improved welfare of calves during transport and at slaughter.

Significant effects of space were found, although the percentage of time animals were lying down was not affected. This is in contrast to other studies in which space allowance did affect time spent lying. For example Uetake *et al.* [18] found that increasing the space allowance from 0.25 m^2 to 0.45 m^2 increased the number of calves that lie down, although they transported calves that were somewhat older at 11–26 days old, with a body weight of 43–58 kg. Todd *et al.* [13] transported 5–10 day old calves at 0.2 m^2 and 0.4 m^2 and also found an increase in lying behaviour with increased space, although those calves were also slightly older and heavier than the current study, which may have inhibited lying at the lower space allowance where space was very limited. Moreover, lying behaviour in the latter study was only casually observed and not specifically measured. Given there is sufficient space, young calves prefer to lie down during transport. In several studies young calves were found to lie down the majority of the time, ranging from 50% [2] to more than 70% [3]. This is similar to the finding in this study, where calves provided with bedding and 0.5 m^2 laid down 71% of the time. There was a trend in our study for space allowance to affect lying during transport, mainly because this effect was only seen when straw was provided. There was however an increase in lying behaviour during the 12 h recovery after transport in calves that were transported with lower space allowances, indicating that these animals may have been more affected by transport. There was also a clear reduction of the number of posture changes during transport in animals provided with the smallest space allowance. This suggests that once animals were lying down they may have found it more difficult to get up and animals standing may have found it more difficult to lie down. This is also reflected in the higher standard deviation of percentage of time spend lying with the smallest space. In turn, it may explain the higher CK activity found with the smallest space allowance of 0.2 m^2, although even calves transported at 0.3 m^2 space allowance had elevated activity of CK compared to calves transported at 0.5 m^2 space allowances. CK increases in the bloodstream as a result of muscle cell damage resulting from exertion [19] or through direct trauma to the muscle such as bruising [20]. Therefore increased activity of CK may either indicate animals standing becoming muscle fatigued or animals lying down being stood on, resulting in bruising. Bruising is often reported at abattoirs. In a study of 16,400 transported calves, 50% were found to have bruised stifles and it was concluded that this bruising probably occurred during transport [21]. No calves were seen to lose their balance during transport, similarly to Grigor *et al.* [7] who also found that increased space allowance did not result in greater loss of stability or risk of injury.

Cortisol was not used as a measure of stress in this study. Due to the incomplete development of the HPA axis in young calves the cortisol response is not a reliable measure of stress during transport in these animals [2,22].

The Australian Animal Welfare Standards and Guidelines for Land Transport of Livestock [1] stipulate that space allowance during transport should be sufficient for all calves to lie down on their sternum during transport however no specific space allowance is specified. Anecdotally, space allowances as low as 0.17 m^2 have been observed on commercial transport trucks, even though only a space allowance of 0.3 m^2 or above provides enough space for all animals to lie down on their sternum. In accordance, the results from this study indicate that space allowance should be at least 0.3 m^2 per calf for calves of average size, while providing more space to 0.5 m^2 would provide even greater benefits. Indeed, regulations within the EU requires that transport times of calves less than 14 days old cannot exceed 8 h, are provided with adequate bedding material which guarantees their comfort and space allowances for animals should be at least 0.30 m^2 to 0.40 m^2 for a 50 kg calf. These figures may vary, depending not only on the animals' weight and size but also on their physical condition, the meteorological conditions and the likely journey time [23].

While mesh flooring is often provided in trucks specifically set up to transport young calves in order to provide a non-slip and dry surface, no clear advantages were found over a solid floor in this study. However no weather extremes of wet and cold weather, when a mesh floor may have an advantage, were encountered. In fact, higher CK activity found in calves transported on mesh flooring in this study may indicate disadvantages of this flooring. Straw bedding however had a large effect on lying behaviour, with calves on straw spending significantly more time lying. As a result straw bedding resulted in lower activity of CK, indicating that these calves may be less fatigued. The PCV measurements were difficult to interpret as they may have been influenced by factors other than the hydration status of the calves. Acute stressors, by stimulating adrenaline release, can cause splenic contraction thereby increasing the numbers of red blood cells in the circulation [24–26]. Glucose concentrations reduced with time as calves were fasted during transport and recovery, as has been reported in previous studies [2,13]. However concentrations stayed within a physiological normal range and did not differ between treatments, other than a slight reduction during recovery in calves transported on a mesh floor. A concurrent increase occurred in BOHB concentration indicating an increase in utilisation of fat reserves for energy, as has also previously been reported [2]. Straw bedding resulted in lower concentrations of BOHB during transport, possibly due to the insulation properties of straw and the lower energy demands while calves were lying down more. The results indicate that calves may be somewhat reluctant to lie down on a metal surface and that this may result in a greater energy expenditure.

Interestingly, there were several interactions of space and flooring found. In general they indicated that the effect of space was less pronounced when straw bedding was provided, overcoming some of the negative effects of reduced space, particularly on lying behaviour. While straw may not be practical under commercial conditions, both from a cost and a biosecurity standpoint, the results indicate that both solid steel or steel mesh are not ideal flooring when transporting bobby calves. Indeed, most European countries require calves up to 2 weeks old to be transported on straw bedding [23]. In addition, in Australia, calves younger than 5 days, who are transported to rearing facilities, must be provided with thick bedding. The guidelines in the Australian Animal Welfare Standards and Guidelines for Land Transport of Livestock [1] also recommend the provision of bedding for calves less than 30 days old to minimise welfare risks. Alternatives such as perforated rubber matting may be investigated to improve the welfare of bobby calves during commercial transport.

5. Conclusions

In conclusion, it was found that many measures were affected by age, which indicates that the physiology and particularly lying behaviour of 3-day old calves is fundamentally different from older calves. It is unclear how this affects the calves' ability to cope with the stressors of transport. However, 3-day old calves did lie down more than older calves, which indicates that a comfortable area to lie down is particularly important for these animals. Space clearly affected the measures during and after transport and the results from this study indicate that space allowance should be at least 0.3 m^2 per calf for calves of average size, while providing more space to 0.5 m^2 would provide even greater benefits. Straw bedding is of benefit to calves during transport, to the extent that it may even reduce some of the negative effects of reduced space. While the use of straw may not be practical under commercial conditions, a more suitable surface for calves to lie on during transport should be investigated, such as perforated rubber mats.

Acknowledgments

We would like to thank technical staff and students at the Animal Welfare Science Centre for assistance in data collection and animal care. This study was funded by DEPI Victoria.

Author Contributions

E.C. Jongman designed and carried out the experiment and drafted the manuscript. K.L. Butler is a biometrician and was responsible for the statistical design and analysis of the experiment and contributed to the writing of the manuscript.

Conflicts of Interest

The authors declare no conflict of interest.

References

1. The Australian Animal Welfare Standards and Guidelines for the Land Transport of Livestock, 1st ed.; Version 1.1, 21 September 2012. Available online: www.animalwelfarestandards.net.au (accessed on 25 August 2013).
2. Knowles, T.G.; Warriss, S.N.; Brown, J.E.; Edwards, J.E.; Watkins, P.E.; Phillips, A.J. Effects of calves less than one month old of feeding or not feeding them during road transport of up to 24 hours. *Vet. Rec.* **1997**, *140*, 116–124.
3. Eicher, S.D.; Morrow-Tesch, J.L. Behavior following subcutaneous electrolyte treatment in transported calves. In Proceedings of 34th International Congress of the International Society for Applied Ethology, Florianópolis, Brazil, 17–20 October 2000.
4. Atkinson, P.J. Investigation of the effects of transport and lairage on hydration state and resting behaviour of calves for export. *Vet. Rec.* **1992**, *130*, 413–416.
5. Cave, J.P.; Callinan, A.P.L.; Woonton, W.K. Mortalities in bobby calves associated with long distance transport. *Aus. Vet. J.* **2005**, *83*, 82–84.
6. Knowles, T.G. A review of post transport mortality among younger calves. *Vet. Rec.* **1995**, *137*, 406–407.
7. Grigor, P.N.; Cockram, M.S.; Steele, W.B.; Le Sueur, C.J.; Forsyth, R.E.; Guthrie, J.A.; Johnson, A.K.; Sandilands, V.; Reid, H.W.; Sinclair, C.; Brown, H.K. Effects of space allowance during transport and duration of mid-journey lairage period on the physiological, behavioural and immunological responses of young calves during and after transport. *Anim. Sci.* **2001**, *73*, 341–360.
8. Fraser, A.F.; Broom D.M. *Farm Animal Behaviour and Welfare*; CAB International: Wallingford, UK, 1997.
9. Thompson, K.V. Behavioral development and play. In *Wild Mammals in Captivity: Principles and Techniques*; Kleiman, D.G., Allen, M.E., Thompson, K.V., Lumpkin, S., Eds.; University of Chicago Press: Chicago, IL, USA, 1996, pp. 352–371.
10. Jongman, E.C.; Butler, K.L. Ease of moving young calves at different ages. *Aus. Vet. J.* **2013**, *91*, 94–98.

11. Animal Husbandry Survey 2010. Dairy Australia. Available online: http://www.dairyaustralia.com.au/~/media/Documents/Animals%20feed%20and%20environment/Animal%20welfare/Cow%20welfare/DA-Animal-Husbandry-Survey-Dec2010.PDF (accessed on 25 August 2013).
12. Hides, S.J.; Hannah, M.C. Drying times of umbilical cords of dairy calves. *Aus. Vet. J.* **2005**, *83*, 371–373.
13. Todd, S.E.; Mellor, D.J.; Stefford, K.J.; Gregor, N.G.; Bruce, R.A.; Ward R.N. Effects of food withdrawal and transport on 5- to 10-day-old calves. *Res. Vet. Sci.* **2000**, *68*, 125–134.
14. Australian Code for the Care and Use of Animals for Scientific Purposes, 8th ed.; 2013. Available online: http://www.nhmrc.gov.au/guidelines/publications/ea28 (accessed on 25 August 2013).
15. Payne, R.W.; Weham, S; Harding, S. *A Guide to REML in Genstat*; VSN International: Hertfordshire, UK, 2012.
16. Hadorn, U.; Hammon, H.; Bruckmaier, R.M.; Blum, J.W. Delaying colostrum intake by one day has important effects on metabolic traits and on gastrointestinal and metabolic hormones in neonatal calves. *J. Nutr.* **1997**, *127*, 2011–2023.
17. Jacob, S.K.; Ramnath, V.; Philmonia, P.T.; Raghunandhanan, K.V.; Kannan, A. Assessment of physiological stress in periparturient cows and neonatal calves. *Indian J. Physiol. Pharmacol.* **2001**, *45*, 233–238.
18. Uetake, K.; Tanaka, T.; Sato, S. Effects of haul distance and stocking density on young suckling calves transported in Japan. *Anim. Sci. J.* **2011**, *82*, 587–590.
19. Warriss, P.D.; Brown, S.N.; Knowles, T.G.; Kestin, S.C.; Edwards, J.E.; Dolan, S.K.; Phillips, A.J. Effects on cattle of transport by road for up to 15 hours. *Vet. Rec.* **1995**, *136*, 319–323.
20. Tarrant, P.V. Transportation of cattle by road. *Appl. Anim. Behav. Sci.* **1990**, *28*, 153–170.
21. McCausland, I.P.; Austin, D.F.; Dougherty, R. Stifle bruising in bobby calves. *N. Z. Vet. J.* **1977**, *25*, 21–72.
22. Mormede, P.; Soisson, J.; Bluthe, R.; Raoult, J.; Legarff, G.; Levieux, D.; Dantzer, R. Effect of transportation on blood serum composition, disease incidence and production traits in young calves. *Ann. Vet. Res.* **1982**, *13*, 369–384.
23. European Commission. Regulation (EC) No 1/2005 on the protection of animals during transport. 2005. Available online: http://eur-lex.europa.eu/LexUriServ/LexUriServ.do?uri=CELEX:32008L0119:EN:NOT (accessed on 25 August 2013).
24. Potocnik, S.J.; Wintour, E.M. Development of the spleen as a red blood cell reservoir in lambs. Reprod. *Fert. Dev.* **1996**, *8*, 311–315.
25. Locatelli, A.; Sartorelli, P.; Agnes, F.; Bondiolotti, G.P.; Picott, G.B. Adrenal response in the calf to repeated simulated transport. *Br. Vet. J.* **1989**, *145*, 517–522.
26. Stewart, M.; Webster, J.R.; Stafford, K.J.; Schaefer, A.L.; Verkerk, G.A. Technical note: Effects of an epinephrine infusion on eye temperature and heart rate variability in bull calves. *J. Dairy Sci.* **2010**, *93*, 5252–5257.

6

Consumer Acceptance of Dry Dog Food Variations

Brizio Di Donfrancesco, Kadri Koppel *, Marianne Swaney-Stueve and Edgar Chambers IV

The Sensory Analysis Center, Department of Human Nutrition, Ice Hall, Kansas State University, Manhattan, KS 66506, USA; E-Mails: briziod@ksu.edu (B.D.); Marianness@ksu.edu (M.S.-S.); eciv@ksu.edu (E.C.)

* Author to whom correspondence should be addressed; E-Mail: kadri@ksu.edu.

Simple Summary: The objectives of this study were to compare the acceptance of different dry dog food products by consumers, determine consumer clusters for acceptance, and identify the characteristics of dog food that drive consumer acceptance. Pet owners evaluated dry dog food samples available in the US market. The results indicated that appearance of the sample, especially the color, influenced pet owner's overall liking more than the aroma of the product.

Abstract: The objectives of this study were to compare the acceptance of different dry dog food products by consumers, determine consumer clusters for acceptance, and identify the characteristics of dog food that drive consumer acceptance. Eight dry dog food samples available in the US market were evaluated by pet owners. In this study, consumers evaluated overall liking, aroma, and appearance liking of the products. Consumers were also asked to predict their purchase intent, their dog's liking, and cost of the samples. The results indicated that appearance of the sample, especially the color, influenced pet owner's overall liking more than the aroma of the product. Overall liking clusters were not related to income, age, gender, or education, indicating that general consumer demographics do not appear to play a main role in individual consumer acceptance of dog food products.

Keywords: appearance; aroma; consumer; dog; liking; pet food

---

1. Introduction

Pet food buyers, despite economic recession challenges and subsequent money-saving trends, seem to be more than willing to spend money on pet food. A recent survey [1] indicated nearly one-third of consumers "preferred to shop at pet product retailers that offer the best products available, even if they are more expensive". Another survey on pet owners showed that 21% of US dog owners spend an average of US $100 or more per month on their dogs [2]. The pet food industry benefits from this consumer behavior and is focusing even more on premium products. In the pet food market, this means natural ingredients and a focus on health issues.

Factors such as brand and package contribute to the formation of expectation, the selection process, and the purchase intention of a product by consumers [3]. For those products that can be experienced only after purchase and in categories where multiple products are available for the consumer, such as the pet food category, brand represents a signal of quality and can help in the selection process [4]. Moreover, considering that pet food will not be directly consumed by owners, and therefore complete feedback cannot be provided, branding can hold a much higher importance. Packaging in the pet food industry conveys information on the particular properties of 'premium' products or natural and healthy ingredients, increasing with humanization of pets by owners. When brand and packaging information are removed, only sensory properties such as appearance and aroma contribute to the consumer's acceptance of the pet food, with the result being important especially for the repurchase of a product by owners [5].

Human sensory analysis with pet foods has not been frequent. A few studies have been conducted with pet food [6] and cat foods [7,8]. Di Donfrancesco *et al.* [9] looked at a variety of dry dog food products are available in the US market with varying appearance, aroma, flavor, and texture sensory properties, demonstrated by recent studies. These authors showed that some common aroma attributes, such as barnyard, grain, brothy, oxidized oil, cardboard, and stale are common sensory characteristics in this category. Other aroma notes such as meaty, liver, or fishy are more product-specific. Dry dog food products also were shown to be different for appearance characteristics such as surface roughness, oily appearance, porousness, and fibrousness.

In the United States and other developed countries most pet dogs and cats are fed commercial food, with about 50% of dogs fed entirely with dry commercial food [10]. Those authors noted that the most common is to feed dogs two times per day and provide one or more treats each day. Laflamme *et al.* [10] also observed that 31% of owners watch their dogs eat. This information suggests a high daily exposure of dog owners to pet food. Pet owners interact with pet food when feeding their pet and because of the lack of linguistic capability of pets, they can often determine pet food acceptability, in the same way parents can do with infants [11]. Understanding the boundaries that industry can push during product development without having a negative impact on pet owners' acceptability can be fundamental.

Sensory analysis techniques, both analytical and hedonic, can help in this process to determine properties such as appearance, texture, aroma and flavor that are important for pet food acceptability. It has been shown that 'taste plus flavor' is considered the most important factor for consumers when experiencing food and beverages [12]. Other sensory characteristics such as aroma and appearance can assume a higher relevance when trying to assess humans' pet food acceptability, since humans wouldn't typically taste pet food.

The objectives of this study were to: (1) understand consumers' acceptance of various different commercial dry dog food products without branding or packaging; (2) identify consumer clusters and determine if these clusters relate to age, income, gender, or education; and (3) isolate drivers of consumers' liking and purchase intent.

2. Materials and Methods

2.1. Samples

Eight samples were purchased from local pet stores, grocery stores, and discount stores. Samples were different in brand, type of kibble, price, and presence of specialty ingredients (Table 1). Sample A (3 kibbles) and sample C (4 kibbles) were each comprised of multiple kibbles, differing in size, shape and color. The samples were chosen based on their aroma and appearance characteristics measured by Di Donfrancesco *et al.* [9]. In that study, samples were small (D, G), medium (A, B, E, F, H), and large (one kibble type of sample A). Some samples were nugget-shaped (A, B, E, G, H), other were oval-shaped (kibble in sample A), 'o-shaped' (D), square-shaped (F), or they showed a miscellaneous shape such as one kibble in sample A. The choice of some of the samples was based on preliminary descriptive data collection in order to have a wide range of aroma profiles within the sample set. Some samples had higher fishy aroma notes (G, H) while others, such as sample E, had higher grain aroma notes. Sample D had high oxidized aroma levels and sample A showed plastic aroma notes. Some samples (F and D) presented higher meaty aroma notes than the others and sample G showed higher levels of liver aroma.

All samples were evaluated within the "best by" date on the package and all sample lots were checked to ensure they had not been subject to a product recall. The products were purchased one week before testing and were stored at room temperature.

2.2. Descriptive Sensory Analysis

Six highly trained panelists from the Sensory Analysis Center, Kansas State University (Manhattan, KS, USA) analyzed the samples for aroma and appearance attributes. Each of the panelists had more than 120 hours of descriptive analysis panel training which included techniques and practice in attribute identification, terminology development, and intensity scoring. Moreover, each assessor had more than 1,000 hours of experience with a variety of food products, including dried dog food, and had conducted studies using the consensus method (used in this study).

Attribute intensities were evaluated on a scale where 0 = none and 15 = very high. Samples were first evaluated individually by panelists, then the final aroma and appearance profile was developed after a discussion led by the panel leader to determine the consensus score for each attribute. Similar procedures have been used recently in other sensory studies [13–15]. The lexicon used in descriptive profiling was developed and used by Di Donfrancesco *et al.* [9].

Each sample was prepared 30 minutes prior to testing and was served in a ~100 mL plastic cup for appearance evaluation. For aroma evaluation, 3 grams of sample was weighed in a medium glass snifter, and covered with a watch glass. Samples were coded with three-digit random numbers. The testing room was maintained at 21 ± 1 °C and 55 ± 5% relative humidity.

Table 1. Dry dog food samples and ingredients.

Sample	Additional information	Ingredients *
A	Multiple kibbles, speciality recipe	Beef, soybean meal, soy flour, animal fat, brewers rice, soy protein concentrate, corn gluten meal, ground yellow corn, glycerin, poultry by-product meal, ground wheat, animal digest, pearled barley, calcium carbonate, calcium phosphate, salt, grilled sirloin steak flavor, dried green beans, dried potatoes, sulfur, Vitamin E supplement, choline chloride, zinc sulfate, ferrous sulfate, added color (Red 40, Blue 2, Yellow 5, Yellow 6), niacin, wheat flour, potassium chloride, L-Lysine monohydrochloride, vitamins, minerals, garlic oil, C-5900.
B	Mature dogs	Whole grain corn, chicken by-product meal, animal fat, soybean mill run, flaxseed, chicken liver flavor, lactic acid, corn gluten meal, potassium chloride, l-lysine, choline chloride, vitamin E supplement, iodized salt, vitamins, calcium carbonate, dicalcium phosphate, minerals, l-tryptophan, taurine, glucosamine hydrochloride, l-carnitine, chondroitin sulfate, phosphoric acid, beta-carotene, rosemary extract.
C	Multiple kibbles	Corn, soybean meal, beef & bone meal, ground wheat, animal fat (BHA used as preservative), wheat middlings, corn syrup, water sufficient for processing, animal digest (source of roasted flavor), propylene glycol, salt, apple, hydrochloric acid, potassium chloride, caramel color, vegetable blend (peas, carrots & green beans), sorbic acid, sodium carbonate, minerals, choline chloride, vitamins, calcium sulfate, titanium dioxide (color), red 40 lake, yellow 5, red 40, BHA, blue 2 lake, yellow 6 lake, blue 1, DL-methionine, yellow 6.
D	Small breed, aging care	Chicken meal, rice, brown rice, corn gluten meal, chicken fat, barley, natural chicken flavor, dried beet pulp (sugar removed), rice flour, dried egg product, anchovy oil, dried brewers yeast, potassium chloride, flaxseed, calcium carbonate, fructo-oligosaccharides (FOS), salt, choline chloride, sodium tripolyphosphate, DL-methionine, vitamins, taurine, salmon meal, trace minerals, glucosamine hydrochloride, tea (green tea extract), L-carnitine, chondroitin sulfate, marigold extract (*Tageteserectal.*), rosemary extract.
E	Affordable cost	Ground corn, wheat middlings, de-fatted rice bran, meat and bone meal, animal fat, salt, potassium chloride, animal digest, corn gluten meal, coline chloride, minerals, vitamins.
F	Easy to digest, grain free	Chicken, potatoes, chicken meal, pea protein, peas, sweet potatoes, poultry fat (preserved with mixed tocopherols), apples, pumpkin, natural flavor, tapioca starch, tomato pomace, salt, potassium chloride, choline chloride, vitamins, minerals, citric acid (used as a preservative), *Yucca schidigera extract*, rosemary extract.
G	Real salmon	Salmon, brewers rice, ground whole grain sorghum, potato, ground whole grain barley, chicken meal, fish meal, chicken fat, dried egg product, dried beet pulp, natural flavor, brewers dried yeast, potassium chloride, salt, sodium hexametaphosphate, calcium carbonate, dl-methionine, choline chloride, fructooligosaccharides, minerals, vitamins, beta-carotene, rosemary extract.
H	Low fat	Turkey, chicken, barley, brown rice, potato, rice, pea fiber, chicken meal, herring, natural flavors, chicken fat, flaxseed, apple, carrot, herring oil, sunflower oil, egg, cottage cheese, alfalfa sprouts, pumpkin, dried chicory root, L-carnitine, vitamins, minerals, direct fed microbials (dried *Lactobacillus acidophilus* fermentation product, dried *Lactobacillus casei* fermentation product, dried *Enterococcus faecium* fermentation product), lecithin, rosemary extract.

* Vitamin and mineral lists of all samples (except for sample B) are not all-inclusive.

The appearance attributes evaluated were brown color, color uniformity, shape uniformity, size uniformity, surface roughness, porous, oily, grainy, and fibrous. For aroma the panelists evaluated ashy, barnyard, broth, brown, cardboard, cooked, dusty/earthy, fish, grain, liver, meaty, musty/dusty, oily, oxidized oil, soy, smoky, spice brown, spice complex, stale, starchy, straw-like, toasted, and vitamin. For multiple kibble samples (A and C) all types of kibbles were combined for the evaluation, to mimic how the product is perceived by the pet owner.

2.3. Consumer Study

A Central Location Test (CLT) was conducted in the Sensory and Consumer Research Center at Kansas State University (Olathe, KS, USA). Participants (n = 100, men = 30, women = 70) were recruited from the Kansas City area. Participants were recruited from the Center's database and were screened for age (>18 years old), dog ownership, not working in the pet food industry, and had to be personally responsible for at least 50% of dog food purchases. Among recruited pet owners, 66% had one dog in the household, 29% had two dogs, and 5% had 3 dogs. Participant demographics are shown in Table 2.

Table 2. Demographics of the participants in the consumer study: gender, age, consumers annual income (US dollars), number of dogs owned.

<table>
<tr><th>Gender</th><th colspan="6">Male</th><th colspan="6">Female</th></tr>
<tr><td>Consumers %</td><td colspan="6">30%</td><td colspan="6">70%</td></tr>
<tr><th>Age</th><th>18–24</th><th colspan="3">25–34</th><th colspan="2">35–44</th><th colspan="2">45–54</th><th colspan="3">55–64</th><th>>55</th></tr>
<tr><td>Consumers %</td><td>2</td><td colspan="3">25</td><td colspan="2">22</td><td colspan="2">35</td><td colspan="3">12</td><td>4</td></tr>
<tr><th>Income (USD)</th><th colspan="2"><25,000</th><th colspan="3">25,000–49,000</th><th colspan="2">50,000–74,000</th><th colspan="3">75,000–100,000</th><th colspan="2">>100,000</th></tr>
<tr><td>Consumers %</td><td colspan="2">3</td><td colspan="3">14</td><td colspan="2">26</td><td colspan="3">33</td><td colspan="2">24</td></tr>
<tr><th>Education level</th><th>Some high school</th><th colspan="3">High school degree</th><th colspan="2">Some college</th><th colspan="2">College degree</th><th colspan="3">Some graduate studies</th><th>Graduate degree</th></tr>
<tr><td>Consumers %</td><td>1</td><td colspan="3">3</td><td colspan="2">14</td><td colspan="2">44</td><td colspan="3">10</td><td>27</td></tr>
<tr><th>Number of dogs</th><th colspan="3">One</th><th colspan="3">Two</th><th colspan="3">Three</th><th colspan="3">Four or more</th></tr>
<tr><td>Consumers %</td><td colspan="3">66</td><td colspan="3">29</td><td colspan="3">5</td><td colspan="3">0</td></tr>
</table>

For the evaluation, each pet owner used a tablet computer and computer questionnaires were administered by Compusense *at-hand* software (Compusense Inc., Guelph, ON, Canada). The number of participants for each session varied from 6 to 8. The samples were served monadically in a randomized order. Samples were presented in brown paper bags, lined with a plastic bag, containing approximately 900 grams of sample, a typical amount sold for purchase in small bags in the US. Bags were labeled with three-digit random codes. All eight samples were served to each participant during a 1-hour session. Participants were asked to open the bag and pour the sample into a ceramic pet bowl and then rate *overall liking, aroma liking, appearance liking, color, size, shape, uniformity,* and *oily appearance*. In addition, the participants were asked to indicate how much they thought their dog would like the sample using a 9-point hedonic scale where 1 = *dislike extremely* and 9 = *like extremely*. Pet owners were also asked about *aroma, oily appearance, uniformity shape, size*, and *color* intensities on a 5-point Just-About-Right (JAR) scale where 1 indicated "too weak", 3 "just about right", and 5 "too strong". Moreover, participants scored their expected purchase intent (5 = *definitely would purchase*, 4 = *probably would purchase*, 3 = *may or may not purchase*, 2 = *probably would not purchase*, 1 = *definitely would not purchase*) and the expected cost of each sample (1 = *not at all expensive* to 5 = *very expensive*). Pet owners were also asked to describe their specific likes and dislikes for each sample using open-ended questions.

2.4. Data Analysis

Clusters among consumers were identified according to their *overall liking* score (Ward's clustering procedure) using SAS® statistical software (Version 9.3, SAS Institute Inc., Cary, NC, USA). Significant differences ($P < 0.05$) among products were determined using two-way analysis of variance and Fisher's protected Least Significant Difference (LSD) in SAS® statistical software (Version 9.3, SAS Institute Inc., Cary, NC, USA) for clusters among consumers according to their overall liking scores and Tukey's HSD test in Compusense *at-hand* (Compusense Inc., Guelph, ON, Canada) for liking scores. Unscrambler software (The Unscrambler X version 10.2, Camo Software AS, Oslo, Norway) was also used to plot a liking map of samples fitted with consumers' liking using Principal Components Analysis. Compusense *at-hand* (Compusense Inc., Guelph, ON, Canada) was used to collect consumer scores and analyze JAR data. For this data, scores 1–2 were grouped as "too low" and scores 4–5 were grouped as "too high". Scores of 3 were considered as "just about right". Correlation among overall liking, appearance, aroma, color, size, shape, uniformity, and oily appearance liking was calculated using Pearson correlation in Unscrambler *vs.* 2014.1.08 (Addinsoft, New York, NY, USA).

3. Results and Discussion

3.1. Descriptive Data

Descriptive sensory analysis showed a wide range of shapes, sizes, aromas, and flavors present in the samples. The aroma attributes common to all of the samples were barnyard and cooked (Table 3). Aroma attributes such as broth, grain, musty/dusty, straw-like, and vitamin, were detected in seven out of eight samples while brown and cardboard were present in six samples. Other attributes found were oxidized oil (B, D, G, H, A), toasted (C, D, E, F, A), meaty (C, D, F, A), soy (C, D, E, A), spice complex (C, D, E, F), stale (B, C, E, A), smoky (C, F, A), oily (C, E, F), fish (G, H), dusty/earthy (B, G), vegetable complex (C, A), burnt (D), liver (G), spice brown (F), starchy (D) and plastic (A).

Most of the scores were within the low intensity range (0–5 on a scale from 0 to 15), indicating the low overall aroma and the blended and complex nature of the product category, as was found by Di Donfrancesco *et al.* [9]. Sample D showed barnyard aroma notes in the moderate intensity range (5.5–10 on a scale from 0 to 15) with attributes such as cooked and oxidized oil scoring low-moderate and low for meaty and toasted notes. Descriptive analysis confirmed the specific characteristics expected to be present in the samples, such as the fishy notes in samples G and H, or the higher meaty notes in samples D and F. Sample D (the sample with no grain notes) had the highest levels of barnyard, broth, burnt, and cooked as well as meaty, musty/dusty, oxidized oil, soy, spice complex, starchy, straw-like, toasted, and vitamin within the sample set. Sample F presented the highest levels for brown and meaty, together with smoky and brown spice notes. Sample H had higher levels for both fish and oxidized oil, and lacked any presence of attributes such as broth or brown, present in most of the other samples. Plastic aroma was only present in sample A, probably due to processing or packaging. Sample C showed grain, smoky, oily, meaty, vegetable complex, and brown notes as well as the highest levels for stale aroma among the sample set. Oxidized oil aroma was not detected in this sample.

Samples G and F were characterized by a darker brown color while sample H was lighter (Table 3). Sample E showed the lowest shape and size uniformity within the sample set. Samples B, G, and E presented higher surface roughness than the other samples. Samples F and D showed low scores for both grainy and fibrous appearance.

Table 3. Aroma and appearance profiles from descriptive analysis (0–15 scale).

Aroma profile from descriptive analysis (0–15 scale)								
Sample # **Atribute**	**A**	**B**	**C**	**D**	**E**	**F**	**G**	**H**
Ashy	0	0	0	0	1.5	0	0	0
Barnyard	3.0	5.0	3.0	5.5	3.0	2.5	3.0	2.5
Broth	2.5	2.5	3.0	3.5	2.5	3.0	2.5	0.0
Brown	3.0	2.0	2.5	0.0	3.0	4.0	3.0	0.0
Burnt	0.0	0.0	0.0	3.0	0.0	0.0	0.0	0.0
Cardboard	3.0	4.0	2.5	0.0	3.0	0.0	3.0	3.0
Cooked	2.0	3.0	2.5	5.0	2.0	3.0	3.0	2.0
Dusty/Earthy	0.0	2.0	0.0	0.0	0.0	0.0	2.0	0.0
Fish	0.0	0.0	0.0	0.0	0.0	0.0	4.0	4.0
Grain	3.0	2.5	3.0	0.0	4.0	2.5	3.0	3.0
Liver	0.0	0.0	0.0	0.0	0.0	0.0	3.0	0.0
Meaty	3.5	0.0	3.0	4.0	0.0	4.0	0.0	0.0
Musty/Dusty	2.0	2.0	2.0	3.0	3.0	2.5	0.0	2.5
Oily	0.0	0.0	2.5	0.0	2.0	2.0	0.0	0.0
Oxodized Oil	2.5	2.5	0.0	5.0	0.0	0.0	3.5	3.0
Plastic	2.0	0.0	0.0	0.0	0.0	0.0	0.0	0.0
Soy	2.5	0.0	1.5	3.0	2.5	0.0	0.0	0.0
Smokey	2.0	0.0	2.0	0.0	0.0	2.0	0.0	0.0
Spice Brown	0.0	0.0	0.0	0.0	0.0	1.0	0.0	0.0
Spice Complex	0.0	0.0	2.5	3.0	1.5	1.0	0.0	0.0
Stale	2.5	2.0	2.5	0.0	2.0	0.0	0.0	0.0
Starchy	0.0	0.0	0.0	2.5	0.0	0.0	0.0	0.0
Straw-like	1.5	2.0	2	2.5	0.0	2.0	2.5	2.0
Toasted	1.5	0.0	1.5	4	2.5	2.0	0.0	0.0
VegetableCompl.	2	0.0	2	0.0	0.0	0.0	0.0	0.0
Vitamin	2.0	2.5	2.0	3.0	2.5	2.5	2.0	0.0

Table 3. *Cont.*

Appearance profile from descriptive analysis (0–15 scale)								
Sample # **Atribute**	**A**	**B**	**C**	**D**	**E**	**F**	**G**	**H**
Brown color	Nd *	6.0	Nd *	7.0	7.0	12.0	12.0	3.5
Shape	Misc.	Nugget	Misc.	Round	Nugget	Square	Nugget	Nugget
Color Uniformity ** Uniformity ** Uniformity **	nd	99%	nd	70%	99%	98%	98%	98%
Shape Uniformity **	nd	93%	nd	60%	80%	95%	85%	95%
Size Uniformity **	nd	0.95%	nd	80%	80%	90%	90%	98%
Surface Roughness	nd	6.5	nd	2.0	6.0	2.0	5.0	3.0
Porous	nd	6.0	nd	2.0	4.0	2.0	6.0	3.5
Oily	nd	3.0	nd	5.0	2.0	3.0	2.5	2.0
Grainy	nd	4.0	nd	2.0	4.5	1.5	6.0	4.0
Fibrous	nd	2.0	nd	2.0	2.0	1.5	4.5	2.0

* Data relative to appearance of sample composed by multiple different kibbles (A and C) are not shown.
** uniformity scores expressed as percentages.

3.2. Consumer Study Results

3.2.1. Acceptability and Intensity Scores

Overall liking was significantly correlated with appearance, color, and aroma liking of the products. Sample C, one of the two samples composed of multiple kibbles, was the sample that was scored the highest overall liking score as well as highest scores for liking of appearance, shape, uniformity, oily appearance, and color (Table 4). The liking score for color in this sample represented the highest liking score observed in the study (average score >7).

Table 4. Consumers' liking scores (1–9 hedonic scale).

Sample # **Atribute**	**A**	**B**	**C**	**D**	**E**	**F**	**G**	**H**
Overall liking	5.26bc **	5.70b	6.77a	5.15bc	5.79b	4.54c	4.83c	5.01bc
Appearance liking	5.24bcd	5.82bc	6.99a	5.24bcd	6.12ab	4.53d	4.86d	4.92cd
Aroma liking	5.00abc	4.69bc	5.56a	4.37c	5.27ab	4.63bc	4.69bc	4.97abc
Color liking	5.97bc	6.20bc	7.05a	6.29ab	6.32ab	5.02de	5.41cd	4.4e
Size liking	5.16bc	6.14a	6.32a	5.52ab	6.42a	4.14d	4.28cd	6.40a
Shape liking	4.98cd	6.55ab	6.84a	5.37cd	6.59ab	4.91d	5.80bc	6.43ab
Uniformity liking	5.02c	6.22ab	6.77a	5.77bc	6.25ab	5.50bc	5.69bc	6.08ab
Oily appearance liking	5.59ab	5.29b	6.08a	5.56ab	5.31b	5.26b	5.38b	5.48ab
Dog liking *	5.76b	5.99b	6.87a	5.85b	5.70b	5.28b	5.40b	5.30b

* Predicted by consumers; ** Different letter within a row indicates a significant difference among the samples ($P < 0.05$).

Table 5. Response to aroma, color, appearance, size, and uniformity intensity as too low, just about right (jar), or too high by % of consumers.

	AROMA			COLOR			OILY APPEARANCE			SIZE			UNIFORMITY		
Sample	Too low	JAR	Too high	Too dark	JAR	Too light	Too low	JAR	Too oily	Too small	JAR	Too large	Too low	JAR	Too high
A	19	48	33	31	58	11	26	73	1	16	46	38	54	44	2
B	9	43	48	6	72	22	11	61	28	6	56	38	5	67	28
C	6	61	33	14	79	7	12	76	12	5	67	28	20	77	3
D	5	34	61	21	72	7	8	65	27	43	53	4	7	69	24
E	11	50	39	2	70	28	34	64	2	24	71	5	8	70	22
F	11	37	52	60	39	1	9	68	23	75	25	0	6	68	26
G	13	43	44	46	52	2	18	68	14	76	24	0	9	65	26
H	33	49	18	0	26	74	36	63	1	27	68	5	2	76	22

Figure 1. Purchase intent (1 = definitely would not purchase by consumers, 3 = may or may not purchase, 5 = definitely would purchase), predicted cost (1 = not at all expensive to 5 = very expensive) Different letters within a variable indicate a significant difference among the samples ($P < 0.05$).

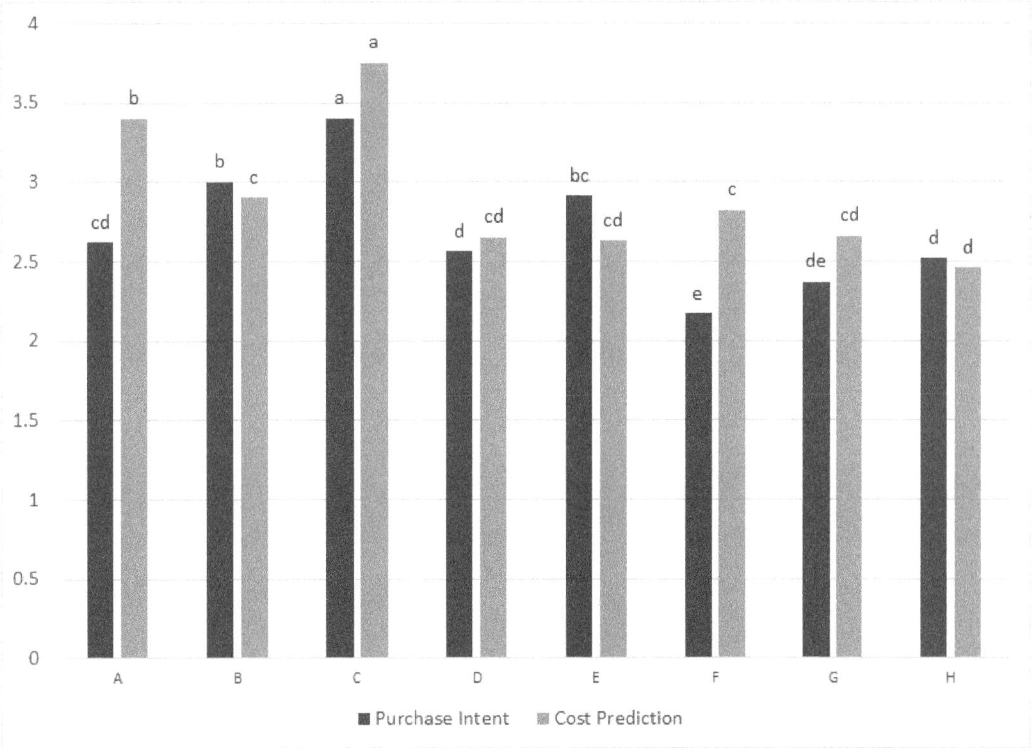

Attributes such as aroma, color, oily appearance, and size also were scored for intensity (Table 5). Color intensity of kibbles in sample C was perceived by most of the consumers (79%) as 'just about right'. In contrast to the other sample with different kibbles (Sample A) which was perceived as low in uniformity of shape by a large portion of consumers (54%), sample C was perceived as 'just about right' for shape uniformity by 77% of consumers. When asked to predict purchase intent and product price, consumers indicated this sample (C) was the one they were more willing to buy despite the fact that this sample also was perceived to be the most expensive product within the sample set (Figure 1). This could be explained by the positive correlation shown between perception of quality and price. Plassmann *et al.* [16] found that when a product was perceived as more expensive, the consumers rate it better than the product perceived as less expensive. Consequently, a low price perception is translated into a lower acceptability by consumers because of expected lower product quality. In this study, the highest predicted prices were earned by the two multi-shaped and multicolored kibbles products (C and A). However, the highest score (C) was 3.75 on a scale where 3 = *neither expensive nor inexpensive* and 5 = *very expensive*. Pet owners also predicted that sample C would be the most appreciated product by their dogs. This data suggest that consumers equate high price with high pet acceptability and appear willing to purchase more expensive dog foods. Except for sample C, the other samples in this study do not show a significant difference for consumers' expectation of liking by their pet dogs and it is not possible to verify if consumers relate low predicted price with low pet acceptability.

Despite the actual low cost on the market, sample (E), characterized by a nugget shape and a moderate brown color, was the second highest in overall liking and appearance liking. However, it scored almost one full point lower than sample C for both of the attributes (Table 4). Sample E also had the highest score for size liking and the second highest score for aroma, shape and uniformity liking (average scores >6).

The least liked product was sample F, which was dark brown and square-shaped and with the highest oily appearance among samples, based on the descriptive analysis. It showed the lowest liking scores for size, shape, and oily appearance. This sample earned the lowest predicted 'dog liking' score, but was only slightly lower than other samples such as G (nugget-shaped and dark brown) or H (nugget-shaped and light brown). The sample perceived as having the lowest cost was the sample that was scored the lowest for color liking (sample H).

Sample F, one of the most expensive products in the market, was not perceived as the most expensive by consumers. This product was grain free, included natural ingredients and was claimed to favor an easy digestion. Sample F received the lowest scores for appearance liking, size liking, shape liking, and oily appearance liking as well as for overall liking. The low-cost sample (E) was not perceived as the lowest cost sample by consumers (Figure 1). Sample E had a remarkably lower cost than other samples in the market, and earned some of the highest scores for attributes such as aroma liking and appearance liking. The low nutritional value and the low protein quality was probably counterbalanced in consumer's perception by the appearance (not too dark and uniform brown color, high surface roughness, moderate porousness, fibrousness, and low oily appearance) and a high level of grain aroma notes with absence of oxidized oil aroma.

When asked to comment on their likes and dislikes for the products, the consumers focused on overall appearance of samples. For instance, consumers' comments indicated that sample C was appreciated mostly because of the variety of colors, shapes, sizes, and textures. To some consumers this was associated with a variety in ingredients and flavors, while others perceived it as an indicator of healthiness or freshness of the product. For sample F, the least liked sample, most of the comments pointed out that the kibbles were too small, it was too dark in color, and had a poor smell. The o-shaped sample (D) was one of the least liked among the set, and earned comments about its similarity with a well-known breakfast cereal product. For some consumers this was a good aspect, while some others considered this shape odd for a dog food product and more appropriate for cat food. Some consumer even considered this shape dangerous because of the possibility for a child to mistake the product for a breakfast cereal. Some consumers appreciated sample A for its variety of colors and sizes. However, other consumers highlighted the low uniformity of the sample together with kibble shapes that was considered strange, especially one kibble that was irregularly shaped and seemed like an imitation of a chunk of meat.

Average aroma liking scores fell in a range between '*dislike slightly*' and '*like slightly*'. Samples E and C were the only samples scored higher than 5 for aroma liking on the average. Although descriptive sensory data showed some unique aroma characteristics that distinguished these samples (e.g., a higher level of grain aroma (4.0) for sample E and vegetable complex notes for sample C) it's possible that the particular combinations of aroma attributes present in these samples, more than a single note, originated the highest aroma liking scores by consumers. In addition to the notes present in their aroma profile, it has to be highlighted that both of the samples did not show any oxidized oil notes. Consumers' comments also indicated that sample C was appreciated because of a mild aroma. Although sample C was not the only sample showing a total absence of oxidized oil aroma, this sample also exhibited a lack of many other attributes such as ashy, dusty/earthy, fish, liver, plastic, spice brown, and starchy. This likely is related to the mild aroma perception noted in the consumers' comments.

3.2.2. Consumer Clusters

Cluster analysis of consumers based on overall liking scores showed six clusters among consumers who participated in the study (Table 6). These clusters, based on individual consumer variation in liking scores showed little or no relation to income, age, gender, or education.

Table 6. Consumer clusters according to overall liking.

Sample#	Cluster 1 (n = 19)	Cluster 2 (n = 17)	Cluster 3 (n = 15)	Cluster 4 (n = 21)	Cluster 5 (n = 10)	Cluster 6 (n = 18)
A	3.7 d *	7.8 a	4.8 c	6.0 b	7.3 a	2.8 d
B	6.8 a	5.6 bc	3.6 d	6.3 ab	6.6 ab	5.2 c
C	7.7 ab	7.8 ab	7.0 bc	6.3 c	8.1 a	4.4 d
D	6.2 a	4.0 c	5.9 ab	6.5 a	4.5 bc	3.3 c
E	6.2 ab	5.3 bc	4.1 d	6.9 a	4.5 cd	6.7 a
F	3.7 cd	3.2 d	5.3 b	6.6 a	3.0 d	4.6 bc
G	3.8 b	4.6 b	4.7 b	6.5 a	1.4 c	6.2 a
H	5.8 a	5.5 ab	4.3 b	5.8 a	2.5 c	4.8 ab

* Different letter within a row indicates a significant difference among the clusters ($P < 0.05$).

Cluster 1 included consumers who did not like the two samples perceived as too small (F and G) and the multiple kibble product with low shape uniformity (sample A). On the contrary this cluster provided one of the highest scores for the other multiple kibble sample (C). Consumers in cluster 2 gave scores below 6 for all of the samples except the two with multiple kibbles. Cluster 3 showed scores below 6 for all of the products except for sample C. On the contrary, cluster 4 (n = 21), the largest cluster, liked all of the products but all of the scores were within the 5.8–6.9 range. The 5.8 average score for sample H was higher than the average score it earned for overall liking by all of the participants (5.0). Cluster 5 (n = 10) seemed to be positively influenced by appearance variety and large dimensions with consumers providing the highest scores to multiple kibbles and products perceived as large in size. The average score for sample C, the most liked overall by consumers in this cluster, was 8.1 (overall data average was 6.8). These consumers also showed the lowest scores for the products perceived as too small (sample F and sample G). Cluster 6 (n = 18) was formed by consumers that provided the lowest scores for the multiple kibble products, samples C and A (multi-colored and multi-shaped), compared to the scores these sample earned in the other clusters. It is possible to consider this consumer cluster as negatively influenced by appearance variety and large kibble dimensions. However, products perceived as too small (consumer intensity score) did not earn the highest score by consumers of this cluster either.

Purchase intent and cost prediction within each of the six clusters also was analyzed confirming that for most of the clusters, purchase intent and cost prediction were linked with overall liking. For example in cluster 2 (Figure 2) both purchase intent and cost prediction followed the overall liking scores of the cluster, with sample C and A earning the highest scores and sample D, F, and G the lowest for purchase intent. In Cluster 6 (Figure 3), although there was not a significant difference related to cost prediction among samples, samples were significantly different for purchase intent and showed a trend similar to the overall liking scores of the cluster. This cluster was the only one where sample C was not preferred over the other samples and, thus, it was possible to observe an potential relationship to purchase intent. The other multiple kibble product (sample A) that earned the lowest overall liking score in this cluster, also earned the lowest purchase intent score.

Figure 2. Cluster 2: purchase intent (1 = definitely would not purchase by consumers, 3 = may or may not purchase, 5 = definitely would purchase), predicted cost (1 = not at all expensive to 5 = very expensive). Different letters within a variable indicate a significant difference among the samples ($P < 0.05$).

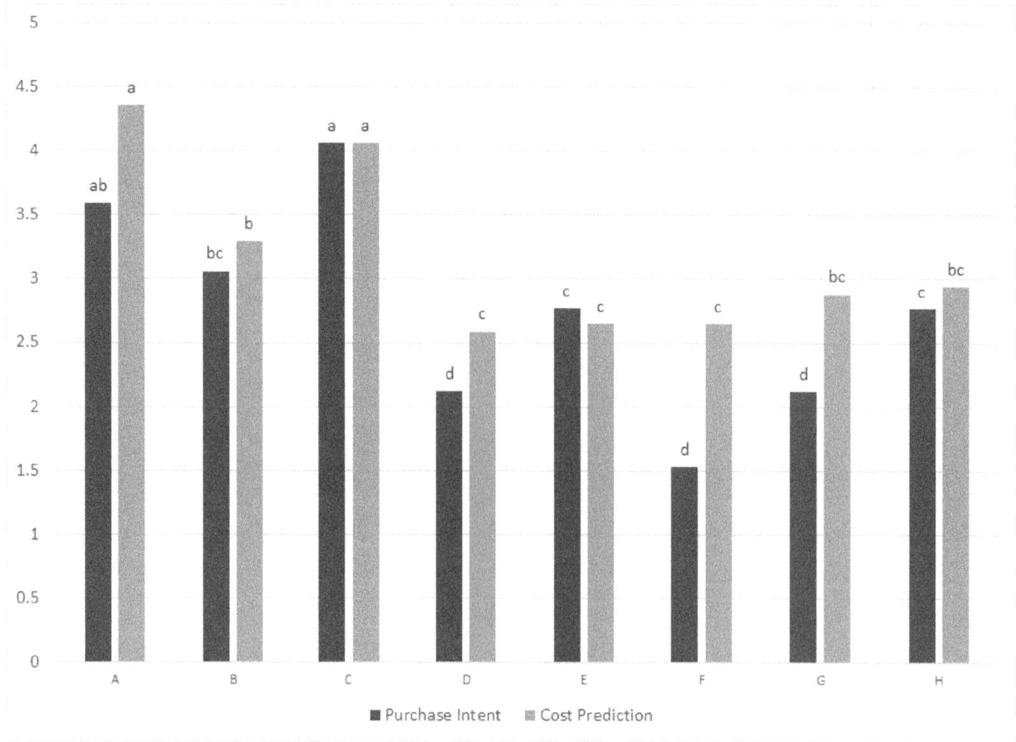

Figure 3. Cluster 6: purchase intent (1 = definitely would not purchase by consumers, 3 = may or may not purchase, 5 = definitely would purchase). Different letters within a variable indicate a significant difference among the samples ($P < 0.05$).

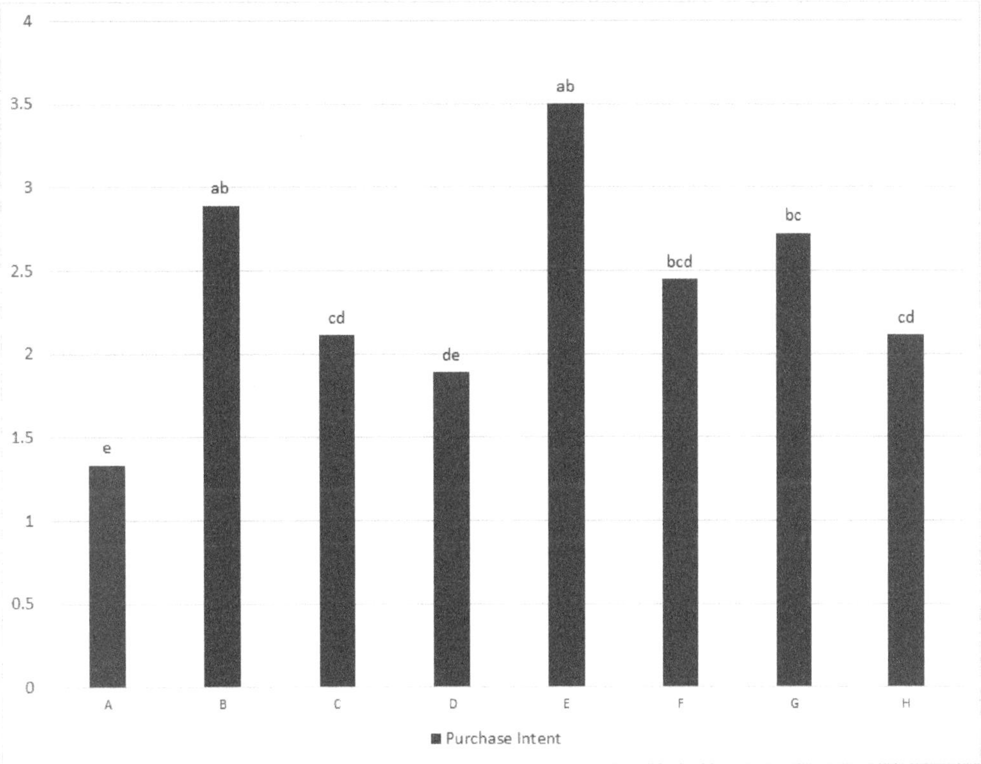

Consumers were asked to indicate the brands that they usually purchased and this information was related to the different clusters. Clearly current consumer purchase behavior can influence consumer acceptance scores. Approximately 50% of consumers in cluster 5 usually purchased the Kibbles 'n Bits brand, a multi-colored, multi-shaped kibble product. The consumers in this cluster provided the highest overall liking score (8.1) to sample C (a multi-colored and multi-shaped product). Finally cluster 6 was characterized by 44% of consumers purchasing Science Diet. Conversely cluster 6, which contained a high proportion (44%) of Science Diet users (a highly uniform product), scored products with low uniformity (A, C) low in overall liking. No other cluster contained such high percentages of brand users. The most purchased brands by consumers in cluster 1 were Iams (21.1%), Purina One (26.3%), Science Diet (31.6%). In cluster 2 there was no brand purchased by more than 20% of consumers with the most purchased brands represented by Science Diet and Purina One (17.6%), Iams, Purina Proplan, and Kibble 'n Bits (11.8%). In cluster 3 the most purchased brands were Purina One (26.7%), Purina Proplan and Purina Beneful (20%). In cluster 4, brands like Science Diet, Purina One (19%), Iams, and Kibble 'n Bits (14.3%) were still the most purchased.

3.2.3. Drivers of Liking and Disliking

The products used were commercially available products and did not attempt to hold specific variables constant. Thus, the aspects that appear to drive liking or disliking are based on overlapping characteristics and with only eight products represent a general overview. Specific aspects would need to be studied in more controlled studies or with larger numbers of products to determine specific relationships.

Generally, overall liking was greatly influenced by the appearance of the samples (Figure 4). Among the different specific appearance characteristics, color liking was highly related to the overall liking scores by dog owners. Overall, the most liked sample was a multiple-colored and -shaped kibble product and the two least liked samples were the two darkest brown samples according to the descriptive analysis. It is also possible to notice that prediction of dog liking was highly correlated with the consumers' overall liking (r = 0.928).

Figure 4. Principal Components Analysis based on consumer liking.

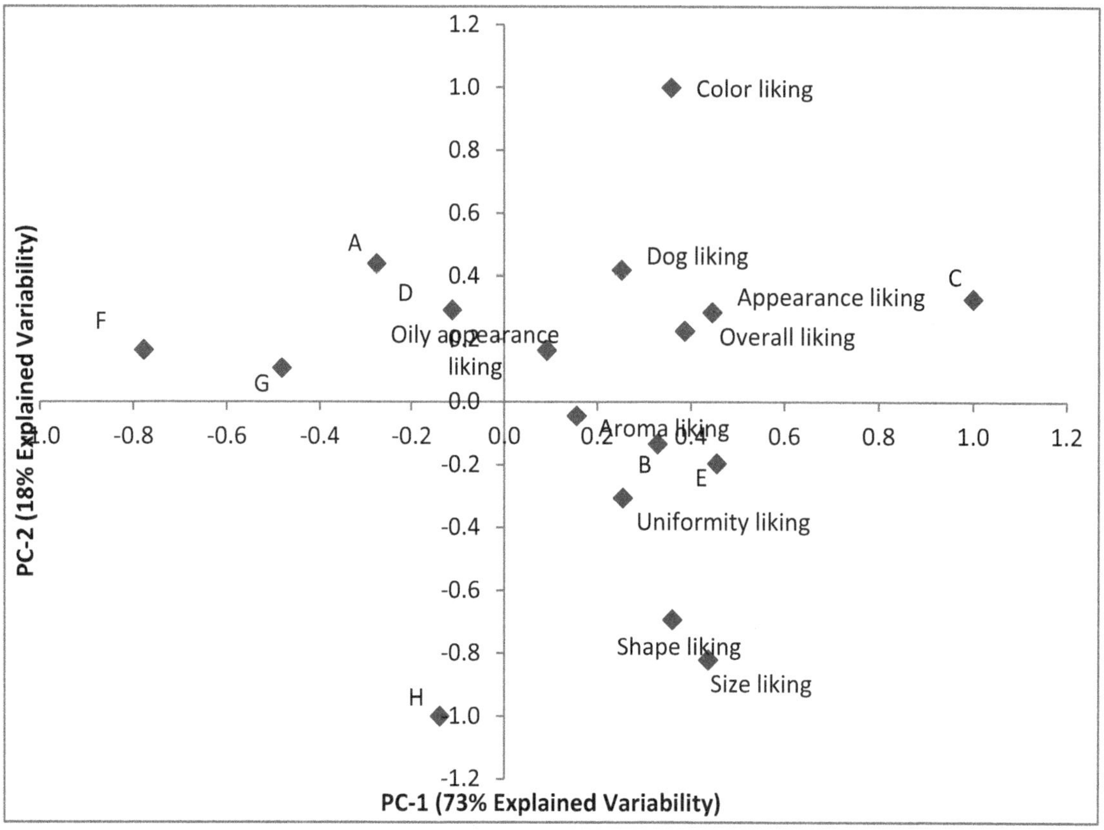

Table 7. Correlation between consumers' overall liking and the other liking scores.

Correlation *r*	Aroma liking	Appearance liking	Color liking	Size liking	Shape liking	Uniformity liking	Oily appearance liking	Dog liking
Overall liking	0.762	0.993	0.809	0.705	0.721	0.754	0.697	0.928
p-value	0.028	<0.0001	0.015	0.051	0.044	0.031	0.055	0.001

Aroma did not drive consumer's overall liking and does not appear to drive acceptance as much as appearance, as shown in the correlation analysis (Table 7). However, aroma may have some impact on individual consumer clusters. For example, consumers in cluster 5 gave the lowest scores (<3 point-scale) to the only two sample showing fish aroma notes from descriptive analysis (G and H). Another example could be sample G that was perceived as too small by owners but also was the only sample that showed liver aroma notes. The aroma component may have contributed to the extremely low score (1.4) earned from owners in cluster 5 with all the other clusters scoring in a 3.8–6.5 range.

Expected cost did not seem to drive overall acceptance as one of the two products that scored highest for expected cost was the fourth most liked sample.

3.3. Discussion

Descriptive analysis showed the tested samples were different from each other and offered a wide range of characteristics to study across the samples. This enabled analysis of these different characteristics with the aim of understanding the aspects that drive consumer's acceptance of dry dog food when brand and packaging are removed. Clearly, appearance is a key driver for acceptance of dry dog food, a product that is not eaten by the actual purchaser. Other examples of aspects that were important for consumer segments were the overall intensity perception of aroma or the presence of particular aroma notes.

Some similarities among products helped clarify if a characteristic influenced consumer liking. An example of this was the influence of appearance and not aroma on overall liking for the sample composed of multiple different colored and shaped kibbles (C). It was also characterized by aroma attributes such as smoky, broth, grain, meaty, toasted, and musty/dusty. Sample C was the most liked among consumers while sample F, with similar aroma characteristics, was the least liked overall within the sample set. This indicates the importance of visual stimulation in overall liking of dry dog foods. When asked about color intensity, sample F was perceived by 60% of consumers as *too dark*. Specific characteristics of samples also highlighted the lower influence of aroma on pet owners liking scores. For instance, the sample with the highest scores for oxidized oil aroma based on descriptive analysis (sample D) showed the lowest score for aroma liking, but was not the least liked overall.

The results indicated that multiple kibbles in a product are not enough to drive consumer's liking, and that an optimal combination in color, shape, size, and oily appearance has to be pursued. Although sample C was highly liked, the other sample with multiple kibbles (A) was one of the least liked by consumers, and was scored the lowest in uniformity liking among the samples. Sample A contained a particular kind of kibble, characterized in descriptive analysis by its large size, highly irregular shape, and high springiness, which was different from sample C.

Pet owners were not accurately able to predict how expensive/inexpensive the dog food was based on appearance and aroma alone. Multiple kibbles were related to cost expectation; the samples composed of multiple kibbles were perceived as the most expensive samples in the set. Sample H was perceived as the least expensive product and it also was the sample earning the lowest color liking scores. These results show that cost prediction is related with color liking but at the same time the cost prediction is not driving the overall liking.

Previous studies have shown that appearance plays a major role, among sensory characteristics, in determining consumers purchase intent [17]. Moreover, for new products and products that consumers have not previously tasted, appearance is even more important in driving consumer preference [18]. Consumers' intensity and liking scores indicated that a too small kibble size may not be appreciated by pet owners. Samples G and F were perceived as too small by consumers (respectively 76% and 75%) and consequently earned the lowest scores for size liking. It was observed from clustering analysis that different consumer clusters like different sized kibbles. This aspect may be related to dog size and breed and future studies can help clarify that relationship.

Based on intensity scores given by consumers, it is possible to observe that consumers did not appreciate a strong aroma in their dog food. Sample D had moderate aroma intensity scores from descriptive analysis, compared to low aroma intensity scores of the other samples and was the only sample not scored for grainy attribute in its aroma profile. This sample was perceived as having too strong aroma intensity by 61% of consumers and earned the lowest score for aroma liking but was only the fourth least liked overall confirming that aroma characteristics did not drive the overall liking as the appearance characteristics did. The information related to the grainy aroma attribute can indicate a primary role of grainy aroma in the aroma liking of dry dog food. When grainy aroma was absent, the aroma liking scores were low. Furthermore, when the grainy aroma was stronger, like was noted with the low-cost product, the aroma liking score was higher as well.

Previous studies have looked at the human-dog relationship and the epidemiological data that can be related to dog obesity [19–21]. According to Suarez *et al.* purchase behavior of commercial dog food is different for owners of normal weight dogs when compared to the owners of overweight dogs [19]. These authors found that owners of overweight dogs are more interested in special prices and promotions and less interested in the correct dog nutrition than were the owners of normal weight dogs. Similar findings regarding the price of dog food were reported by Kienzle *et al.* [20]. These authors also found that the owners of overweight dogs tended to overhumanize their pet, thus, some of the needs of their pets, such as exercise, were ignored. This was confirmed by Courcier *et al.* [21] who found a correlation among dog obesity and exercise hours per week. Furthermore, they found that feeding snacks and treats to the dog is a risk factor for being overweight. Pet obesity is a serious issue and sensory properties of dog food as perceived by the owner and as perceived by the pet have not been studied in relation to being overweight. Future studies should address the possible associations among aroma, flavor, and texture and quantities served and consumed, further.

4. Conclusions

Eight dry dog food samples, with different appearance and aroma characteristics, were evaluated by a descriptive panel and by pet owners. The study indicated that consumers' liking was most influenced by the appearance of the products. Product color intensity, especially darker brown colors, seems to have a negative relation with pet owners' liking. In addition, kibble size also influenced product liking, with products where kibbles are perceived as too small showed the lowest overall liking scores. Cluster analysis showed a group of consumers who liked large kibble size more than other participants, but the same was not seen for small kibbles. Uniformity of shape within a product can also play an important role in dry dog food acceptance. Of the two multi-colored and multi-shaped kibbles products, one resulted the most liked and the other, perceived as too low in uniformity of shape (particularly related to one of its kibbles), earned a score almost 2 points lower for appearance liking. The brands consumers usually purchased seem to be associated with overall liking at least for some consumer segments.

Aroma of dry dog food seems to have less of a role in driving consumers liking and their willingness to purchase specific dry dog foods than appearance. However, for products where the aroma was perceived as too strong, was disliked, or had higher the presence of off-flavor notes (e.g., oxidized oil, musty/dusty), overall liking was impacted negatively. This indicates that pet owners are generally accepting of "dog food aroma" or specific flavor notes associated with the product.

Interestingly, the presence of grain-type aroma notes seemed to increase liking by consumers and a lack of that note seemed to penalize the product. This may be related to the modulation of aroma by that relatively bland aroma characteristic.

Based on this research, dry dog food products will be well liked by pet owners if the kibbles vary in color and shape with high uniformity within a single kibble type, and a low aroma that includes grain-type notes. Including different colors and shapes of kibbles also can increase the perception of a more expensive product.

Author Contributions

The study was planned by Kadri Koppel, Edgar Chambers IV, and Marianne Swaney-Stueve. The study was executed by Kadri Koppel and Marianne Swaney-Stueve. Data was analyzed and the manuscript was composed by Brizio Di Donfrancesco. The manuscript was reviewed by Kadri Koppel, Marianne Swaney-Stueve, and Edgar Chambers IV.

Conflicts of Interest

The authors declare no conflict of interest.

References

1. Taylor, J. Market Update: The Premium Petfood Shopper Survives. Petfood Industry, May 2013. Available online: http://www.petfoodindustry.com/Market_update__The_premium_petfood_shopper_survives.html (accessed on 11 April 2014).
2. Phillips-Donaldson, D. Humanization Still Driving Petfood Industry Growth. *Petfood Industry*, November 2011. Available online: http://www.petfoodindustry.com/Default.aspx?pageid=5306&id=8131&terms=dog+food (accessed on 11 April 2014).
3. Gadioli, I.L.; De Oliveira Pineli, L.D.L.; Quintiliano Rodrigues, J.D.S.; Bezerra Campos, A.; Quieroz Gerolim, I.; Chiarello, M.D. Evaluation of packing attributes of orange juice on consumers' intention to purchase by conjoint analysis and consumer attitudes expectation. *J. Sens. Stud.* **2013**, *28*, 57–65.
4. Cuellar, S.S.; Claps, M. Differential effects of brand, ratings and region on willingness to pay: A hedonic approach. *J. Wine Res.* **2013**, *24*, 138–155.
5. Koppel, K. Sensory Analysis of pet foods. *J. Sci. Food Agr.* **2014**, doi:10.1002/jsfa.6597.
6. Lin, S.; Hsieh, F.; Heymann, H.; Huff, H.E. Effects of lipids and processing conditions on the sensory characteristics of extruded dry pet food. *J. Food Qual.* **1998**, *21*, 265–284.
7. Pickering, G.J. Optimisation of dried cat food using a human taste panel: Methodology and characterization of flavor. *Food Aust.* **2009**, *61*, 30–36.
8. Pickering, G.J. Optimizing the sensory characteristics and acceptance of canned cat food: Use of a human taste panel. *J. Anim. Physiol. Anim. Nutr.* **2009**, *93*, 52–60.
9. Di Donfrancesco, B.; Koppel, K.; Chambers, E., IV. An initial lexicon for sensory properties of dry dog food. *J. Sens. Stud.* **2012**, *27*, 498–510.

10. Laflamme, D.P.; Abood, A.K.; Fascetti, A.J.; Fleeman, L.M.; Freeman, L.M.; Michel, K.E.; Bauer, C.; Kemp, B.L.E.; Van Doren, J.R.; Willoughby, K.N. Pet feeding practices of dog and cat owners in the United States and Australia. *J. Am. Vet. Med. Assoc.* **2008**, *5*, 687–694.
11. Day, J.E.L.; Kergoat, S.; Kotrschal, K. Do pets influence the quantity and choice of food offered to them by their owners: Lessons from other animals and the pre-verbal human infant? *CAB Rev. Perspect. Agr. Vet. Sci. Nutr. Nat. Resour.* **2009**, *42*, 1–12.
12. Rabino, S.; Moskovitz, H.; Katz, R.; Maier, A.; Paulus, K.; Aarts, P.; Beckley, J.; Ashman, H. Creating databases from cross-national comparison of food mind-sets. *J. Sens. Stud.* **2006**, *22*, 550–586.
13. Koppel, K.; Adhikari, K.; Di Donfrancesco, B. Volatile compounds in dry dog foods and their influence on sensory aromatic profile. *Molecules* **2013**, *18*, 2646–2662.
14. Suwonsichon, S.; Chambers, E., IV.; Kongpensook, V.; Oupadissakoon, C. Sensory lexicon for mango as affected by cultivars and stages of ripeness. *J. Sens. Stud.* **2012**, *27*, 148–160.
15. Chambers, E., IV; Lee, J.; Chun, S.; Miller, A. Development of a lexicon for commercially available cabbage (baechu) kimchi. *J. Sens. Stud.* **2012**, *27*, 511–518.
16. Plassmann, H.; O'Doherty, J.; Shiv, B.; Rangel, A. Marketing actions can modulate neural representations of experienced pleasantness. *Proc. Natl. Acad. Sci. USA* **2008**, *105*, 114–131.
17. Herrera-Corredor, J.A.; Saidu, J.E.P.; Khachatryan, A.; Prinyawiwatkul, W.; Carballo-Carballo, A.; Zepeda-Bautista, R. Identifying drivers for consumer acceptance and purchase intent of corn tortilla. *J. Food Sci.* **2007**, *72*, S727–S731.
18. Rocha, M.C.; Deliza, R.; Corrêa, F.M.; Carmo, M.G.F.; Abboud, A.C.S. A study to guide breeding of new cultivars of organic cherry tomato following a consumer-driven approach. *Food Res. Int.* **2013**, *51*, 265–273.
19. Suarez, L.; Peña, C.; Carreton, E.; Juste, M.C.; Bautista-Castaño, I.; Montoya-Alonso, J.A. Preferences of owners of overweight dogs when buying commercial pet food. *J. Anim. Physiol. Anim. Nutr.* **2012**, *96*, 655–659.
20. Kienzle, E.; Bergler, R.; Mandernach, A. A comparison of the feeding behavior and the human-animal relationship in owners of normal and obese dogs. *J. Nutr.* **1998**, *128*, 2779S–2782S.
21. Courcier, E.A.; Thomson, R.M.; Mellor, D.J.; Yam, P.S. An epidemiological study of environmental factors associated with canine obesity. *J. Small Anim. Pract.* **2010**, *51*, 362–367.

7

Welfare of Pigs Being Transported over Long Distances Using a Pot-Belly Trailer during Winter and Summer

Jorge A. Correa [1,2,†], Harold Gonyou [3], Stephanie Torrey [4,‡], Tina Widowski [5], Renée Bergeron [6], Trever Crowe [7], Jean-Paul Laforest [2] and Luigi Faucitano [4,*]

[1] F. Ménard Inc., Ange Gardien, QC, J0E 1E0, Canada

[2] Département de sciences animales, Université Laval, Quebec City, QC, G1K 7P4, Canada; E-Mail: Jean-Paul.Laforest@fsaa.ulaval.ca

[3] Prairie Swine Centre, Saskatoon, SK, S7H 5N9, Canada; E-Mail: hgonyou@shaw.ca

[4] Dairy and Swine and Development Research Centre, Agriculture and Agri-Food Canada, Sherbrooke, QC, J1M 0C8, Canada

[5] Department of Animal & Poultry Science, University of Guelph, Guelph, ON, N1G 2W1, Canada; E-Mail: twidowsk@uoguelph.ca

[6] University of Guelph, Alfred Campus, Alfred, ON, K0B 1A0, Canada; E-Mail: RBergeron@alfredc.uoguelph.ca

[7] Department of Mechanical Engineering, University of Saskatchewan, Saskatoon, SK, S7N 59, Canada; E-Mail: trever.crowe@usask.ca

† Present address: Canadian Meat Council, Ottawa, ON, K1Z8P9, Canada; E-Mail: jorge@cmc-cvc.com.

‡ Present address: Department of Animal and Poultry Science, University of Guelph, Guelph, ON, N1G 2W1, Canada; E-Mail: storrey@uoguelph.ca.

* Author to whom correspondence should be addressed; E-Mail: luigi.faucitano@agr.gc.ca.

Simple Summary: The pot-belly trailer, which can transport large loads in a single journey, is commonly used for swine transportation in Canada. However, it is generally acknowledged that pot-belly trailers and some specific compartments within this vehicle are worse than others in terms of animal losses. The objective of this study was to evaluate the effects of pot-belly design on animal welfare and meat quality in pigs being transported long distance in two different seasons of the year.

Abstract: A total of 2,145 pigs were transported for 8 h in summer (six trips) and winter (five trips) using a pot-belly trailer accommodating pigs in four locations (upper deck or UD, bottom-nose or BN, middle deck or MD and bottom deck or BD). Heart rate of pigs during loading and transportation and lactate and creatine kinase (CK) concentrations in exsanguination blood were measured. Meat quality was evaluated in the *Longissimus thoracis* (LT), *Semimembranosus* (SM) and *Adductor* (AD) muscles. During summer, pigs loaded in the UD and MD had higher ($P < 0.05$) heart rate at loading compared to those located in the BD and BN. Blood lactate and CK concentrations were higher ($P < 0.001$) in winter than in summer. Lactate concentration was higher ($P = 0.01$) in the blood of pigs transported in the BN. Pigs transported in the BN had higher pHu values in the LT, SM and AD muscles ($P = 0.02$, $P < 0.001$ and $P = 0.002$, respectively) and lower ($P = 0.002$) drip loss values in the SM muscle. This study confirms that some locations within the PB trailer have a negative impact on the welfare of pigs at loading and during transport with more pronounced effects in the winter due to the additive effect of cold stress.

Keywords: blood metabolites; heart rate; pigs; pork quality; season; transport

1. Introduction

In Western Canada, the large extension of the territory coupled with the centralization of the slaughter industry, with more pigs being killed in fewer larger plants, forces producers to transport pigs for long distances [1]. This has resulted in the increased use of pot-belly (PB) trailers that can transport large loads (up to 230 pigs) in a single journey. However, due to the presence of multiple steep internal ramps, pigs are more difficult to handle while loading and unloading this vehicle type [2], resulting in higher risk of animal losses during transport compared to other vehicle types [3,4]. In North America, a higher percentage of in-transit deaths and non-ambulatory pigs have been both recorded in summer (+0.15% and +2%, respectively) and in winter (+0.10% and +0.20%, respectively) compared to winter and summer, respectively [3,5–7]. These increases have been associated with the use of the PB trailer compared to a double-decked truck or a flat-deck trailer that are equipped with hydraulic decks [4,6,7]. Both cold and heat stress have an impact on *ante-* and *post-mortem* muscle glycogen stores leading to higher incidence of DFD (dark, firm, dry) and PSE (pale, soft, exudative) pork, respectively [8,9]. Recently, a greater percentage of PSE loins was found in the summer compared to winter (3% *vs.* 1%) and a greater incidence of DFD loins was reported in winter than in summer (8% *vs.* 4%) under Eastern Canadian transport conditions [4]. In two previous studies [4,10], the animal location (deck and/or compartment position in the truck) in the PB trailer during summer trasportation has an impact on pig body temperature and meat quality variation, with higher gastro-intestinal tract temperature in pigs in the upper deck and a greater percentage of pale pork being found in the upper and bottom decks compared to other locations. These effects are very likely the result of the physical exertion required by pigs to negotiate the ramps to get to these compartments under warm ambient conditions. However, these results were obtained in short distance transportation trials (2 h trip). Sutherland *et al.* [6] and Weschenfelder *et al.* [11] reported no detrimental effects on animal welfare when the PB trailer was used for a 9- and 7-h trip, respectively. However, in the former study [6] no interaction between trailer type and season was found, while in the latter one [11] these results were obtained under mild environmental conditions (11.2 °C on average). There is no evidence of the effects of the season and animal location on stress response and meat quality of pigs transported long distance in a PB trailer.

Because there is a gap in the knowledge on the role of ambient temperature and long-distance transportation on the variation of physiological variables and pork quality of pigs transported with a PB trailer, the objective of this study was to examine the physiological response (heart rate and exsanguination blood stress indicators) as well as skin bruise score and meat quality of pigs transported 8 h to slaughter in different transport compartments during both summer and winter.

2. Experimental Section

2.1. General

All experimental procedures performed in this study were approved by the AAFC Animal Care Committee in Sherbrooke (QC) based on the current guidelines of the Canadian Council on Animal Care [12]. A total of 2,145 crossbred pigs (BW = 115.2 ± 6.8 kg) were transported for 8 h (565 km) in summer (June and July, 2008; average temperature of 18.4°C, ranging from 9.1 to 20.7 °C) and winter (January to March, 2008; average temperature of −10.4°C, ranging from −22.3 to −9.7 °C) seasons from the Prairie Swine Center Elstow Research growing-finishing unit in Saskatchewan to a slaughter plant located in Brandon (Manitoba) using a dual-purpose (cattle and pig) pot-belly (PB) trailer.

Pigs were transported in 5 weeks in winter and 6 weeks in summer, in terms of one load of 195 pigs per week in each season, at an average density of 0.42 and 0.41 m^2/pig, respectively. During the experiment, the transport schedules changed between the seasons to concur with the current transport practices of the region. In summer, the transporter only had two short stops (15 and 30 min each) after an initial transport phase of 190 min. These stops were considered short enough to protect pigs from the temperature and humidity rise inside a stationary PB trailer [11]. In winter, the transporter only had a single stop, lasting 180 min, before continuing the journey to the abattoir. Pigs were transported on three decks and distributed into 9 out of 10 compartments (four on the upper deck, three in the middle deck and two in the bottom deck of the vehicle; Figure 1). Compartment 6 was not filled due to load limitations. The trailer included three internal ramps: a 22° ramp going to the upper level (compartments 1, 2, 3 and 4), a 32° ramp going to compartment 5 ("bottom-nose" or BN), and a 22° ramp giving access to the bottom level (compartments 9 and 10; Figure 1). The trailer was bedded with wood shavings in the summer and straw and wood shavings in the winter. The side panels were open 100% in the summer, but only 10% in the winter. The trailer compartments were loaded in the following order: 5, 1, 2, 4, 3, 9, 10, 7, and 8. At loading, pigs were moved along an alley, up the chute into the trailer and then through ramps in groups of four or five using boards and the electric prod as necessary. The loading crew did not change between seasons.

Figure 1. The location of compartments and distribution of pigs by compartment in the pot-belly trailer. Internal ramps are solid lines in compartments 5, 8, and 10.

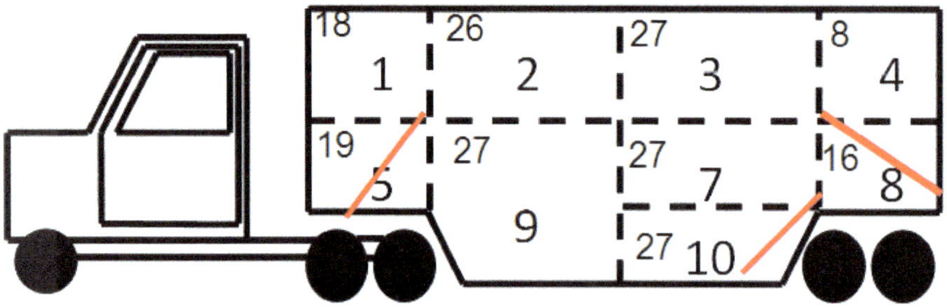

Within a group of six pigs in each compartment, one pig (30 pigs/trip or replicate: total of 330 pigs) was chosen for physiological evaluation (heart rate and blood analysis). This pig plus another one selected out of every four pigs (45 pigs/replicate: total of 495 pigs) within the same group were also used for the meat quality assessment. Only barrows were chosen for these evaluations. Feed was withdrawn from the pigs 5–6 h prior to transport. Pigs were transported for 8 h and unloaded at the plant using boards and electric prods as necessary. After 1.5 to 2 h in lairage, pigs were driven in a single line to stunning, were electrically stunned (head-to-chest electrical stunning) and exsanguinated in the prone position.

2.2. Physiological Measurements

Heart rates were recorded by Polar heart rate monitors (Polar Electro Canada) at 5 s intervals for the duration of loading and transportation. For protection and stable positioning, heart rate monitors were covered by leather or nylon weight-lifting belts buckled around the pig's chest. These were installed 24 h prior to transportation to allow animals to recover from the stress of this handling procedure. Belts were removed immediately after unloading. Data were downloaded and the average heart rate for each pig was determined for each of the experimental periods up to and including unloading.

At exsanguination, 2 mL of blood were collected in a tube (BD Vacutainers®, VWR International Ltd., Montreal, Canada) containing 6 mg of NA_2 EDTA and 3 mg of NaF solution to extract plasma for lactate analysis and 10 mL of blood were put in a tube (BD Vacutainers®, VWR International Ltd., Montreal, Canada) to extract serum for creatine-kinase (CK) analysis. The 2-mL blood tubes were immediately centrifuged at 4 °C for 10 min at 1,400 × g. Plasma was then transferred into 1.5 mL Eppendorf tubes and stored at −80 °C until lactate determination. Serum samples were kept at room temperature (~23 °C) for 1 h before refrigeration at 4 °C. The following day, serum samples were centrifuged at 4 °C for 10 min at 1,400 × g, transferred to 1.5 mL Eppendorf tubes, and stored at −80 °C until analysis. Plasma lactate concentrations were measured with a microplate reader using a commercially available kit (Lactate Assay Kit, Biomedical Research Service Center, University of Buffalo, Buffalo, NY, USA) whereas CK concentrations were measured with a spectrophotometer using a creatine kinase-sl kit (Creatine Kinase-SL Assay of Chemicals Diagnostic Limited, Vancouver, Canada). All analyses were done in triplicate. The intra-assay coefficients of variation for CK and lactate concentration data were 3.43 and 3.40%, respectively.

2.3. Measurement of Carcass Quality Traits

Following slaughter, carcasses were eviscerated, split and blast chilled for 2 h. Hot carcass weight (HCW) and lean meat yield were recorded to characterize the population under study.

Skin damage was assessed on the day of slaughter in the cooler using the 5-point, photographic scale (1 = none to 5 = severe) [13], whereas bruises were classified as fighting-type bruises (score 1 = less than 5 bruises; 2 = 6 to 10 bruises; and 3 = greater than 10 bruises) and mounting-type bruises (score 1 = less than 5 bruises; 2 = 6 to 10 bruises) by visual assessment of shape and size according to the photographic standards of the Institut Technique du Porc [14]. According to the ITP scale, bruises due to biting during fighting are recognized as being of 5–10 cm in length, comma shaped and concentrated in high number in the anterior (head and shoulders) and posterior (ham) regions of the carcass. Long (10 to 15 cm), thin (0.5 to 1 cm wide) comma shaped bruises densely concentrated on the back of pigs typically caused by the fore claws were classified as mounting-type bruises. Lacerations and scratches normally produced when pigs are handled aggressively and run in closed and tight spaces were also noted and classified as "other bruise types".

2.4. Meat Quality Measurements

Measurements of pH were made at 6 h *post-mortem* (after blast chilling) in the *longissimus thoracis* (LT) muscle at the third/fourth last rib level and *Semimembranosus* (SM) muscle and at 24 h (pHu) *post-mortem* in the LT, SM and *Adductor* (AD) muscles using a temperature-compensating, spear-type probe (Cole-Palmer Instrument Co., Vernon Hills, IL, USA) attached to a pH meter (pH 100 series; Oakton Instruments, Vernon Hills, IL, USA). At 24 h *post-mortem*, color data were collected on the LT and SM muscle after a 45 min bloom period. Visual color was evaluated using the Japanese color standards [15] in the LT muscle only, whereas instrumental color (L^*, a^*, and b^* values) was measured with a Minolta Chromameter (CR-300; Minolta Canada Inc., Mississauga, Canada) equipped with a 25 mm aperture, 0° viewing angle, and D65 illuminant in the LT and SM muscles. Drip loss was measured in the LT muscle using the modified EZ-driploss method of Correa *et al.* [16]. Briefly, three 25 mm diameter cores were removed from the center of 2.5 cm thick LT (removed at the third/fourth last rib level) chop, weighed, and placed into plastic drip loss containers (Christensen Aps Industrivaengetand, Hilleroed, Denmark), before being stored for 48 h at 4 °C. At the end of the 48 h storage period, muscle cores where removed from their containers, surface moisture was carefully dabbed, cores were reweighed, and drip loss percentage was calculated by dividing the difference between initial and final core weights by the initial core weight.

2.5. Statistical Analysis

The experimental design was a one-way factorial (with the compartments as the levels of the factor to be compared) in a randomized complete block design (weeks as blocks) using the SAS software (SAS 2002) and repeated mixed model analyses (for heart rate data only) to test for any effects of season, compartment, transport event and their interactions. Considering the difference in transport schedule between seasons, for a reliable comparison only heart rate data recorded in the initial transport phase, which was of the same length in each season, were considered in the analysis. Carcass and meat quality data were analyzed by analysis of variance of SAS (SAS Institute Inc., Cary, NC, USA). A probability level of $P < 0.05$ was chosen as the limit for statistical significance in all tests.

3. Results and Discussion

No significant effect of the trailer compartment as a single factor or in interaction with the season was found on any physiological or meat quality variable (data not shown). Hence, data were pooled across compartments in order to study the effects of the deck (upper deck or UD = compartments 1+2+3+4; middle deck or MD = compartments 7+8; bottom deck or BD = compartments 9+10) or trailer section (bottom-nose or BN = compartment 5) on these variables.

Figure 2. Heart rate from loading at the farm to 8 h transit time of pigs transported in a pot belly trailer in summer (six journeys) and winter (five journeys).

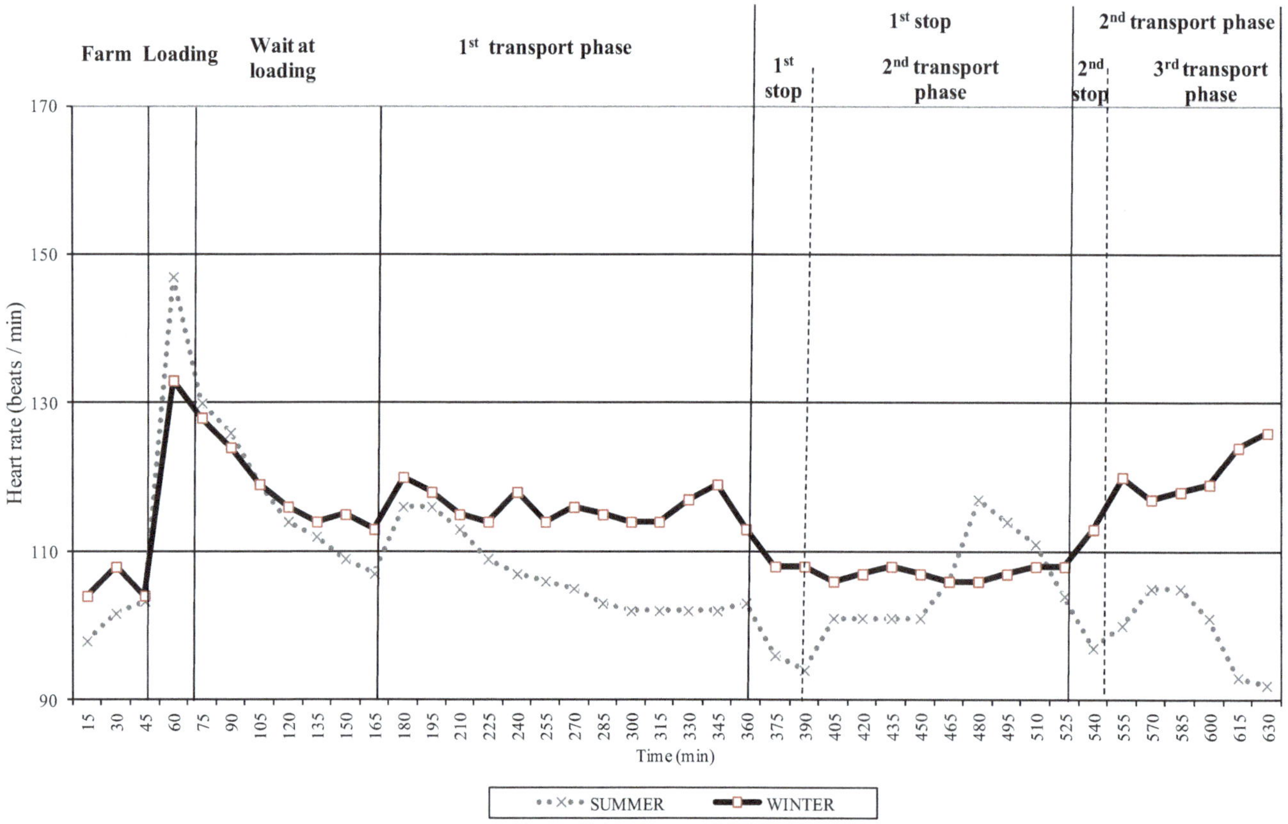

The significant differences are from the least square mean in every event, where at farm: $P < 0.001$; loading: $P < 0.001$; Transport: $P < 0.001$; first stop: $P < 0.001$. From the first stop, transport schedules changed between the seasons (statistical differences were not considered): in winter, first stop lasted 180 min and heart rate recording ends after the second transport phase, and in summer, first stop lasted 30 min. Second transport phase 140 min, second stop 15 min and heart rate recording ends after the third transport phase.

3.1. Physiological Response to Transport

As shown in Figure 2, heart rate was higher ($P < 0.001$) at loading in the summer, which may be explained by the increased frequency of slips, balks and vocalizations on the loading chute and truck ramp observed in this season compared to winter in a companion study [17]. A higher ($P < 0.001$) heart rate was also recorded during the first transport phase in winter. The increased heart rate in the initial transport phase during winter transports may be explained by the animal's need to maintain the body temperature and to maintain balance while the truck was in motion as in a companion study pigs stood more at the beginning of the journey in winter than in summer transports [17]. More recently, Goumon *et al.* [18] reported higher heart rates and more pigs standing during the initial phase of transport using a similar PB trailer in winter. It is usually reported that pigs mostly stand in the initial phase of transport as they usually need time to acclimate in the truck after the departure from the farm [19,20].

An interaction was found between animal location in the PB trailer and season on pigs' heart rate, with pigs in the UD and MD showing a greater heart rate during the wait after loading in summer ($P = 0.01$; Table 1). The higher heart rate recorded in pigs loaded on the UD may result from their physical effort to negotiate the steep ramp to have access to this location. Whereas, the loading order may explain the higher heart rates in pigs located in the MD as this was the last deck to be loaded and pigs were still under the effects of loading stress at the time of departure from the farm.

Table 1. Effects of animal location during transport on the pot-belly (PB) trailer on heart rate [1] average values in summer.

		Truck location[2]					
Transport phase	**Total time (min)**	**UD**	**BN**	**MD**	**BD**	**SE**	***P*-value**
N		78	18	36	48		
Farm	120	95	96	98	96	2.19	0.74
Loading	5	152	154	147	146	5.23	0.54
Waiting at loading	120	124^a	115^b	129^a	126^a	2.61	0.01
First transport phase	190	109	106	109	104	2.32	0.29
First stop	30	95	97	94	95	2.09	0.88
Second transport phase	140	108	105	107	103	2.01	0.22
Second stop	15	97	94	97	96	2.57	0.93
Third transport phase	45	104	106	107	101	3.20	0.51

[1] Units of average values are in beats per minute; [2] UD: upper deck (compartments 1,2,3,4); BN (compartment 5); MD (compartments 7,8); BD (compartments 9,10); [a,b] Within a row, least squares means lacking a common superscript differ at $P < 0.05$.

Table 2. Effects of animal location during transport in the PB trailer on heart rate average values [1] in winter.

		Truck location [2]					
Transport phase	**Total time (min)**	**UD**	**BN**	**MD**	**BD**	**SE**	***P*-value**
N		65	15	30	40		
Farm (rest)	120	107	102	103	105	2.06	0.27
Loading	5	135	139	128	133	2.96	0.15
Waiting at loading	120	120	126	125	122	2.86	0.25
First transport phase	190	118	118	112	116	2.20	0.15
First stop	180	108^b	112^a	102^c	110^{ab}	2.11	0.02
Second transport phase	90	122^a	125^a	114^b	123^a	2.84	0.06

[1] Units of average values are in beats per minute; [2] UD: upper deck (compartments 1,2,3,4); BN (compartment 5); MD (compartments 7,8); BD (compartments 9,10); [a,b,c] Within a row, least squares means lacking a common superscript differ at $P < 0.05$.

Although a couple of companion papers reported a greater behavioral response (more slips and vocalizations) [17] to loading on the UD and colder temperatures in this deck during winter transports [21], heart rates of pigs did not differ between truck locations at any time in this season in this study (Table 2).

As no interaction was found for blood variables between season and animal location in the trailer, data were pooled and presented for each variable separately. Consistent with heart rates, both blood lactate and CK concentrations were higher ($P < 0.001$) in winter than in summer (Table 3). Higher lactate and CK concentrations are usually observed in blood of pigs subjected to rigorous physical exertion as a result of muscle tissue damage [22]. As such, both blood parameters are indicators of muscle fatigue, but in response to different types of stressors. Based on the relatively rapid rate of plasma lactate concentration increase (4 min) and return to basal levels (2 h) after physical exercise [23], the greater blood lactate concentrations at slaughter in winter than in summer may reflect the greater activity (longer latency to rest) in the lairage pen observed in a companion study in this season [17]. In this season pigs were thus more fatigued at slaughter as they stood more than lying in lairage and could not recover from transport and handling stress. Ávcros *et al.* [24] and Seddon *et al.* [25] also found elevated exsanguination blood lactate concentrations in winter compared to summer.

Table 3. Lactate and creatine kinase (CK) concentrations in exsanguination blood of pigs (n = 329) transported on the PB trailer according to the season and the truck location.

	Season			**Truck location** [1]					***P*–value**	
	Summer	**Winter**	**SE**	**UD**	**BN**	**MD**	**BD**	**SE**	**Season**	**Location**
CK (UI/L) [2]	4,605.8	6,865.8		5,695	5,892	4,760	6,327		<0.001	0.20
Lactate (mmol/L)	10.4	13.3	0.5	12.2 [b]	14.2 [a]	10.1 [c]	11.9 [b]	0.7	<0.001	0.01

[1] UD: upper deck (compartments 1,2,3,4); BN (compartment 5); MD (compartments 7,8); BD (compartments 9,10); [2] CK: Creatine kinase (SE is not presented because CK data have been calculated with inverse transformation); [a,b,c] Within a row, least squares means lacking a common superscript differ at $P < 0.05$.

Higher ($P = 0.01$) blood lactate concentrations were also observed in pigs transported in the BN compartment. This increase may be associated to the response to *peri-mortem* handling in pigs having experienced a previous physical stress while negotiating the two ramps, of which one was very steep (32°), to access to this truck location [17].

Similar to blood lactate concentrations, blood CK levels were greater ($P < 0.001$) in winter than in summer. Correa *et al.* [4] also reported higher blood CK levels in winter than in summer. Differently from blood lactate, CK concentration in blood is strongly correlated with long-term physical stress as it reaches a maximum concentration peak 6 h after the physical effort and does not return to basal levels until 48 h afterward [23]. Based on its dissipation pattern in blood after stress, the higher blood CK concentrations in winter in this study may reflect the greater fatigue of pigs at slaughter in this season. In this study, fatigue may be associated to the higher incidence of slips and falls at loading recorded in winter [17]. All these events may have resulted in muscle tissue damage and increased CK release into the blood flow. Similar to Correa *et al.* [4], animal location within a PB trailer had no effect on blood CK concentrations at slaughter.

3.2. Carcass Quality Traits

On average, HCW of the population under study was 95.7 kg (ranging from 65.5 to 129.8 kg) and the carcass lean percentage was 61.2% (ranging from 55.1 to 66.6%).

Overall, skin damage score and the proportion of carcasses showing fighting-type bruises were higher ($P = 0.02$ and $P < 0.001$, respectively) in the summer transports compared to the winter ones (Table 4). The higher skin damage score in summer may be associated with the increased frequency of slips on the loading chute and truck ramp and slips, falls and overlaps observed at unloading in a companion study [17]. The reduced proportion of bruises in winter in this study contradicts the results from previous studies which either reported a higher incidence of bruised carcasses in this season due to increased fighting or mounting behavior in pigs huddling to maintain their body temperature [26,27] or which failed to find a seasonal variation in skin bruise scores [28].

Table 4. Skin damage score and percentage of bruised carcasses of pigs transported on the PB trailer according to the season and the truck location.

	Season			Truck location [1]					*P*-value	
	Summer	**Winter**	**SE**	**UD**	**BN**	**MD**	**BD**	**SE**	**Season**	**Location**
N	257	215		185	55	104	129			
Skin damage [a]	2.3	2.1	0.046	2.2	2.3	2.1	2.2	0.1	0.02	0.42
Fighting type bruise [b], **%**	46.5	24.7		36.8	38.2	35.6	35.7		<0.001	0.80
Mounting type bruise [c], **%**	0.8	1.4		1.1	0.00	1.0	1.5		0.99	0.68
Other type of bruises [d], **%**	21.3	21.9		23.2	21.8	17.3	23.3		0.96	0.75

[1] UD: upper deck (compartments 1,2,3,4); BN (compartment 5); MD (compartments 7,8); BD (compartments 9,10); [a] Based on the MLC scale from 1 (none) to 5 (severe) [13]; [b] Percentage of carcasses with more than 10 fighting-type bruises according to the ITP scale [14]; [c] Percentage of carcasses with more than 5 mounting-type bruises according to the ITP scale [14]; [d] Percentage of carcasses presenting bruises of different origin (lacerations, scratches, *etc.*).

The greater proportion of fighting-type bruises recorded in the summer compared to winter is hard to explain considering that pigs laid more during transport and took shorter time to rest in the lairage pen after transport in summer compared to winter [17].

Despite the variation in pig postures observed between truck compartments at unloading, with pigs from the top compartments being slower to move out and those from the bottom compartments overlapping more [17], bruise score did not vary between truck locations in this study. This discrepancy between pigs' posture observation in the truck and bruise scores has been also reported by Scheeren *et al.* [29] using a similar PB trailer model.

3.3. Meat Quality

It is known that cold and heat stress have an impact on *ante-* and *post-mortem* muscle glycogen stores leading to higher incidence of DFD and PSE pork, respectively [8,9]. As expected, pH24 values were greater ($P < 0.001$) in the LT, and SM and AD muscles in winter than in summer (Table 5). Consistently, in winter the LT muscle had lower ($P = 0.001$) drip loss and higher ($P = 0.02$) subjective color score (darker color). However, in the SM muscle pH6 value was lower ($P < 0.001$) and drip loss value was higher ($P = 0.03$) in winter than in summer. Both meat quality traits are indicative of increased muscle acidification which may result in PSE pork. O'Neill *et al.* [30] also reported a higher prevalence of PSE meat in winter compared to summer and hypothesized that it was related to faster slaughter rates in winter. To maintain fast slaughter speeds, handlers push pigs to walk at a faster pace resulting in acute physical stress immediately before slaughter. It is not surprising that this effect is more pronounced in a locomotory muscle, such as the SM, as this muscle is more susceptible to physical exercise [11,18,31].

Table 5. Meat quality variation as measured in the *Longissimus thoracis* (LT), *Semimembranosus* (SM) and *Adductor* (AD) muscles of pigs transported on a PB trailer according to the season and the truck location.

	Season			Truck location [1]					*P*-value	
	Summer	Winter	SE	UD	BN	MD	BD	SE	Season	Location
N	270	225		198	55	110	132			
LT muscle										
pH 6 h	6.02	6.02	0.02	6.04	5.99	6.02	6.00	0.03	0.84	0.75
pH 24 h	5.64	5.73	0.01	5.69 [a]	5.70 [a]	5.66 [b]	5.66 [b]	0.02	<0.001	0.02
L*	49.19	49.04	0.26	49.32	48.29	49.09	49.12	0.36	0.67	0.34
a*	8.43	8.16	0.09	8.34	8.16	8.30	8.25	0.13	0.03	0.81
b*	4.91	4.90	0.08	4.96	4.62	4.95	4.92	0.12	0.94	0.29
JCS [2]	2.94	3.11	0.06	3.02	3.18	3.00	2.98	0.08	0.02	0.42
EC [3]	6.99	7.49	0.17	7.57 [a]	7.21 [a]	7.20 [a]	6.87 [b]	0.23	0.03	0.04
Drip loss (%)	4.05	3.39	0.14	3.70	3.21	3.89	3.83	0.20	0.001	0.19
SM muscle										
pH 6 h	6.32	6.07	0.02	6.18	6.21	6.19	6.21	0.03	<0.001	0.86
pH 24 h	5.63	5.71	0.01	5.66	5.76	5.65	5.69	0.02	<0.001	<0.001
L*	46.84	46.19	0.21	46.86 [a]	46.24 [ab]	46.69 [a]	45.97 [b]	0.29	0.03	0.03
a*	7.90	8.64	0.10	8.28	7.85	8.47	8.27	0.14	<0.001	0.08
b*	3.69	4.08	0.07	3.96 [a]	3.68 [b]	4.01 [a]	3.79 [a]	0.09	<0.001	0.007
EC [3]	6.88	6.98	0.18	7.17	6.62	6.86	6.67	0.26	0.68	0.30
Drip loss (%)	3.77	4.15	0.13	4.17 [a]	3.76 [b]	3.98 [ab]	3.96 [ab]	0.18	0.03	0.002
AD muscle										
pH 24 h	5.81	6.01	0.02	5.91 [a]	5.97 [a]	5.84 [b]	5.92 [a]	0.03	<0.001	0.002

[1] UD: upper deck (compartments 1,2,3,4); BN (compartment 5); MD (compartments 7,8); BD (compartments 9,10); [2] According to Japanese Color Scales (from 1 = pale to 6 = dark) [15]; [3] Electrical conductivity measured by the PQM (Pork Quality Meter, Aichach, Germany); [a,b,c] Within a row, least squares means lacking a common superscript differ at $P < 0.05$.

Meat quality was also affected by animal location during transport, with pigs located in the BN and UD having higher ($P = 0.02$) pH24 values (Table 5). Similar to the effects of the season, the effects of transporting pigs in the BN were more pronounced in locomotor muscles, with SM and AD muscles of these pigs showing higher ($P < 0.001$ and $P = 0.002$, respectively) pH24 values. Lower L* values and drip loss percentages ($P = 0.03$ and $P = 0.002$, respectively) were also reported in the SM muscle of pigs transported in the BN. These meat characteristics indicate that pigs loaded in the BN area may become fatigued and be prone to produce DFD pork.

4. Conclusions

This study shows that some pot-belly trailer locations, such as the upper deck and bottom- nose, impose a certain level of stress on pigs during transport resulting from the use of internal ramps at loading and unloading. Additional studies are needed to determine means of reducing the stress of moving pigs into and out of such trailer locations. Although in this study the effect of the season may have been confounded by the different transport schedule between seasons, which reflects the commercial practice in the Canadian Prairies, the greater physical exhaustion (higher blood lactate and CK levels, and pH24 values) of pigs transported long distance in winter which is due to the additive effect of cold stress confirms results that have been previously reported in the literature [4,25,32].

Acknowledgments

This research project was funded by NSERC, Alberta Pork, SaskPork, Manitoba Pork, Ontario Pork and Maple Leaf Foods. We appreciate the technical assistance of Sophie Horth, Frederic Morel, Thusith Samarakone, Stephanie Hayne, Crystal Kappel, Megan Bouvier, Brenda Sawatzky, José Rodolfo Ciocca, Angela Vanelli Weschenfelder and Andreanne Bornais for the data collection at the slaughter plant, blood sampling, meat quality measurements and laboratory analysis, and Steve Méthot for the statistical analysis. The authors are grateful to Steve's Livestock for providing the transport and Maple Leaf Foods for providing manpower and facilities. J. A. Correa thanks Fulgence Ménard Inc. for allowing him pursue his Ph.D. studies during the working hours.

Author Contributions

Conceived and design the experiments: HG; obtained the financial support: HG; prepared pigs at the farm: JAC and HG; performed the physiological data collection and analysis: JAC and LF; performed the carcass and meat quality data collection and analysis: JAC and LF; performed the statistical analysis: JAC; wrote the paper: JAC, HC, ST, TW, RB, TC, JPL, LF.

Conflicts of Interest

There are no conflicts of interest issues concerning this submission.

References

1. Bench, C.; Schaefer, A.L.; Faucitano, L. The welfare of pigs during transport. In *The Welfare of Pigs—From Birth to Slaughter*; Faucitano, L., Schaefer, A.L., Eds.; Wageningen Academic Publishers: Wageningen, The Netherlands, 2008; pp. 161–195.
2. Torrey, S.; Bergeron, R.; Gonyou, H.W.; Widowski, T.; Lewis, N.; Crowe, T.; Correa, J.A.; Brown, J.; Faucitano, L. Transportation of market-weight pigs 1. Effect of season and truck type on behaviour with a 2 hour transport. *J. Anim. Sci.* **2013**, *91*, 2863–2871.
3. Ritter, M.J.; Ellis, M.; Bowman, R.; Brinkmann, J.; Curtis, S.E.; DeDecker, J.M.; Mendoza, O.; Murphy, C.M.; Orellana, D.G.; Peterson, B.A.; Rojo, A.; Schlipf, J.M.; Wolter, B.F. Effects of season and distance moved during loading on transport losses of market-weight pigs in two commercially available types of trailer. *J. Anim. Sci.* **2008**, *86*, 3137–3145.
4. Correa, J.A.; Gonyou, H.W.; Torrey, S.; Widowski, T.; Bergeron, R.; Crowe, T.G.; Laforest, J.P.; Faucitano, L. Welfare and carcass and meat quality of pigs being transported for 2 hours using two vehicle typcs during two seasons of the year. *Can. J. Anim. Sci.* **2013**, *93*, 43–55.
5. Schwartzkopf Genswein, K.; Faucitano, L.; Dadgar, S.; Shand, P.; Gonzàlez, L.A.; Crowe, T. Road transport of cattle, swine and poultry in North America and its impact on animal welfare, carcass and meat quality: A review. *Meat Sci.* **2012**, *92*, 227–243.
6. Sutherland, M.A.; McDonald, A.; McGlone, J.J. Effects of variations in the environment, length of journey and type of trailer on the mortality and morbidity of pigs being transported to slaughter. *Vet. Rec.* **2009**, *165*, 13–18.
7. Kephart, K.B.; Harper, M.T.; Raines, C.R. Observations of market pigs following transport to a packing plant. *J. Anim. Sci.* **2010**, *88*, 2199–2203.
8. Guàrdia, M.D.; Estany, J.; Balash, S.; Oliver, M.A.; Gispert, M.; Diestre, A. Risk assessment of PSE meat due to pre-slaughter conditions and RYR1 gene in pigs. *Meat Sci.* **2004**, *67*, 471–478.
9. Guàrdia, M.D.; Estany, J.; Balash, S.; Oliver, M.A.; Gispert, M.; Diestre, A. Risk assessment of DFD meat due to pre-slaughter conditions and RYR1 gene in pigs. *Meat Sci.* **2005**, *70*, 709–716.
10. Tamminga, E.; Bergeron, R.; Correa, J.A.; Crowe, T.; Dewey, C.; Faucitano, L.; Gonyou, H.W.; Lewis, N.; Torrey, S.; Widowski, T. Core body temperatures of market swine transported to slaughter. *Can. J. Anim. Sci.* **2009**, *89*, 176.
11. Weschenfelder, A.V.; Torrey, S.; Devillers, N.; Crowe, T.; Bassols, A.; Saco, Y.; Piñeiro, M.; Saucier, L; Faucitano, L. Effects of trailer design on animal welfare parameters and carcass and meat quality of three Pietrain crosses being transported over a long distance. *J. Anim. Sci.* **2012**, *90*, 3220–3231.
12. *Guidelines on: The Care and Use of Farm Animals in Research, Teaching and Testing*; Canadian Council on Animal Care: Ottawa, Canada, 2009.
13. *Concern at Rindside Damage in Pigs*; Meat and Marketing Technical Notes No. 4; Meat and Livestock Commission: Bletchley, Milton Keynes, UK, 1985.
14. ITP. *Notation des hématomes sur couenne—porcs vivant ou carcasse*; Institute Technique du Porc: Rennes, France, 1996.
15. Nakai, H.; Saito, F.; Ikeda, T.; Ando, S.; Komatsu, A. Standard models of pork colour. *Bull. Nat. Inst. Anim. Ind.* **1975**, *30*, 69–74.

16. Correa, J.A.; Méthot, S.; Faucitano, L. A modified meat juice container (EZ-DripLoss) procedure for a more reliable assessment of drip loss and related quality changes in pork meat. *J. Muscle Foods* **2007**, *18*, 67–77.
17. Torrey, S.; Bergeron, R.; Gonyou, H.W.; Widowski, T.; Lewis, N.; Crowe, T.; Correa, J.A.; Brown, J.; Faucitano, L. Transportation of market-weight pigs 2. Effect of season and animal location in the truck on behaviour with a 8 hour transport. *J. Anim. Sci.* **2013**, *91*, 2872–2878.
18. Goumon , S.; Brown, J.A.; Faucitano, L.; Bergeron, R.; Widowski, T.M.; Crowe, T.; Connor, M.L.; Gonyou, H.W. Effects of transport duration on maintenance behavior, heart rate and gastrointestinal tract temperature of market-weight pigs in 2 seasons. *J. Anim. Sci.* **2013**, *91*, 4925–4935.
19. Barton-Gade, P.; Christensen, L. Effect of different stocking densities during transport on welfare and meat quality in Danish slaughter pigs. *Meat Sci.* **1998**, *48*, 237–247.
20. Bradshaw, R.H.; Hall, S.J.G.; Broom, D.M. Behavioural and cortisol response of pigs and sheep during transport. *Vet. Rec.* **1996**, *138*, 233–234.
21. Brown, J.A.; Samarakone, T.S.; Crowe, T.; Bergeron, R.; Widowski, T.; Correa, J.A.; Faucitano, L.; Torrey, S.; Gonyou, H.W. Temperature and humidity conditions in trucks transporting pigs in two seasons in eastern and western Canada. *Trans. ASABE* **2011**, *54*, 2311–2318.
22. Knowles, T.G.; Warriss, P.D. Stress physiology of animals during transport. In *Livestock Handling and Transport*; Grandin, T.A., Ed.; CAB International: Wallingford, UK, 2000; pp. 385–407.
23. Anderson, D.B. Relationship of blood lactate and meat quality in market hogs. Available online: http://fass.acrobat.com/p86799506/ (accessed on 21 June 2013).
24. Averós, X.; Herranz, A.; Sanchez, R.; Comella, J.X.; Gosálvez L.F. Serum stress parameters in pigs transported to slaughter under commercial conditions in different seasons. *Vet. Med.* **2007**, *52*, 333–342.
25. Seddon, Y.M.; Brown, J.; Crowe, T.; Bergeron, R.; Widowski, T.; Correa, J.A.; Faucitano, L.; Gonyou, H.W. Truck compartment and trip duration affect stress of pigs transported under Canadian conditions. *J. Anim. Sci.* **2012**, *90*(Suppl. 3), 255.
26. Gosálvez, L.F.; Averós, X.; Valdevira, J.J.; Herranz A. Influence of season, distance and mixed loads on the physical and carcass integrity of pigs transported to slaughter. *Meat Sci.* **2006**, *73*, 553–558.
27. dalla Costa, O.A.; Faucitano, L.; Coldebella, A.; Ludke, J.V.; Peloso, J.V.; dalla Roza, D.; Paranhos da Costa, M.J.R. Effects of the season of the year, truck type and location on truck on skin bruises and meat quality in pigs. *Livest. Sci.* **2007**, *107*, 29–36.
28. Guàrdia, M.D.; Estany, J.; Balash, S.; Oliver, M.A.; Gispert, M.; Diestre, A. Risk assessment of skin damage due to pre-slaughter conditions and RYR1 gene in pigs. *Meat Sci.* **2009**, *81*, 745–751.
29. Scheeren, M.B.; Gonyou, H.W.; Brown, J.; Weschenfelder, A.V.; Faucitano, L. Effects of season, transport time and compartment in the pot-belly trailer on skin bruises and meat quality in pigs. *Can. J. Anim. Sci.* **2014**, *94*, 1–8.
30. O'Neill, D.J.; Lynch, P.B.; Troy, D.J.; Buckley, D.J.; Kerry, J.P. Influence of time of year on the incidence of PSE and DFD in Irish pigmeat. *Meat Sci.* **2003**, *64*, 105–111.

31. Hambrecht, E.; Eissen, J.J.; Newman, D.J.; Smits, C.H.M.; den Hartog, L.A.; Verstegen, M.W.A. Negative effects of stress immediately before slaughter on pork quality are aggravated by suboptimal transport and lairage conditions. *J. Anim. Sci.* **2005**, *83*, 440–448.
32. Fortin, A. The effect of transport time from the assembly yard to the abattoir and resting time at the abattoir on pork quality. *Can. J. Anim. Sci.* **2002**, *82*, 141–150.

8

The Effects of Cooking Process and Meat Inclusion on Pet Food Flavor and Texture Characteristics

Kadri Koppel [1,*], Michael Gibson [2], Sajid Alavi [2] and Greg Aldrich [2]

[1] Sensory Analysis Center, Department of Human Nutrition, Kansas State University, 1310 Research Park Drive, Manhattan, KS 66502, USA

[2] Department of Grain Science and Industry, Kansas State University, Manhattan, KS 66506, USA; E-Mails: michael.gibson171@gmail.com (M.G.); salavi@ksu.edu (S.A.); aldrich4@ksu.edu (G.A.)

* Author to whom correspondence should be addressed; E-Mail: kadri@ksu.edu.

Simple Summary: The results of this research indicate that processing (baked *vs.* extruded) plays an important role in determining pet food product texture. In addition, raw ingredients (fresh meat *vs.* meal-based) did not consistently affect product sensory characteristics. These results may help pet food technologists better understand factors that affect palatability.

Abstract: The pet food industry is an important portion of the food and feed industries in the US. The objectives of this study were (1) to determine cooking method (baking or extrusion), meat inclusion (0 or 20%), and extrusion thermal to mechanical energy ratios (low, medium, and high) effects on sensory and volatile properties of pet foods, and (2) to determine associations among sensory and volatile characteristics of baked and extruded pet foods. Descriptive sensory analysis and gas chromatography-mass spectrometry were used to analyze the pet food samples. It was found that baked samples were lighter in color (2.0–2.6 baked *vs.* 3.5–4.3 extruded, color intensity scale 0–15), and had lower levels of attributes that indicated rancidity (*i.e.*, fishy flavor; 0.3–0.6 baked, 0.6–1.5 extruded, scale 0–15), whereas extruded pet foods were more cohesive in mass, more friable, hard, and crisp, but less powdery than baked samples. Fresh meat inclusion tended to decrease bitterness and increase fishy flavor and cohesiveness of pet foods. High thermal to mechanical energy ratio during extrusion resulted in less musty and more porous kibbles. The main volatile compounds included aldehydes, such as hexanal and heptanal, ketones, and alcohols. Extruded samples did not contain methylpyrazine, while baked samples did not contain 2-butyl furan. Future studies should consider evaluating the relationship between sensory results and animal palatability for these types of foods.

Keywords: aroma; baked; dog food; extruded; sensory analysis

---

1. Introduction

The pet food industry in the US continues to grow at a rate of approximately 4% per year, with a current estimated size of $19.7 billion [1]. Growth in this industry is driven by new product entries, such as naturally preserved diets; raw foods; "novel" ingredients like bison, potato, and peas; addition of nutraceuticals such as kelp, algae, acai berries; and an emphasis on fatty acid nutrition with foods containing fatty acids from fish and various seeds. While ingredients in pet foods are constantly changing, pet owners expect similar quality kibbles manufactured from any ingredient source. Most of the information in the pet food industry has been highly proprietary and, as a result, few publications have examined specific formulation or ingredient effects on pet food sensory properties.

Pet food processing has previously been evaluated from an extrusion perspective [2–4], and several studies have evaluated the effects of raw ingredients on pet food physical characteristics, palatability, and digestibility [5–7]. Other than extrusion, another popular processing technique used in dry pet food manufacturing is baking, mainly used in manufacturing pet treats. Gibson and Alavi described the effects of baking and extrusion on starch properties in pet foods [8]. However, to date, no studies have been found in which baked pet foods sensory characteristics have been characterized in comparison to extruded pet foods.

Sensory analysis of pet foods provides an additional tool in helping to understand both consumer and pet behavior. For example, Lin *et al.* studied selected processing effects such as fat source and moisture content with sensory analysis techniques [9]. These authors focused on selected pet food sensory properties such as aroma and appearance. Other studies have developed vocabularies to aid in a more thorough description of pet food sensory properties such as aroma, flavor, appearance, and texture. Examples are available on commercial dry dog food [10] and dry and canned cat foods [11,12]. Another study characterized volatile compounds in commercial pet foods and related those to sensory attributes [13]. Some associations, such as aldehydes and rancidity were detected among sensory qualities and various volatile molecules; however an approach that includes controlled ingredient composition and processing information would provide further insight.

The objectives of this study were (1) to determine processing, meat inclusion, and extrusion thermal and mechanical energy ratio level effects on sensory and volatile properties of pet foods, and (2) to determine associations among sensory and volatile characteristics of baked and extruded pet foods. The primary hypothesis being tested was that meat inclusion, processing method (baking *vs.* extrusion), and thermal to mechanical energy ratio during extrusion had an effect on pet food appearance, aroma, flavor, and texture properties. More specifically, it was hypothesized that baked pet food products would have a harder texture than extruded products, as the former are typically dense, while the latter are more expanded and porous in structure. Extensive scientific literature is available relating density to mechanical strength and hardness of porous or cellular products in general and extruded foods in particular [14,15]. It was also hypothesized that higher thermal to mechanical energy level ratios during extrusion would lead to harder products (due to reduced macromolecular degradation) and meat inclusion would result in dog food with less barnyard flavor.

2. Experimental Section

2.1. Diet Formulation

Two maintenance dog food diets were formulated to be iso-nutritional based on carbohydrate, lipid, and protein content. Major variations within the diets were fresh meat inclusion (0 and 20%), chicken fat, and chicken by-product meal (Table 1). Dry ingredients were procured from Lortscher Agri Service, Inc. (Bern, KS, USA). Mechanically deboned chicken was acquired from C J Foods (Bern, KS, USA). Chicken fat was procured from American Dehydrated Foods (Springfield, MO, USA).

Table 1. Sample ingredients and nutritional composition.

Ingredients, %	**0% Fresh Meat**	**20% Fresh Meat**
Mechanically Deboned Chicken	0.00	20.00
Chicken Fat	5.32	2.34
Chicken By-Product Meal	20.94	10.91
Brewers Rice	21.21	18.84
Corn	21.21	18.84
Wheat	21.21	18.84
Beet Pulp	4.00	4.00
Corn Gluten Meal, 75%	3.00	3.00
Calcium Carbonate	0.75	0.75
Potassium Chloride	0.49	0.42
Sodium Chloride	0.46	0.43
Dicalcium Phosphate	0.87	1.12
Choline Chloride	0.20	0.20
Natural antioxidant, Dry	0.07	0.07
Natural antioxidant, Liquid	0.02	0.01
Trace Mineral Premix	0.10	0.10
Vitamin Premix	0.15	0.15
Nutritional Composition in the final product *		
Crude Protein	21.69–22.36	20.24–21.58
Crude Fat	5.42–8.86	5.35–9.65
Ash	6.53–10.74	6.36–6.75
Crude Fiber	1.84–2.95	2.15–7.86
Moisture	4.20–6.67	4.23–6.25

* Nutritional Composition analyzed at University of Missouri Experiment Station Chemical Laboratories, w/w%.

2.2. Grinding and Mixing

Whole grains (corn and wheat) were ground using a Fitz mill (Model D, Fitzpatrick Company, Elmhurst, IL, USA) to pass through a 1532-0040 screen with a round hole opening of 1.02 mm. Dry ingredients (Table 1) were mixed together in a double-ribbon horizontal mixer (Wenger Manufacturing, Sabetha, KS, USA). Major ingredients (brewer's rice, corn, wheat, beet pulp, chicken by-product meal, and corn gluten meal) were mixed for three minutes, and then minor ingredients (calcium carbonate, potassium chloride, sodium chloride, dicalcium phosphate, choline chloride, dry antioxidant, trace mineral and vitamin premixes) were added into the mixer for an additional two minutes. Post mixing, the entire batch was ground through the same milling system in order to achieve a more uniform particle size for the entirety of dry ingredients (major and minor ingredients).

2.3. Processing

Two cooking methods—extrusion or baking—were used to manufacture the pet food samples. For extruded samples three thermal energy input levels (Low; LE, Medium; ME, and High; HE) and 0 or 20% meat inclusion were used resulting in six pet food treatments: 0LE, 20LE, 0ME, 20ME, 0HE, and 20HE. For baked samples one processing time (11 min) was used with 0 and 20% meat inclusion resulting in two baked samples (0B and 20B). The extrusion and baking processes are described in detail below.

2.4. Extrusion

Diets were processed on a single screw extruder (X-20, Wenger Manufacturing, Sabetha, KS, USA) with the screw profile displayed in Figure 1. Processing conditions, e.g., extruder screw RPM (350 425 RPM as Medium, and 500 RPM) and preconditioner steam input (8 kg/h, 12 kg/h, and 16 kg/h as High) were varied to achieve different thermal to mechanical ratios. The specific ratios used were 500 RPM and 8 kg/h steam input for Low thermal to mechanical energy ratio, 425 RPM and 12 kg/h steam input for Medium, and 350 RPM and 16 kg/h steam input for High thermal to mechanical energy ratios.

The extruder screw profile, starting at the feed throat, was a single flight single pitch screw and tapered down to a double flight half pitch screw element. Shear locks increased in size, from small to large, in between each screw element after the inlet screw element. The extruder screw profile was selected to convey and compress material as the pet food mash passed through the extruder.

The natural liquid antioxidant was mixed into chicken fat prior to being pumped into the middle section of the preconditioner using a Seepex pump (Range, MO, USA). Mechanically deboned chicken was pumped into the final zone of the preconditioner using a Waukesha Sanitary pump (Delavan, WI, USA). Each pump was calibrated to the required set points for each formulation prior to extrusion.

Processing moistures were calculated prior to extrusion to achieve 27% in-barrel moisture. The introduction of fresh meat and oil changed flow rates of the dry feed rate and moisture additions.

After extrusion, kibbles were pneumatically conveyed to a double pass dryer and single pass cooler (4800 series, Wenger Manufacturing, Sabetha, KS, USA). Dryer settings were 104 °C for 10 min per pass, followed by cooling with room temperature air for 10 minutes. The dryer and cooler were both continuous, perforated belt type, and were part of an integrated system. Samples were collected at the end of the cooler and stored in hermetically sealed bags at ambient temperature. All samples were stored for similar periods of time until further testing.

Figure 1. Schematic showing pilot scale single screw extruder profile and barrel temperature setting. The screw element codes a:b:x imply the following: a = 1 (full pitch screw), 0.5 (half pitch screw), SL (steam lock element); b = element length (mm); x = SF (single flighted screw), DF (double flighted screw), SM (small diameter steam lock), M (medium diameter steam lock), L (large diameter steam lock). The last screw element is a conical shaped segment.

Zone Number	**1**	**2**	**3**
Barrel Temperature (°C)	**60**	**75**	**90**

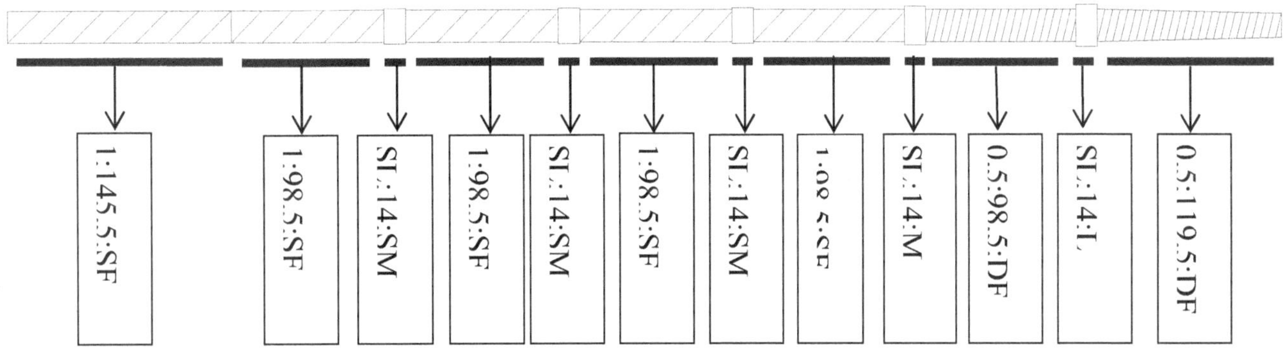

2.5. Baking

The baked treatments were mixed together in a planetary mixer (HL800 Hobart, Troy, OH, USA) at the American Institute of Baking (Manhattan, KS, USA). The mixes were comprised of the dry mix described above, mechanically deboned chicken, chicken fat, and water. The final dough moisture levels were targeted to be 33–34% on a wet basis (w.b.). The dough was passed through a rotary molder (RM14B81, Weidenmiller Company, Itasca, IL, USA) to make frustum-shaped kibbles.

The rotary molded kibbles were placed into a rack oven (Model 626, Revent, Inc., Somerset, NJ, USA) preheated to 220 °C and baked for 11 min. Post baking, kibbles were placed in a drying oven at 50 °C for 5 h to drive off excess moisture. To confirm the dog food achieved the final target moisture level below 10% w.b., moisture content was measured following AOAC method 930.15.

2.6. Descriptive Sensory Analysis

2.6.1. Panelists

Five highly trained panelists from the Sensory Analysis Center, Kansas State University (Manhattan, KS, USA) participated in this study. All of the panelists had completed 120 h of general descriptive analysis training with a variety of food products. The training included techniques and practice in attribute identification, terminology development, and intensity scoring. Each of the panelists had more than 1,000 h of testing experience with a variety of food products. For this project, the panelists received further orientation on dried dog food using samples that may or may not be included in the study. Panels of similar size and training have been reported in other recent research [16–19].

2.6.2. Sample Presentation and Evaluation

Each sample was served in a ~100 mL plastic cup for appearance, texture, and flavor evaluation, and in a medium snifter covered with a watch glass for the evaluation of aroma. The amount of product in the snifter was 3 g. Samples were prepared 30 min prior to the testing and were coded with three-digit random numbers. All of the samples were evaluated in a randomized order in duplicate for appearance, texture, flavor, and aroma using attributes selected from a lexicon developed for this product category by Di Donfrancesco *et al.* [10]. Barnyard, brothy, toasted, brown, grain, vitamin, stale, meaty, musty, oxidized oil, cardboard, liver, and fish aroma, flavor, and aftertaste attributes were evaluated in all samples. In addition sour, salty, sweet, and bitter taste and aftertaste and metallic aftertaste attributes were evaluated. Brown color intensity, porous, grainy, and fibrous appearance characteristics and cohesiveness of mass, fracturability, hardness, powdery, crispness, and mouth-coating texture attributes (powdery and mouthcoat) were evaluated. Six 2-hour sessions were held for the evaluation phase. For the evaluation, a numeric scale of 0–15 with 0.5 increments where 0 represents none and 15 extremely high was applied to each attribute to provide a measure of intensity. Each panelist individually assigned intensities to the attributes present in the sample according to their perception of the appearance, aroma, flavor, and texture references included in the lexicon. The panelists were provided with a definition sheet with the list of attributes and their definitions as well as reference materials for each attribute according to Di Donfrancesco *et al.* [10].

The panelists were asked to chew one kibble for flavor and texture evaluation. The panelists were instructed to expectorate samples after evaluation. Panelists were provided with apple slices, unsalted crackers, purified water, and toothbrushes for palate cleansing in between the evaluations. The testing room was at 21 ± 1 °C and 55 ± 5% relative humidity.

2.7. Volatile Compounds Measurement

2.7.1. Extraction Procedure of Volatile Aroma Compounds

The extraction method chosen for studying the aroma profile in the dry dog foods was headspace-solid phase microextraction (HS-SPME) as described by Koppel *et al.* [13]. The samples were ground in pestle & mortar, then a 0.5 g samples was weighed into a 10 mL screw-cap vial with a polytetrafluoroethylene/silicone septum. Exactly 0.48 mL distilled water was added to the ground sample in the vial. To this an internal standard consisting of 0.02 mL 1,3-dichlorobenzene (98%, Sigma Aldrich, St. Louis, MO, USA) dissolved in hexane (mixture of isomers, optima grade, Fisher Scientific; Pittsburgh, PA, USA), with final concentration in the sample of 0.2 mg/kg was added. The vials were equilibrated for 10 min at 40 °C in the autosampler (Pal system, model CombiPal, CTC Analytics, Zwingen, Switzerland) and agitated at 250 rpm. After the equilibration, a 50/30 μm divinylbenzene/carboxen/polydimethylsiloxane fiber was exposed to the sample headspace for 30 min at 40 °C. The fiber method was chosen for its high capacity of trapping volatile compounds in food products [20].

After sampling, the analytes were desorbed from the SPME fiber coating prior in the GC injection port at 270 °C for 3 min in splitless mode.

2.7.2. Chromatographic Analyses

The isolation, tentative identification, and semi-quantification of the volatile compounds were performed on a gas chromatograph (Varian GC CP3800; Varian Inc., Walnut Creek, CA, USA), coupled with a Varian mass spectrometer (MS) detector (Saturn 2000). The GC-MS system was equipped with an RTX-5MS (Crossbond® 5% diphenyl/95% dimethyl polysiloxane) column (Restek, U.S., Bellefonte, PA, USA; 30 m × 0.25 mm × 0.25 μm film thickness). The initial temperature of the column was 40 °C held for 4 min; the temperature was then increased by 5 °C per min to 260 °C, and held at this temperature for 7 min. All samples were analyzed in triplicates. The quantities of volatile compounds were calculated against the internal standard peaks.

Most of the compounds were identified using two different analytical methods: (1) mass spectra (>80%) and (2) Kovats indices (NIST/EPA/NIH Mass Spectral Library, Version 2.0, 2005). Identification was considered tentative when it was based on only mass spectral data. The retention times for a C7–C40 saturated alkane mix (Supelco Analytical, Bellefonte, PA, USA) was used to determine experimental Kovats indices for the volatile compounds detected.

2.8. Data Analysis

Significant treatment effects ($P < 0.05$) were determined for meat inclusion (all samples), processing (all samples), and thermal input level (extruded samples only) using SAS Glimmix procedure (Version 9.3, SAS Institute Inc., Cary, NC, USA).

Partial least squares regression (PLSR) study is a multivariate statistical technique that has been used by several researchers for creating external preference maps for determining relationships between descriptive data (X-matrix) and consumer acceptability data (Y-matrix) [21]. PLSR can be used to correlate the instrumental volatile data (X-matrix) and descriptive sensory data (Y-matrix), an approach similar to the one reported by Koppel *et al.* [13]. This procedure using sensory flavor attributes data as the Y-matrix and volatile compounds data as the X-matrix was conducted in our study using Unscrambler (version 10.2; Camo Software; Oslo, Norway).

3. Results and Discussion

3.1. Descriptive Sensory Analysis

Most aroma, flavor, and aftertaste attributes were scored at low intensity levels (0–5 on a scale from 0 to 15; Table 2(a,b)). According to Di Donfrancesco *et al.* most commercial dry dog food samples exhibit low flavor intensities [10]. The same authors reported meaty flavor in dry dog foods to be a complex attribute usually detected at low levels. In our study, meaty flavor was not identified by the panelists, although it was included in the attribute list. This indicates that meaty flavor probably results from a surface flavoring applied to commercial products that was not included in our formulas. A similar situation was observed for sweet taste; wherein, sweetness in dry dog foods may result from added dextrose, cane syrup or other flavoring agents such as sweet-tasting amino acids to enhance overall sweetness.

Fresh meat inclusion tended to affect pet food bitterness (P = 0.03) and fish flavor (P = 0.008; Table 2a). Pet foods manufactured with fresh meat tended to be less bitter but higher in fish flavor than samples manufactured without fresh meat. The fish flavor may be related to rancid fatty acid flavor notes. Rancidity in foods, including pet foods, is recognized by volatile compounds that result from the oxidation of fatty acids (e.g., hexanal, heptanal, octanal). In pet foods manufactured with animal by-product meals these volatiles are likely to be present at a lower level because the rendering process includes cooking the materials at 115–145 °C [22]. Fresh meat inclusion was also observed to increase cohesiveness of mass characteristics in pet food samples. This is probably related to the enhanced binding properties of meat fibers in the fresh meat treatment.

Thermal to mechanical energy ratio had an effect on sensory characteristics among the extruded pet food samples. A higher ratio tended to decrease brown color intensity and increase porous, grainy, and fibrous appearance; these results are in line with findings by Cheng *et al.* [23]. Musty flavor was more pronounced in pet food samples manufactured at lower thermal input. In addition some texture characteristics, such as fracturability, hardness, and crispness were affected by thermal input. Fracturability (defined as "the force with which the sample ruptures") was highest for medium thermal input samples, while hardness (defined as "the force required to bite completely through the sample with molar teeth") was scored at highest intensity for low thermal samples. Initial crispness, defined as "the intensity of audible noise at first chew with molars" was scored as more intense for medium and high thermal input samples. This is consistent with the hypothesis stated earlier that increased thermal energy as compared to mechanical energy input leads to lesser macromolecular degradation and a product with a stronger solid matrix.

Baking is a process that involves only thermal energy (heat), while extrusion involves both thermal and mechanical energy (friction) under pressure [24]. Intuitively one would expect the texture characteristics of baked and extruded products to be different. This was substantiated by our study. Cooking process (baked *vs.* extruded) effects were different for all sensory attributes shown in Table 2(a,b) except for grainy appearance and musty flavor. Baked pet food samples resulted in a more porous appearance and were lower in brown color intensity. According to Cowell *et al.* baking would result in more uniform products when compared to extrusion, and this may have an influence on consumer perception [25]. In addition, baked pet foods were found to be lower in almost all flavor attributes than extruded samples except for bitter taste and aftertaste. Furthermore baked samples were lower in cohesiveness of mass (P = 0.0003), hardness (P < 0.0001), and initial crispness (P < 0.0001), but more intense in powdery (P < 0.0001) and mouthcoat attributes (P < 0.0001). The lower hardness of baked products was contrary to the hypothesis stated earlier that these higher density products would have a greater hardness. The primary reason was the limited gelatinization of starch in the baked products due to absence of mechanical energy input as compared to almost complete gelatinization in extruded products [8]. Lower starch gelatinization would lead to a lesser binding of various components in the formulation and weaker solid matrix, which in turn would result in reduced overall product hardness. According to Houpt and Smith, dogs have certain preferences when it comes to food flavor and texture, such as moist and canned food is preferred over dry, and beef may be preferred over pork, chicken, and other meats [26]. No information was found in the scientific literature on baked *vs.* extruded texture preferences, and this presents an opportunity for future research.

Table 2a. Descriptive sensory analysis attributes (mean values) for pet foods differing in cooking technique, extrusion thermal input, and amount of fresh meat included in the formula reported on an intensity scale of 0 to 15 with 1 being none to 15 extremely intense.

Attribute	Sample									Fresh Meat effect	TI effect	Proc. effect
	0B	20B	0LE	20LE	0ME	20ME	0HE	20HE	STDEV			
Brown ap	2.7	2.9	4.3	3.9	4.0	3.7	3.6	3.5	0.860	NS	0.003	<0.0001
Porous ap	3.9	3.3	1.9	1.8	2.1	2.2	3.2	3.1	1.136	NS	<0.0001	<0.0001
Grainy ap	2.4	2.3	2.2	2.3	2.6	2.3	2.9	2.7	0.776	NS	0.004	NS
Fibrous ap	0.8	1.0	1.5	1.0	1.7	1.5	1.7	1.9	0.839	NS	0.03	0.0007
Toasted ar	1.4	1.6	1.6	1.6	1.7	1.8	1.7	1.8	0.467	NS	NS	0.018
Brown ar	0.5	0.5	0.3	0.3	0.1	0.5	0.2	0.3	0.597	NS	NS	0.02
Stale ar	1.5	1.3	1.6	1.9	1.9	1.9	1.6	1.6	0.746	NS	NS	0.018
Fish ar	0.0	0.3	0.4	0.6	0.3	0.5	0.5	0.5	0.622	NS	NS	0.017
Toasted fl	1.4	1.6	1.9	1.8	1.7	1.7	1.9	2.1	0.509	NS	NS	0.004
Grain fl	2.9	3.2	3.3	3.3	3.5	3.5	3.4	3.3	0.665	NS	NS	0.01
Vitamin fl	0.4	0.7	1.1	0.8	1.0	0.6	0.8	0.8	0.689	NS	NS	0.03
Stale fl	2.1	2.0	2.2	2.4	2.2	2.1	2.4	2.4	0.774	NS	NS	0.02
Bitter	4.6	4.2	4.3	4.2	4.3	3.9	4.0	3.9	0.740	0.03	NS	0.03
Musty fl	1.3	1.2	1.6	1.2	1.1	1.1	1.0	1.0	0.890	NS	0.03	NS
Ox oil fl	2.6	2.6	2.7	3.0	3.0	2.8	3.0	2.8	0.625	NS	NS	0.007
Fish fl	0.3	0.7	1.0	1.2	1.0	1.1	0.6	1.5	0.938	0.008	NS	0.001

TI: thermal:mechanical energy ratio; L: Low; M: Medium; H: High; B: baked; E: Extruded; Proc.: processing; Ox. Oil: oxidized oil; ap: appearance; ar: aroma; fl: flavor; STDEV: standard deviation.

Table 2b. Descriptive sensory analysis attributes mean values, formulation and processing effects.

Attribute	Sample									Fresh Meat effect	TI effect	Proc effect
	0B	20B	0LE	20LE	0ME	20ME	0HE	20HE	STDEV			
Barn. at	2.7	2.5	2.9	2.9	3.1	2.8	2.8	2.7	0.711	NS	NS	0.03
Salty at	1.3	1.2	1.7	2.0	1.9	1.6	1.5	1.8	0.827	NS	NS	0.004
Bitter at	4.8	4.5	4.5	4.5	4.3	4.5	4.1	4.1	0.896	NS	NS	0.04
Vitamin at	0.1	0.4	1.1	0.5	1.0	0.4	0.5	0.7	0.707	NS	NS	0.003
Musty at	1.2	1.2	0.8	0.9	0.8	1.2	0.7	0.8	0.992	NS	NS	0.005
Ox oil at	2.4	2.2	2.5	2.5	2.6	2.5	2.5	2.8	0.735	NS	NS	0.01
Liver at	0.7	0.9	1.5	1.3	1.5	1.4	1.2	1.5	1.052	NS	NS	0.0003
Fish at	0.2	0.4	1.0	0.8	0.9	1.0	0.8	1.0	0.799	NS	NS	0.0004
Coh. mass	2.5	3.0	3.6	3.8	3.7	4.9	3.4	4.3	1.552	0.01	NS	0.0003
Fractu-rability	5.3	5.0	6.9	6.8	7.9	8.0	7.7	7.3	2.087	NS	0.048	<0.0001
Hardness	5.1	5.1	8.5	8.3	8.0	8.0	7.9	7.5	1.791	NS	0.001	<0.0001
Powdery	3.7	3.8	2.3	2.5	2.5	2.4	2.1	2.3	1.111	NS	NS	<0.0001
Crispness	6.0	5.9	9.9	9.8	10.7	10.7	10.7	10.5	2.409	NS	0.04	<0.0001
Mouthcoat	2.9	2.4	2.1	2.2	1.8	2.1	2.0	1.9	0.581	NS	NS	<0.0001

TI: thermal:mechanical energy ratio; L: Low; M: Medium; H: High; B: baked; E: Extruded; Proc.: processing; Ox. Oil: oxidized oil; Barn: barnyard; at: aftertaste; STDEV: standard deviation.

Table 3a. Volatile compounds in samples (µg/kg).

No	Volatile	KI Exp	KI Lit	Sample							
				0B	20B	0LE	20LE	0ME	20ME	0HE	20HE
	Alcohols										
A1	Octen-3-ol	960	961d	1.61±0.70	1.80±0.47	3.15±0.74	2.69±0.57	3.07±0.43	3.62±0.26	2.17±0.28	2.30±0.37
A2	2-Decen-1-ol	1187	*1101c*	ND	ND	0.32±0.02	0.32±0.10	0.30±0.00	0.45±0.02	0.20±0.02	0.32±0.04
A3	2-Butyl octanol	1298	*1201c*	2.44±0.71	3.34±0.94	0.76±0.05	2.63±0.38	2.52±0.29	2.94±0.35	0.85±0.07	2.13±0.13
	Total alcohols			**4.06**	**5.15**	**4.23**	**5.64**	**5.89**	**7.02**	**3.22**	**4.75**
	Aldehydes										
A4	3-Methylbutanal	NA	654c	1.41±0.82	1.74±0.30	1.06±0.04	0.70±0.28	1.28±0.23	0.99±0.15	1.13±0.30	0.89±0.14
A5	Hexanal	NA	800a	21.34±11.53	23.89±5.24	54.47±7.34	67.03±20.77	50.21±6.98	85.77±13.68	39.06±5.91	54.46±6.52
A6	3-Furaldehyde	NA	829b	0.50±0.30	0.55±0.23	0.34±0.01	0.36±0.14	0.38±0.03	0.40±0.05	0.45±0.05	0.40±0.08
A7	2-Hexenal(E)	NA	854b	0.30±0.13	0.31±0.08	0.35±0.02	0.45±0.05	0.33±0.03	0.48±0.07	0.24±0.03	0.31±0.03
A8	Heptanal	872	872d	1.96±0.89	2.24±0.49	3.90±0.70	3.46±1.17	4.07±0.63	4.95±0.73	3.21±0.43	3.63±0.58
A9	3-Methylthiopropanal	NA	902c	0.31±0.18	0.49±0.14	0.25±0.05	0.16±0.02	0.26±0.03	0.22±0.04	0.26±0.02	0.20±0.04
A10	2-Heptenal(Z)	902	904d	1.31±0.66	1.77±0.64	1.65±0.29	1.81±0.19	1.54±0.21	2.50±0.11	0.90±0.03	1.21±0.10
A11	Benzaldehyde	909	910d	4.56±2.62	4.30±1.06	6.34±1.10	5.36±2.28	6.42±1.02	6.08±0.90	5.16±0.93	4.98±1.18
A12	Octanal	976	977d	1.09±0.47	1.22±0.28	3.05±0.57	3.16±1.00	3.02±0.25	4.55±0.61	2.52±0.36	3.34±0.51
A13	2-Ethyl-2-hexenal	979	NA	ND	ND	0.29±0.05	0.12±0.03	0.38±0.05	0.25±0.04	0.33±0.02	0.25±0.07
A14	Benzeneacetaldehyde	1006	1006d	1.24±0.52	1.59±0.39	1.31±0.10	1.02±0.02	1.56±0.23	1.57±0.39	1.58±0.02	1.00±0.06
A15	2-Octenal	1010	1010d	1.20±0.35	1.36±0.31	1.81±0.10	2.04±0.22	1.03±0.05	1.47±0.20	1.56±0.05	0.95±0.14
A16	Nonanal	1082	1082d	1.77±0.64	2.03±0.41	4.22±0.62	5.21±1.66	17.47±3.62	6.13±0.59	3.46±0.45	4.95±0.77
A17	2-Nonenal	1119	1142c	0.34±0.12	0.38±0.11	0.39±0.03	0.54±0.07	0.36±0.05	0.52±0.07	ND	0.45±0.02
A18	2-Butyl-2-octenal	1366	1366d	0.15±0.02	0.09±0.02	0.22±0.04	0.23±0.11	0.23±0.09	0.13±0.04	0.22±0.09	0.14±0.01
	Total aldehydes			**37.49**	**41.96**	**79.66**	**91.65**	**88.54**	**115.97**	**60.09**	**77.16**
	Ketones										
A19	2-Heptanone	864	865d	1.24±0.65	1.26±0.31	1.23±0.16	0.90±0.25	1.56±0.03	1.15±0.04	1.34±0.30	1.24±0.24
A20	2,5-Octanedione	962	983c	1.16±0.63	1.83±0.46	3.32±0.42	4.59±0.97	2.41±0.21	5.19±0.77	2.02±0.18	3.63±0.24
A21	6-Methyl, 5-hepten-2-one	963	965d	0.31±0.17	0.26±0.02	0.86±0.22	0.65±0.15	0.76±0.12	0.87±0.07	0.46±0.13	0.77±0.10
A22	3-Octen-2-one	998	999d	ND	ND	0.75±0.07	1.24±0.30	0.72±0.10	2.49±0.38	0.83±0.03	1.73±0.11
A23	2-Nonanone	1071	1072d	0.08±0.03	0.07±0.02	0.40±0.03	0.30±0.08	0.54±0.02	0.50±0.06	0.57±0.04	0.45±0.02
	Total ketones			**2.79**	**3.42**	**6.56**	**7.68**	**5.99**	**10.20**	**5.24**	**7.81**

ND: not detected; NA: not available; a: [27]; b: [28]; c: [29]; d: [13]; italic: different column; KI exp: Kovacs Indice calculated experimentally; KI lit: Kovacs Indice from literature.

Table 3b. Volatile compounds in samples (µg/kg).

No	Volatile	KI Exp	KI Lit	Sample							
				0B	20B	0LE	20LE	0ME	20ME	0HE	20HE
	Esters										
A24	Methyl butyrate	NA	724c	0.30±0.13	0.22±0.06	0.16±0.05	0.17±0.07	0.16±0.03	0.16±0.05	0.16±0.03	0.14±0.06
A25	Methyl hexanoate	883	*916c*	0.33±0.20	0.45±0.17	0.43±0.18	0.50±0.25	0.40±0.10	0.55±0.16	0.32±0.08	0.42±0.10
A26	Methyl octanoate	1092	*1107c*	0.03±0.02	0.06±0.03	ND	ND	ND	ND	ND	ND
A27	Propanoic acid 2-methyl butylester	1142	NA	3.70±0.37	2.93±1.20	1.50±1.26	2.96±2.72	1.10±0.58	2.22±2.39	2.04±1.31	1.53±1.10
	Total esters			**4.36**	**3.66**	**2.09**	**3.62**	**1.66**	**2.94**	**2.52**	**2.09**
	Pyrazines										
A28	Methylpyrazine	NA	828b	0.28±0.17	0.39±0.20	ND	ND	ND	ND	ND	ND
A29	Pyrazine, 2,5-dimethyl	NA	911c	0.34±0.14	0.39±0.09	0.26±0.05	0.18±0.04	0.29±0.03	0.23±0.04	0.19±0.02	0.14±0.02
	Total pyrazines			**0.62**	**0.78**	**0.26**	**0.18**	**0.29**	**0.23**	**0.19**	**0.14**
	Furans										
A30	2-Butylfuran	893	895d	ND	ND	0.25±0.04	0.34±0.08	0.28±0.03	0.28±0.05	0.27±0.11	0.39±0.10
A31	2-Pentylfuran	993	994d	1.00±0.38	1.01±0.14	4.81±0.56	3.90±1.58	5.87±1.19	4.98±0.92	7.14±1.19	6.00±0.82
	Total furans			**1.00**	**1.01**	**5.07**	**4.24**	**6.15**	**5.26**	**7.42**	**6.38**
	Acids										
A32	4-Methyl pentanoic acid	770	NA	0.35±0.24	0.36±0.20	0.69±0.14	0.37±0.17	0.73±0.26	0.47±0.20	0.40±0.08	0.30±0.01
	Terpenes										
A33	1-R-α-pinene	929	932d	ND	ND	0.25±0.01	0.16±0.05	0.34±0.04	0.28±0.04	0.30±0.06	0.26±0.03
A34	Limonene (L)	1040	1041d	0.08±0.06	0.43±0.17	0.56±0.04	0.34±0.08	1.12±0.19	0.94±0.22	0.77±0.07	0.78±0.07
	Total terpenes			**0.08**	**0.43**	**0.81**	**0.50**	**1.46**	**1.22**	**1.08**	**1.04**
	Alkenes										
A35	3-Dodecene(E)	914	NA	1.51±0.22	1.43±0.20	1.99±0.16	1.84±0.08	1.91±017	2.23±0.24	2.10±0.22	1.76±0.39
	Other compounds										
A36	3-Hydroxytoluene	953	NA	ND	ND	2.68±0.47	2.48±0.65	3.15±0.26	2.16±0.41	3.15±0.22	3.12±0.39
A37	Indole	1120	1136c	0.23±0.09	0.14±0.04	0.33±0.03	0.22±0.05	0.39±0.02	0.33±0.01	0.34±0.04	0.29±0.03
	Total other compounds			**0.23**	**0.14**	**3.01**	**2.70**	**3.54**	**2.48**	**3.49**	**3.41**
	Total volatiles			**52.50**	**58.34**	**104.36**	**118.42**	**116.16**	**148.02**	**85.73**	**104.84**

ND: not detected; NA: not available; a: [27]; b: [28]; c: [29]; d: [13]; italic: different column; KI exp: Kovacs Indice calculated experimentally; KI lit: Kovacs Indice from literature.

3.2. Volatile Compounds

Overall 37 volatile compounds were found in the pet food samples (Table 3(a,b)). These volatiles included alcohols (three compounds), aldehydes (15 compounds), ketones (five compounds), esters (four compounds), pyrazines (two compounds), furans (two compounds), alkenes (one compound), acids (one compound), and terpenes (two compounds). Koppel *et al.* looked at volatiles in commercial dry dog food samples and identified 54 volatile compounds [13]. Those samples were manufactured with a variety of grains, proteins, and added flavorings that likely contributed to the greater number of volatiles detected than we found in this study.

The cooking process and meat level in the formulation seemed to have an effect on the volatiles content. Total concentration of volatiles was higher in the extruded samples (85–148 μg/kg) when compared to the baked samples (52–58 μg/kg). In addition, the meat-added samples seemed to be more aromatic (58–148 μg/kg) when compared to the no meat-added samples (52–116 μg/kg). Overall the most aromatic sample was the meat-added medium thermal input extruded pet food.

Some compounds were found only in baked or extruded samples. For example 2-decen-1-ol, 2-ethyl-2-hexenal, 3-octen-2-one, 2-butylfuran, 3-hydroxytoluene, and 1-R-α-pinene (tentative identification) were present in extruded samples, but were not detected in baked foods. Several of these compounds are probably odor-active, although the concentrations found in extruded pet foods were low. According to Eyres *et al.* 2-decen-1-ol could have wet dog aromatics [30]; 1-R-α-pinene may have musty and pungent characteristics (Pherobase); 3-octen-2-one was found in poultry byproduct meal and was claimed to contribute to the fatty, hay, and cardboard-like aromatics [31]. Methylpyrazine and methyl octanoate were present in baked foods, but were not detected in extruded samples, and thus may be processing related in their formation. Methylpyrazine may carry popcorn aromatics [29]. The aromatics that these compounds may have could be further studied using a gas-chromatograph olfactometer (GC-O).

According to Mottram, aldehydes are common lipid oxidation products [32]. Pet food samples in this study contained chicken fat, chicken meat, and chicken byproduct meal. Aldehydes were the most abundant group of volatiles identified, with concentrations ranging from 37–115 μg/kg, and hexanal was found at the highest concentration among aldehydes (21–85 μg/kg). Hexanal is known to be associated with rancid, fatty, and oxidized oil aromatics [13]. According to Greenberg poultry byproduct meal lacks the necessary volatiles to give the meal savory and pleasant meat odor characteristics [31]. In pet foods this can be turned around using meat-like flavorings and coatings.

3.3. Associations between Sensory Attributes and Volatile Compounds

Partial Least Squares Regression (PLS-R) maps (Figures 2 and 3) show associations between sensory flavor attributes and with the instrumental volatile composition. From the first four partial least squares factors 85% volatile compound variation explained 72% of descriptive sensory analysis data variation. Koppel *et al.* found lower percentages of data explained between descriptive sensory aroma attributes and volatile compounds data [13]. Better explanation of data variation may be caused by less variation within the dataset as well as using sensory flavor information instead of aromatics information to detect associations with instrumental volatile compounds concentration. This approach was considered more suitable as for both flavor evaluation and solid phase micro extraction (SPME) the sample is prepared in a similar manner: moisture is added first and next the sample is warmed to enhance aromatics extraction.

Some associations were found among sensory flavor and aftertaste attributes and volatile compounds. Vitamin flavor (Vitfl) and vitamin aftertaste (Vitat) seemed to be related to limonene (A34), 4-methyl pentanoic acid (A32), and nonanal (A16). In addition associations were found among the attributes toasted (Toastfl), grain (Grainfl), stale (Stalefl), and oxidized oil flavor (Oxoilfl), oxidized oil (Oxoilat), metallic (Metat), liver (Liverat), fish (Fishat), and barnyard (Barnat) aftertaste, and volatiles 3-dodecene (A35, tentative identification), 2-butylfuran (A30), benzaldehyde (A11), 3-hydroxytoluene (A36), 2-nonanone (A23), 1-R-α-pinene (A33, tentative identification), and 2-pentylfuran (A31). Furthermore, stale aftertaste (Staleat) and fish flavor (Fishfl) were associated with volatiles hexanal (A5), 3-octen-2-one (A22), octen-3-ol (A1), 2-decen-1-ol (A2), and octanal (A12). This cluster of volatiles and sensory attributes are likely to indicate oxidation processes and rancid aromatics. Similar associations were found by Koppel *et al.* [13].

Figure 2. Partial Least Squares Regression Factors 1 and 2. Suffixes: ap – appearance; ar – aroma; fl – flavor; at – aftertaste.

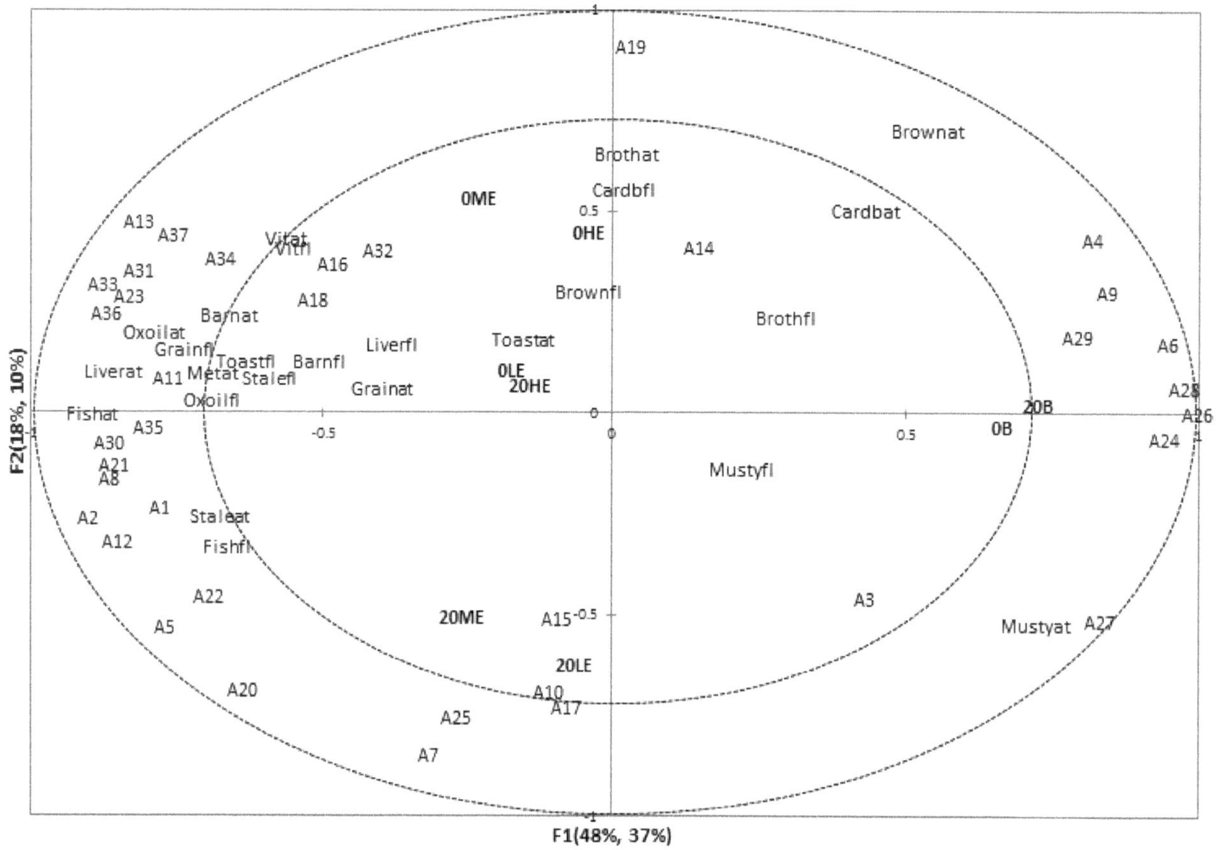

Figure 3. Partial Least Squares Regression Factors 3 and 4. Suffixes: ap – appearance; ar – aroma; fl – flavor; at – aftertaste.

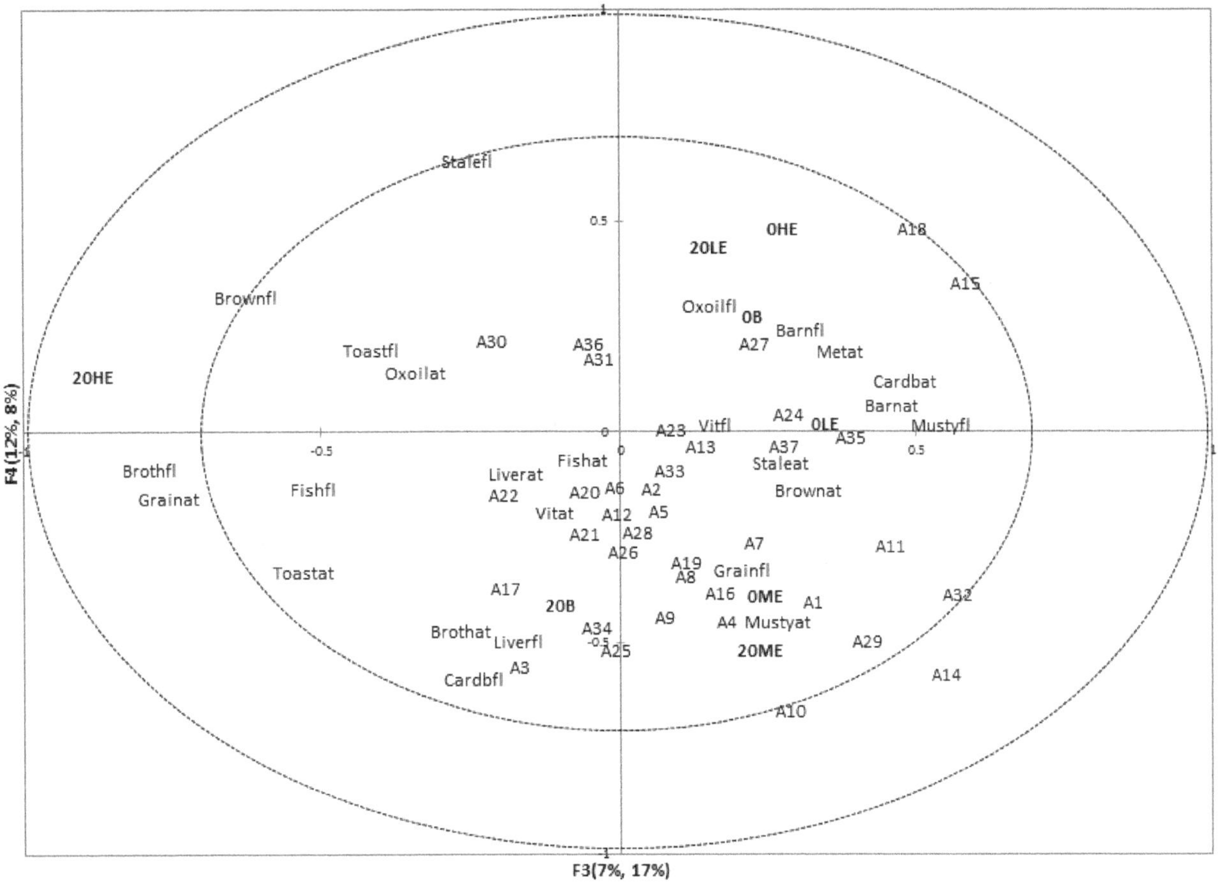

Baked samples (0B and 20B) were associated with volatiles methyl butyrate (A24), methyl octanoate (A26), methylpyrazine (A28), 3-furaldehyde (A6), and 2,5-dimethyl pyrazine (A29). Methylpyrazine may have popcorn-like, 2,5-dimethyl pyrazine roasted odors, 3-furaldehyde bread-like odors, and esters fruity odors [29]. The concentrations of these volatiles were small, grainy, and toasted, and brown flavor attributes were lower in intensity in baked than in extruded samples. This may address why the extruded samples were more related to these sensory characteristics. Similar associations were found among samples 20ME and 20LE and volatiles 2-octenal (A15), 2-heptenal(Z) (A10), 2-nonenal (A17), 2-hexenal(E) (A7), and methyl hexanoate (A25).

This study established a clear difference in sensory characteristics of baked and extruded pet foods not found in previous literature. Although this study has some limitations, such as the small number of samples included, there were sufficient unique characteristics between extruded and baked pet foods to show differences in sensory flavor and texture attributes. Texture is an important factor in determining pet food palatability. According to Gibson and Alavi, extruded pet foods differ from baked pet foods by the proportion of gelatinized starch, and this may be related to pet food texture properties [8]. Furthermore, according to a review by Houpt and Smith, dogs have a preference towards canned and semi-moist meats when compared to dry foods, but no palatability studies have compared baked and extruded pet foods [26]. Anecdotal evidence from the pet trade would suggest that differences among extruded kibbles could influence product acceptability. It would be of interest to determine whether cooking type (extrusion vs. baking) would influence dog food choice.

As an interim step to that question, a human sensory panel was used instead of a panel of animals for sensory evaluation in this study. In part because the animal panel, unfortunately, is not able to describe food aromatics, flavor sensations, or texture attributes, while a trained human panel can. Ideally, these two sensory evaluations would complement each other and so animal preference could be translated via humans into usable information for the industry and scientists. Furthermore, instrumental measurements capable of identifying volatile compounds and then relating this to animal preferences would be of great interest.

4. Conclusions

This study demonstrated differences in baked and extruded pet foods appearance, texture, and flavor characteristics. Baked samples were lighter in color and had lower levels of attributes that indicated rancidity (*i.e.*, fish flavor) than extruded pet foods. Extruded pet foods were more cohesive in mass, more fracturable, hard, and crisp, but less powdery than baked samples. Fresh meat inclusion tended to affect bitterness, fishiness, and cohesiveness of mass of pet foods regardless of processing method. High thermal to mechanical energy ratio during extrusion resulted in less musty and more porous kibbles. The main volatile compounds included aldehydes, such as hexanal and heptanal, ketones, and alcohols. Extruded samples did not contain any methylpyrazine, while baked samples did not contain any 2-butyl furan. Overall, extruded samples seemed to result in greater flavor intensity and aftertaste attributes in comparison to baked samples. Flavor, odor, and texture characteristics associations with palatability should be of interest to future studies.

Acknowledgments

The authors would like to acknowledge Lotus Petfood for funding the ingredients and preparation for samples.

Author Contributions

Kadri Koppel, Sajid Alavi, Greg Aldrich, and Michael Gibson planned the study. Sajid Alavi, Greg Aldrich, and Michael Gibson formulated and manufactured the samples. Kadri Koppel planned and executed the descriptive sensory analysis and the volatile aromatics analysis. Kadri Koppel prepared the manuscript and Sajid Alavi, Greg Aldrich, and Michael Gibson reviewed and provided guidance with manuscript preparation.

Conflicts of Interest

The authors declare no conflict of interest.

References and Notes

1. Mintel. Pet Food–US–March 2013. Available online: http://store.mintel.com/pet-food-us-march-2013 (accessed on 16 April 2014).
2. Mathew, J.M.; Hoseney, R.C.; Faubion, J.M. Effects of corn sample, mill type, and particle size on corn curl and pet food extrudates. *Cereal Chem.* **1999**, *76*, 621–624.

3. Rokey, G.J.; Baldwin, D. Extrusion temperature: A critical control point in pet food processing. AllAboutFeed.net. Available online: http://www.allaboutfeed.net/Processing/Extruding--Expanding/2013/9/Extrusion-temperature-A-critical-control-point-in-pet-food-processing-1359454W (accessed on 16 April 2014).
4. Tran, Q.D.; Hendriks, W.H.; van der Poel, A.F.B. Effects of extrusion processing on nutrients in dry pet food. *J. Sci. Food Agr.* **2008**, *88*, 1487–1493.
5. Felix, A.P.; Carvalho, M.P.; Alarca, L.G.; Brito, C.B.M.; Oliveira, S.G.; Maiorka, A. Effects of the inclusion of carbohydrases and different soybean meals in the diet on palatability, digestibility, and faecal characteristics in dogs. *Anim. Feed Sci. Technol.* **2012**, *174*, 182–189.
6. Carciofi, A.C.; Domingues de-Oliveira, L.; Valerio, A.G.; Borges, L.L.; de Carvalho, F.M.; Brunetto, M.A.; Vasconcellos, R.S. Comparison of micronized whole soybeans to common protein sources in dry dog and cat diets. *Anim. Feed Sci. Technol.* **2009**, *151*, 251–260.
7. Sa, F.C.; Vasconcellos, R.S.; Brunetto, M.A.; Filho, F.O.R.; Gomes, M.O.S.; Carciofi, A.C. Enzyme used in kibble diets formulated with wheat bran for dogs: Effects on processing and digestibility. *J. Anim. Physiol. Anim. Nutr.* **2013**, *97*, 51–59.
8. Gibson, M.; Alavi, S. Pet food processing—Understanding transformations in starch during extrusion and baking. *Cereal Foods World* **2013**, *58*, 232–236.
9. Lin, S.; Hsieh, F.; Heymann, H.; Huff, H.E. Effects of lipids and processing conditions on the sensory characteristics of extruded dry pet food. *J. Food Qual.* **1998**, *21*, 265–284.
10. Di Donfrancesco, B.; Koppel, K.; Chambers, E., IV. An initial lexicon for sensory properties of dry dog food. *J. Sens. Stud.* **2012**, *27*, 498–510.
11. Pickering, G.J. Optimizing the sensory characteristics and acceptance of canned cat food: Use of a human taste panel. *J. Anim. Physiol. Anim. Nutr.* **2009**, *93*, 52–60.
12. Pickering, G.J. Optimisation of dried cat food using a human taste panel: Methodology and characterization of flavor. *Food Aust.* **2009**, *61*, 30–36.
13. Koppel, K.; Adhikari, K.; Di Donfrancesco, B. Volatile compounds in dry dog foods and their influence on sensory aromatic profile. *Molecules* **2013**, *18*, 2646–2662.
14. Agbisit, R.; Alavi, S.; Cheng, E.; Herald, T.J.; Trater, A.M. Relationships between microstructure and mechanical properties of cellular corn starch extrudates. *J. Texture Stud.* **2007**, *38*, 199–219.
15. Gibson, L.G.; Ashby, M.F. *Cellular Solids: Structure and Properties*; Cambridge University Press: Cambridge, UK, 1997.
16. Lee, J.; Chambers, D.H.; Chambers, E., IV. A comparison of the flavor of green teas from around the world. *J. Sci. Food Agr.* **2013**, doi:10.1002/jsfa.6413. Available online: http://onlinelibrary.wiley.com/doi/10.1002/jsfa.6413/pdf (accessed on 16 April 2014).
17. Cherdchu, P.; Chambers, E., IV; Suwonsichon, T. Sensory lexicon development using trained panelists in Thailand and the United States: Soy sauce. *J. Sens. Stud.* **2013**, *28*, 248–255.
18. Vázquez Araújo, L.; Chambers, E., IV; Adhikari, K.; Hough, G.; Carbonell-Barrachina, Á.A. Influence of various traditional seasonings on beef flavor: United States, Spanish, and Argentinian practices. *Meat Sci.* **2013**, *93*, 61–66.
19. Ledeker, C.; Chambers, D.; Chambers, E., IV; Adhikari, K. Changes in the Sensory Characteristics of Mango Cultivars during the Production of Mango Purée and Sorbet. *J. Food Sci.* **2012**, *77*, S348–S355.

20. Ceva-Antunes, P.M.N.; Bizzo, H.R.; Silva, A.S.; Carvalho, C.P.S.; Antunes, O.A.C. Analysis of volatile compounds of siriguela (Spondias purpurea L.) by solid phase microextraction (SPME). *LWT - Food Sci. Technol.* **2006**, *39*, 436–442.
21. Adhikari, K.; Dooley, L.; Chambers, E., IV.; Bhumiratana, N. Sensory characteristics of commercial lactose-free milks manufactured in the United States. *LWT - Food Sci. Technol.* **2010**, *43*, 113–118.
22. Meeker, D.L.; Hamilton, C.R. Essential rendering. All about the animal by-products industry. 2006. Available online: http://assets.nationalrenderers.org/essential_rendering_book.pdf (accessed on 16 April 2014).
23. Cheng, E.M.; Alavi, S.; Pearson, T.; Agbisit, R. Mechanical-acoustic and sensory evaluations of cornstarch-whey protein isolate extrudates. *J. Texture Stud.* **2007**, *38*, 473–498.
24. Dzanis, D.A. Petfood types, quality assessment and feeding management. In *Petfood Technology*; Kwamme, J.L., Phillips, T.D., Eds.; Watt Publishing: Morris, IL, USA, 2003; pp. 68–73.
25. Cowell, C.S.; Stout, N.P.; Brinkman, M.F.; Moser, E.A.; Crane, S.W. Making commercial petfoods. In *Small Animal Clinical Nutrition*, 4th ed.; Mark Morris Institute: Topeka, KS, USA, 2000; pp. 127–146.
26. Houpt, K.A.; Smith, S.L. Taste preferences and their relation to obesity in dogs and cats. *Can. Vet. J.* **1981**, *22*, 77–81.
27. Goodner, K.L. Practical retention index models of OV-101, DB-1, DB-5, and DB-Wax for flavor and fragrance compounds. *LWT - Food Sci. Technol.* **2008**, *41*, 951–958.
28. The Flavornet. Available online: http://www.flavornet.org (accessed on 16 April 2014).
29. The Pherobase. Available online: http://www.pherobase.com (accessed on 16 April 2014).
30. Eyres, G.; Dufour, J.-P.; Hallifax, G.; Sotheeswaran, S.; Marriott, P.J. Identification of character-impact odorants in coriander and wild coriander leaves using gas chromatography-olfactometry (GCO) and comprehensive two-dimensional gas chromatography-time-of-flight mass spectrometry (GCxGC-TOFMS). *J. Sep. Sci.* **2005**, *28*, 1061–1074.
31. Greenberg, M.J. Characterization of poultry byproduct meal flavor volatiles. *J. Agr. Food Chem.* **1981**, *29*, 831–834.
32. Mottram, M. Meat Flavour. In *Understanding Natural Flavors*; Piggott, J.R., Paterson, A., Eds.; Chapman & Hall: London, UK, 1994; pp. 140–163.

9

Comparison of Performance, Meat Lipids and Oxidative Status of Pigs from Commercial Breed and Organic Crossbreed

Giuseppe Martino [1], Cecilia Mugnai [1,*], Dario Compagnone [1], Lisa Grotta [1], Michele Del Carlo [1] and Francesca Sarti [2]

[1] Faculty of Biosciences and Agro-Food Technologies and Environmental, University of Teramo, via C. Lerici 1, 64023, Mosciano S.A., Italy; E-Mails: gmartino@unite.it (G.M.); dcompagnone@unite.it (D.C.); lgrotta@unite.it (L.G.); mdelcarlo@unite.it (M.D.C.)

[2] Department of Agricultural, Food and Environmental Science, University of Perugia, Borgo XX Giugno, 74, 06121, Perugia, Italy; E-Mail: francesca.sarti@unipg.it

* Author to whom correspondence should be addressed; E-Mail: cmugnai@unite.it.

Simple Summary: In recent years, the development of alternative rearing methods, capable of satisfying requests regarding product quality, yet also taking animal welfare and environmental protection into consideration, is becoming an increasingly important consumer demand. When pigs are reared in free range and organic systems, outdoor access is given to pigs; and such rearing conditions increases energy demand for activity and thermoregulation, which reduces growth rate, but improves some meat quality characteristics, such as leaner meat with lower C14:0 and higher C20:1n9, and oxidative stability.

Abstract: The aim of this research was to determine the effect of rearing systems for pig production, as concerns performance, meat lipid content, the fatty acid profile, histidinic antioxidants, coenzyme Q10, and TBARs. One hundred pigs were assigned to one of three treatments: intensively reared commercial hybrid pig (I), free range commercial hybrid pig (FR) or organically reared crossbred pig (O), according to organic EU Regulations. I pigs showed the best productive performance, but FR and O increased: C20:1n9, Δ9-desaturase (C18) and thioesterase indices in meat. Lipid, dipeptides and CoQ10 appeared correlated to glycolytic and oxidative metabolic pathways. We can conclude that all studied parameters were influenced by the rearing system used, and that differences were particularly evident in the O system, which produced leaner meat with higher oxidative stability. In this respect, the organic pig rearing system promotes and enhances biodiversity, environmental sustainability and food quality.

Keywords: pig; rearing system; performance; meat quality; oxidative status

---

1. Introduction

The increased interest in reducing intensity of pork production has led to the implementation of systems aware of animal welfare and without impairment of environmental sustainability, economy and food security [1]. Intensive rearing systems commonly use commercial hybrids selected for their rapid growth rate and adaptability to limited space allowance. However, these genotypes are characterized by low capacity to cope with certain environmental conditions due to their low immune-competence and high susceptibility to environmental stress. In contrast, alternative rearing systems require animals characterized by a slow growth rate and high adaptability to various environments, which may lead to favorable productive performance. In Italy, the extensive rearing system of pigs is quite diffuse and linked to autochthonous pig breeding traditions oriented towards typical meat products [2]. These already existing systems (autochthonous genotypes/outdoor rearing), can be easily adapted to organic pig production matching: consumers opinion, which needs to be adjusted to lower input farming approaches [3], Council Regulation 1804/99/EC [4] and the Network for Animal Health and Welfare in Organic Agriculture's final recommendations [5]. The latter suggests the housing of local, slow-growing breeds for their higher rusticity and capacity to utilize outdoor areas and pasture.

The effect of the rearing system on meat quality is still under debate, and, in particular for pigs, conflicting evidences are found in the literature on the effect of rearing system on the meat quality [6–13]. The contradictory data are probably due to large variations in the design of the production systems [11]. In this context, however, few data were reported on oxidative stability with respect to histidinic antioxidant and CoQ_{10} content of meat. Moreover no information is available on differences between rearing systems for the activity of the Δ9-desaturase complex in the synthesis of the LCMUFA (Long Chain Monounsaturated Fatty Acids). Since the quality of the product is crucial for consumer health, the study reported in here was planned, in order to integrate the issue of a high quality product with those related to animal biodiversity and welfare, and environmental sustainability of livestock production. Thus, the aim of the present study was to evaluate performance, lipids, the fatty acid profile and different indices together with the oxidative status of pork meat produced by different rearing systems, using different analytical techniques.

2. Materials and Method

2.1. Animals, Rearing Systems and Productive Traits Procedures

Two hundred pigs of Commercial hybrid and 100 F1 pig of crossbreed Cinta Senese X Large White (CSXLW), were used for the study. Cinta Senese was selected for F1 pig production, because they are well adapted to outdoor environmental conditions as reported by Council Reg. 1804/99/EC [4].

All animals were reared at the facilities of Soc. Coop Agricoltura Nuova Cooperativa s.r.l. farm, located at Gessopalena (CH, 450 mt above sea level), in the Maiella mountains, Italy. All pigs (gender ratio 50:50), were held and fed in the same conditions from birth until 40 kg of bodyweight (indoor pen group housed; 5 pigs per pen/group). The experiments were performed in the 40–150 kg range of bodyweight. The experimental phase began in April and pigs were slaughtered in August (130 day of experimental phase).

Pigs were assigned to either of the following rearing systems:

- Intensive (I): 100 piglets of Commercial hybrid, housed in two (3.1 m^2/pig, half concrete area, half metal slats) environmentally controlled buildings (22 °C and 60 to 70% relative humidity);
- Free Range (FR): 100 piglets of Commercial hybrid, were raised outdoors in a 1 ha extension land in two pens of 5000 m^2 each (100 m^2/pig of pasture), with access to igloos (4 × 2 × 1.4 m^2/pigs) with barley straw bedding;
- Organic (O): 100 crossbred piglets (CSXLW) were raised outdoors in a 25,000 m^2 extension land in two pens of 12,500 m^2 each (250 m^2/pig of pasture), according to Council Reg. 1804/99/EC [4], with access to igloos (4 × 2 × 1.4 m^2/pigs) with barley straw bedding.

Two repetitions of 50 pigs each per group were carried out; for I pigs, the building was considered as repetition; whereas for outdoor reared pigs, the pen was considered as repetition.

Indoor pigs were placed in temperature-controlled buildings where temperatures did not fall below 18 °C. The average air temperature for the outdoor pigs during this trial was 21 °C (range: 3 to 38 °C) and the average relative humidity was 60%. The air temperature was within normal ranges during this study period.

From 23 to 70 kg BW, and from 70 to 150 kg BW, I, FR and O groups had free access to water and *ad libitum* access to the same organic grower and finisher diets (Table 1), certified by a National agency.

Table 1. Chemical composition (g/100 g DM) and Ingredients of diets.

Diets	Grower	Finisher
Chemical composition		
Crude protein	17.82	17.73
Ether extract	5.30	5.65
Crude fiber	5.33	3.92
Ash	5.21	5.49
Digestible energy *	3665.51	3772.88
Ingredients †		
Barley, wheat, starch wheat flour, roasted soybean, corn, fats, molasses, sunflower extraction meal, calcium carbonate, dicalcium phosphate, sodium chloride.		

* (kcal/kg d.m.); † ingredients are presented in decreasing order.

Pigs were weighed and feed disappearance was recorded weekly. No castration of male piglets, teeth clipping, ear tattooing or tail docking was conducted.

2.2. Slaughter and Sampling Proceedings

When pigs achieved a BW of 150 ± 10.0 kg, they were slaughtered on two consecutive days (N = 150 pigs slaughtered/day, N = 50 per group replication) at the communal abattoir of Casoli (CH), situated less than 10 km from the breeding site. All travel organization followed the rules of Council Regulation (EC) No 1/2005 of 22 December 2004 [14]. FR and O pigs were brought inside the abattoir holding pens 16 h before slaughter, to ensure that no additional feed was consumed by the pigs. I pigs were slaughtered, 16 h after feed withdrawal.

All pigs were stunned electrically (300 V, 3 s) with a pair of stunning tongs, after which they were shackled by the hind leg and exsanguinated. Five minutes after exsanguination samples (N = 25 per replication/day per group) were taken with a cork bore from the *Longissimus dorsi* (LD) between 13th and 14th ribs after approximately 5 min of blooming time. Muscle cubes (0.5 cm^3) were cut from the LD muscle sample. All fresh meat samples, were packed under modified atmosphere and stored at −80 °C till analysis. Muscle samples and measurements were taken from a total of 50 pigs/group.

2.3. Chemical Analysis of Meat

2.3.1. Lipids, Fatty Acid Profile and Indices

Total meat lipids (samples of about 5 g) were extracted [15] in a homogenizer with 50 mL of 2:1 (*vol/vol*) chloroform-methanol, followed by filtration through Whatman No. 1 filter paper.

Lipid extract was trans methylated to fatty acyl methyl esters (FAMEs) at room temperature by using KOH 2 M in anhydrous methanol. Fatty acid methyl esters (FAMEs) composition was determined by gas chromatography using gas chromatograph (Fisions Mega 2 Carlo Erba, Gas Chromatograph, model HRGC, Milan, Italy) with flame ionization detection (FID) equipped with a VARIAN capillary column CP-SIL 88 of 100 m the carrier gas was hydrogen. Oven temperature programming was as follows: 160 °C held for 1 min; 175 °C at 4 °C/min, held for 28 min; 215 °C at 3 °C/min, held for 30 min; 160 °C at 10 °C/min.

The identification of fatty acids (FA) was based on the comparison of retention times of individual FA with standard mixture (Sigma-Aldrich) and FA values were expressed as percentage of the sum of total FA determined. The FA percentages were calculated with the Chrom-Card software.

The activities of Δ9-desaturase and elongase were estimated by relating the amount of product to that of precursor [16]. Particularly, the Δ9-desaturase (16) index was calculated as the relative amount (%) of palmitoleic acid (C16:1) with respect to C16:1 and palmitic acid (C16:0). The Δ9-desaturase (18) index was expressed as the relative amount of C18:1 (C18:1n7+C18:1n9) with respect to the total amount of C18:1 (C18:1n7+C18:1n9) and stearic acid (C18:0). Consequently, the Δ9-desaturase (16+18) index was calculated as the relative amount of the sum of C16:1, C18:1n7 and C18:1n9 *vs.* the amount of C16:1, C16:0, C18:1n7, C18:1n9, and C18:0. The elongase index was calculated as the ratio of C18:0 to C16:0. The thioesterase index was calculated as the ratio of C16:0 to myristic acid (C14:0).

2.3.2. Antioxidant Compounds Analysis

Meat samples were analyzed for anserine and carnosine determination using the method from Aristoy and Toldrà [17], with minor modifications. A procedure for the determination of the histidinic antioxidants was optimized using ion-exchange chromatography on a Bonus RP 3.5 µm, 4.6 × 150 mm column. After removing blood, connective tissue, and subcutaneous fat, meat samples were weighed (2.0 ± 0.1 g) and homogenized with 20 mL of 0.01M trichloracetic acid (TCA) for about two minutes. The homogenate was then centrifuged at 4000 × g for 60 min at +4 °C. The supernatant was collected and filtered on 0.45 µm nylon filter. Before injection, samples underwent a 20 fold dilution in mobile phase. Optimal separation of carnosine and anserine was achieved using a Bonus RP 3.5 µm, 4.6 × 150 mm column in 10 mM acetate buffer at pH 5.0 plus 5% acetonitrile and using 5 mM of sodium Octanesulphonic acid as ion pairing agent with isocratic elution. The flow rate was 1 mL/min. Alanine-Phenylalanine was selected as internal standard because its chromatographic behavior is similar to carnosine and anserine but the retention time is in a "blank window" interval of the chromatogram obtained with meat samples extracts, where no peaks are observed. Optimal pH for the use of Ala-Phe was 5.0, at this pH peak tailing of the internal standard was absent and good separation of anserine and carnosine was obtained at retention times of, 5.8 min for Anserine and 6.4 min for carnosine. Due to its more hydrophobic nature Ala-Phe exhibited a retention time of 8.3 min. Calibration curves for anserine and carnosine obtained in the 0–100 µg/mL range with the use of internal standard were linear using a 20 µg/mL carnosine and anserine standard solution. These values were compared with those reported by Gil-Agustì *et al.* [18], with correlation coefficient r = 0.997.

Ubiquinone (CoQ_{10}) analysis was carried out according to the method of Martino *et al* [19], with modification. Samples (2 g) were minced and homogenized in 10 mL of methanol containing 4% pyrogaroll; saponification at 80 °C for 15 min after adding 1 mL of 59% KOH solution, and extraction was done using 20 mL of hexane; after evaporation under a nitrogen stream, the extract was dissolved in 1 mL of methanol and 10 µL of solution was injected into the liquid chromatograph (Varian, Model 9010, Walnut Creck, CA, USA). For HPLC determination, an LC18 column (4.6 × 250 mm, 5 m) and UV detector (Varian, Model 9050, Walnut Creck, CA, USA), adjusted to 275 nm and detection set at 0.0001 AUFS, were used. For the separation, HPLC grade 2-propanol:methanol (40:60) mobile phase was employed at flow rate of 2 mL/min. For the determination of the CoQ_{10} an appropriate calibration curve was built with standard (Sigma, St Louis, MO, USA).

2.3.3. Fat Oxidation

The extent of intra muscular fat oxidation was evaluated by measuring thiobarbituric acid reactive substances (TBARS) [20]. The TBA distillation method was performed as described by Tarladgis *et al.* [21] except that butylated hydroxytoluene (BHT) was added before homogenization. Meat samples (3.5 g) were homogenized with 50 mL of (5%) TCA and 500 µL of BHT, with Ultra Turrax T25 at 4000 × g, for 5 min. Two mL of 0.02 M TBA in acetic acid were added to 2 mL of distilled Homogenate. This solution was heated in a water bath at 80 °C for 1 h and then cooled for 10 min with cold tap water. The absorbance was determined by Perkin Elmer Lambda 20 UV/vis spectrophotometer a 534 nm against a blank containing 2 mL of distilled TCA and 2 mL of 0.02 M TBA solution. This value was calculated from standard curves and known dilutions.

2.4. Statistical Analysis

The effect of treatment were tested with the procedure SAS/GLM [22], using the following model:

$$yijk = \mu + ai + ei$$

where μ = overall average; ai = fixed effect rearing system (i = 1 … 3); ei = error.

For each of the three rearing systems, two repetitions (50 pigs each rearing system/per replication for productive performance records; and 25 samples of *Longissimus dorsi* of pig for each rearing system per replication for chemical analysis), were used. In a preliminary analysis the effect of gender and replicate was verified; however, they didn't reach the significance level and therefore these two factors and their interactions in the final analysis of the data, were not considered. The significance of differences was estimated by the multiple Student's *t*-test. Differences were considered significant for $P < 0.0001$ and $P < 0.05$.

3. Results and Discussion

A total of 300 pigs (50 for each repetition/rearing system) completed the production period according to the experimental plan, and 150 (25 for each repetition/rearing system) *Longissimus dorsi* of pigs completed all the meat quality measurements.

3.1. Productive Performance

Independently of the rearing system, the overall performance of the pigs was good (Table 2). Mean daily gain was 847 g, and carcass dressing out was 81%. Although in I husbandry practice the mix of pigs in a confined space can result in significant stress reactions and aggressive behavior because of frustration or restriction of natural behavior [23,24], no mortality or health problems occurred during the experimental period, starting from 40 kg live weight until slaughter at a live weight around 150 kg.

Table 2. Effect of rearing system on productive performance of pigs.

Rearing System		I	FR	O	SED
Starting BW †	Kg	39.42	39.48	37.18	5.15
ADG *	Kg	0.92	0.86	0.76	0.12
Feed:Gain Ratio		2.70 ^{a}	3.11 ^{b}	3.90 ^{c}	0.90
Slaughter BW †	Kg	159.02 ^{b}	151.28 ^{ab}	135.98 ^{a}	4.02
Dressing out	%	83 ^{b}	80 ^{ab}	78 ^{a}	2.39

N = 100/group; ^{ac} Means in the same row with the same superscript do not differ significantly ($P < 0.05$); † Body Weight; * Daily Weight Gain.

I pigs showed the best ($P < 0.05$) performance (Feed:Gain Ratio and slaughter BW). The main physical differences among treatments were in climate control and degree of exercise. Thus, the activity level of FR and O pigs is expected to rise respect I pigs. Close and Poorman [25] calculated an additional energy expenditure of 1.67 kcal ME/kg bodyweight per km walked in growing pigs. The higher energy requirements for activity and thermoregulation in outdoor pig rearing [26], therefore, increased requirements of FR and O pigs. Thus, as expected, O pigs had the higher ($P < 0.05$)

Feed:Gain Ratio, even higher than the FR group [6,7,9], because of the larger access area and the lower potential for growth of Cinta Senese [27]. Accordingly, O pigs showed the lower ($P < 0.05$) slaughter BW (159.02 vs 151.28 and 78%, or O, FR and I, respectively) and dressing out percentage (78 *vs.* 80 and 83%, for O, FR and I, respectively).

3.2. Meat Characteristics

Lipid content, fatty acid profile and indices of *Longissimus dorsi* of pig are reported in Table 3.

Table 3. Effect of rearing system on lipid content (g/100 g of muscle), fatty acid profile (g/100 g of total lipids) and fatty acid indices of *Longissimus dorsi*.

Rearing System	I	FR	O	SED
Lipid content	4.23 [c]	3.50 [b]	2.16 [a]	0.52
Fatty acid Profile				
C14:0	1.48 [b]	1.56 [b]	1.20 [a]	0.24
C16:0	27.01	26.66	26.77	1.51
C18:0	13.03	12.57	12.77	1.36
SFA	41.52	40.79	40.74	2.33
C16:1n7	3.16	3.47	3.42	0.57
C18:1n7	3.87	4.07	4.08	0.42
C18:1n9	42.32	41.50	41.02	2.58
C20:1n9	0.86 [a]	1.24 [b]	1.62 [c]	0.32
MUFA	49.35	49.03	48.52	2.76
C18:2n6	6.26	7.28	7.05	1.59
C18:3n3	0.74	0.70	0.67	0.12
PUFA	7.00	7.97	7.73	1.57
Fatty acid indices				
Δ9-desaturase (C16) [1]	10.47	11.52	11.33	0.98
Δ9-desaturase (C18) [2]	458.46 [a]	478.38 [b]	478.88 [b]	2.50
Δ9-desaturase (C16+C18) [3]	55.21	55.56	55.10	0.19
Elongase [4]	0.48	0.47	0.48	0.12
Thioesterase [5]	18.25 [a]	17.09 [a]	22.31 [b]	2.23

N = 50/group; [ac] Means in the same row with the same superscript do not differ significantly ($P < 0.05$); [1] Calculated as 100 × [16:1n-9/(16:1n-9 + 16:0)]; [2] Calculated as 100 × [(18:1n7 + 18:1n-9)/(18:1n7 + 18:1n-9 + 18:0)]; [3] Calculated as 100 × [(16:1n-9 + 18:1n7 + 18:1n-9)/(16:1n-9 + 16:0 + 18:1n7 + 18:1n-9 + 18:0)]; [4] Calculated as 16:0/14:0; [5] Calculated as 18:0/16:0.

A significant ($P < 0.001$) effect of rearing system was found for muscle lipid content with I pigs having the higher amount followed by FR and O pigs. This was due to the greater energy demand (activity and temperature regulation) of outdoor reared pigs, thus producing leaner meat.

Regarding the effect of rearing system on meat lipid content, literature data are conflicting. Our results agree with Enfalt *et al.* [6] and Sather *et al.* [7] that found increased carcass lean meat contents in free-range pigs. Also Bee *et al.* [28] found a decreased lipid content in outdoor/free-range reared pigs.

On the contrary, other Authors [12,29,30] found a greater lipid content of pigs reared with outdoor access compared with the confined.

Considering fatty acid profile, rearing system showed significant ($P < 0.05$) effect only on myristic (C14:0) and gondoic acids (C20:1n9) content. C14:0 was found higher ($P < 0.05$) in I and FR; whereas for C20:1n9: O > FR > I, ($P < 0.05$). With respect to C14:0, Bellizzi and Coworkers [31], found a positive correlation with coronary heart disease mortality. Moreover, the same Authors noted that myristic acid was the major cause of hypercholesterolemia induction. This effect was related both to repression of hepatic low density lipoprotein (LDL) receptor synthesis and to direct stimulation hepatic LDL synthesis. C20:1n9 is a long-chain monounsaturated fatty acids (MUFA), biosynthesized from oleic acid, and was found to alleviate metabolic syndrome partly by regulating genes involved in lipid metabolism, energy expenditure, and inflammation in obese mice [32] and to lower risk of HIV transmission through breast milk [33]. Moreover some Authors [34,35] suggested a correlation between plasma levels of long-chain MUFA and metabolic parameters as hyperglycemia and hyperlipidemia.

The rearing system was a significant source of variation ($P < 0.05$) for Δ9-desaturase (C18), while elongase index appeared to be affected by genotype. These data are in accordance with Zhang *et al.* [36], which found a higher thioesterase index in Landrace, Yorkshire, Hampshire, and Spotted pigs with respect to Duroc and Chester White pigs. Thioesterase in the fatty acid synthase complex terminates the fatty acid synthesis and the release of the newly synthesized fatty acids. Both C14-acyl ACP (Acil Carrier Protein) and C16- acyl ACP are substrates for thioesterase, C16:0 being the major product. The ratio of C16:0 to C14:0 was utilized to reflect the selective cleavage of thioesterase on C14-acyl ACP or C16-acyl ACP; the greater the thioesterase index, the less cleavage of C14-acyl ACP.

In Table 4 the effect of rearing system on anserine, carnosine, CoQ10 and TBARs of meat contents is presented.

The anserine values showed a decreasing trend in meats: I > FR > O pigs, ($P < 0.05$). This trend is in agreement with data published in the literature, which suggests that the anserine content of meat is closely related to the glycolytic metabolism of muscle [37]. Accordingly, outdoor reared pigs showed the lower content, probably due to the more pronounced oxidative metabolism for higher activity.

Table 4. Effect of rearing system on histidyl dipeptides, TBARs and CoQ10 contents of *Longissimus dorsi* of pork.

Rearing system		**I**	**FR**	**O**	**SED**
Anserine	ppm	825.34 ^{b}	567.56 ^{ab}	275.41 ^{a}	551.60
Carnosine	ppm	8594.50 ^{b}	8746.63 ^{b}	3581.25 ^{a}	1006.82
CoQ10	ppm	7.19 ^{a}	9.51 ^{b}	17.99 ^{b}	1.21
TBARs	ppm	0.32 ^{c}	0.23 ^{b}	0.16 ^{a}	0.06

N = 50/group; ^{ac} Means in the same row with the same superscript do not differ significantly ($P < 0.05$).

Considering carnosine content, I and FR pigs exhibited higher values ($P < 0.0001$). Carnosine reacts with simple sugars and blocks the glycation process of proteins, and therefore behaves like a competitive acceptor in the glycoxidation reaction. Some studies have shown that carnosine and its related molecules are capable of acting as antioxidants [38]. Our results are consistent with previous studies [39] demonstrating that white muscle had higher carnosine content than dark muscle. Sewell *et al.* [40] found a strong positive correlation between carnosine content and type II fiber surface area in the equine middle gluteal muscle. These authors showed that carnosine can contribute as much as 46% to the buffering of H+ produced by equine type IIB fibers and concluded that this dipeptide is important in stabilizing the pH in anaerobic contraction.

Our data on O carnosine content suggest a kind of genotype effect. In fact, carnosine content is affected not only by kinetic activity, fiber type, but also by breed, gender, age and breeding [41]. Kanok-Orn *et al* [42], demonstrated that carnosine contents in chicken fresh meat of both breast and thigh meats were significantly different among breeds. Oxidative intermediate and oxidative slow twitch muscle fibers have been found in the *Longissimus dorsi* muscle of wild pigs compared to domesticated pig breeds [43]. Thus, the lower concentration of anserine in O pigs is probably correlated to more pronounced oxidative metabolism, both for the performed kinetic activity and for the crossbreed used. This may explain the similar content of carnosine found in I and FR meat with respect to O meat.

Significantly higher values for CoQ_{10} were found in O and FR pigs than in I pigs ($P < 0.05$). It is now well established that CoQ_{10} (Coenzyme Q_{10}) is a lipid soluble, endogenous hydroxybenzoquinone compound found in the majority of aerobic organisms [44] in two redox forms, and varying length of the isoprenoid side chain. Coenzyme Q_{10} plays an important role as an essential electron carrier in the mitochondrial respiratory chain linked to cellular oxidative metabolism and that is able to prevent lipid peroxidation in most subcellular membranes. Accordingly, we found greater value of CoQ_{10} in O and FR pigs, with outdoor access and increased kinetic activity.

According to CoQ_{10} and lipid contents (that represent the substrate for peroxidative processes), we found TBARS content ($P < 0.05$) in meat, in decreasing order: I, FR and O.

The outdoor rearing system induced the decrease of anserine dipeptide meat content, accompanied by the increase in CoQ_{10} meat content. In fact, when oxidative stress is reported, CoQ10 biosynthesis is increased [45].

TBARS content followed the same trend ($P < 0.05$) found for lipids; higher values were found for I, followed by FR and O meat samples. Lipid oxidation is one of the primary causes of quality deterioration in meat and generates compounds potentially dangerous for human health. The conversion of muscle to edible meat after slaughter can unbalance the equilibrium between pro-oxidative and anti-oxidative factors, resulting in initiation and propagation of lipid oxidation [46].

Possibly, the larger amount of CoQ10 together with the lower oxidation substrate (lipid), repressed the formation of end products of oxidation in O meat, thus reducing food deterioration [47]. Anyhow, TBARS content of meat for all studied systems was very low.

4. Conclusions

Extensive rearing systems of farm animals are perceived by consumers as strongly linked to health, animal welfare, sustainability, and safety; for these reasons, free range and organic rearing systems are highly desirable. Organic farming is the most regulated of the alternative rearing systems, with minimum environmental impact, increased welfare of production animals, and with no use of polluting agents, including antibiotics [48]. The issue is whether these new systems indeed improve welfare and sustainability of farmed pigs and whether, since they replace systems that already produce high-quality meat, they affect production characteristics and meat. On the basis of the reported results, we can conclude that rearing system influences all studied parameters, and when outdoor access is given to pigs, activity and thermoregulation reduce growth rate, but improve some meat quality characteristics (lean meat with lower C14:0, and higher C20:1n9 and oxidative stability). It is evident that for lipid, thioesterase and antioxidant dipeptides of meat, differences could be attributed also to the used genotype.

Differences were particularly evident in O system, with greater outdoor availability and the used crossbred. In our case the CSxLW crossbreed in organic rearing system produced very lean meat with higher oxidative stability. Thus, the aims of the organic production system were fully achieved, both the rearing and diffusion of local genotypes, and the improvement of the role of agriculture in environment preservation.

Further studies should be carried out in the future to deeply investigate the relationships between rearing system, used genotype, muscle energy metabolism and meat quality.

Acknowledgements

The authors would like to acknowledge the financial and in-kind support provided by the CIPE (Comitato Interministeriale per la Programmazione Economica), Progetto di ricerca D.M. 28496, resolution 81/2004: "Alimentazione e qualità delle produzioni zooteniche".

Author Contributions

Conceived and designed the experiments: Giuseppe Martino. Performed the experiments: Giuseppe Martino. Analyzed the data: Francesca Sarti. Contributed reagents/materials/analytical tools: Michele Del Carlo, Lisa Grotta and Dario Compagnone. Wrote the paper: Cecilia Mugnai.

Conflicts of Interest

The authors declare no conflict of interest.

References

1. Hervieu, B.; Hansen, B. *How can Research on Food and Agriculture in Europe Better Respond to Citizens' Expectations and Demands?*; Science for Society-Science with Society: Brussels, Belgium, 2002; p. 32.
2. Maiorano, G. Swine production in Italy and research perspectives for the local breeds. *Slovak J. Anim. Sci.* **2009**, *42*, 159–166.
3. Beharrell, B.; MacFie, J.H. Consumer Attitudes to Organic Foods. *Brit. Food J.* **1991**, *93*, 25–30.
4. European Economic Community. Council Regulation (EC) n. 1804/99 of July 1999 Supplementing Regulation (ECC) n. 2092/91 on Organic Production of Agricultural Products. *Off. J.* **1999**, *L 222*, 1–28.
5. Hovi, M.; Sundrum, A.; Thamsborg, S.M. Animal health and welfare in organic livestock production in Europe: Current state and future challenges. *Livest. Prod. Sci.* **2003**, *80*, 41–53.
6. Enfalt, A.C.; Lundstrom, K.; Hansson, I.; Lundeheim, N.; Nystrom, P.E. Effects of outdoor rearing and sire breed (Duroc or Yorkshire) on carcass composition and sensory and technological meat quality. *Meat Sci.* **1997**, *45*, 1–15.

7. Sather, A.P.; Jones, S.D.M. Schaefer, A.L.; Colyn, J.; Robertson, W.M. Feedlot performance, carcass composition and meat quality of free-range reared pigs. *Can. J. Anim. Sci.* **1997**, *77*, 225–232.
8. Claudi-Magnussen, C. *Organic Pig Production, Comparison of Organic and Conventional Retail Meat Products Meat and Eating Quality*; Technical Report Ref. No. 17.258/01 (0071.wpd); Danish Meat Research Institute: Roskilde, Denmark, 1999.
9. Danielsen, V.; Hansen, L.L.; Møller, F.; Bejrholm, C.; Nielsen, S. Production results and sensory meat quality of pigs fed different amounts of concentrate and ad lib. Clover grass or clover grass silage. In *Ecological Animal Husbandry in the Nordic Countries. Proceedings from NJF Seminar No. 303, Horsens, Denmark 16–17 September 1999*; Hermansen, J.E., Lund, V., Thuen, E., Eds.; CABI Publishing: Wallingford, UK, 2000; pp. 79–86.
10. Nilzen, V.; Babol, J.; Dutta, P.C.; Lundeheim, N.; Enfalt, A.C.; Lundstrom, K. Free range rearing of pigs with access to pasture grazing effect on fatty acid composition and lipid oxidation products. *Meat Sci.* **2001**, *58*, 267–275.
11. Olsson, V.; Andersson, K.; Hansson, I.; Lundström, K. Differences in meat quality between organically and conventionally produced pigs. *Meat Sci.* **2003**, *64*, 287–297.
12. Lebret, B.; Meunier-Salaün, M.C.; Foury, A.; Mormède, P.; Dransfield, E.; Dourmad, J.Y. Influence of rearing conditions on performance, behavioral, and physiological responses of pigs to preslaughter handling, carcass traits, and meat quality. *J. Anim. Sci.* **2006**, *84*, 2436–2447.
13. Lebret, B. Effects of feeding and rearing systems on growth, carcass composition and meat quality in pigs. *Animal* **2008**, *2*, 1548–1558.
14. European Economic Community. Council Regulation (EC) No 1/2005 of 22 December 2004 on the Protection of Animals during Transport and Related Operations and Amending Directives 64/432/EEC and 93/119/EC and Regulation (EC) No 1255/97. *Off. J.* **2005**, *L 3*, 1–44.
15. Folch, J.; Lees, M.; Stanley, G.H.S. A simple method for the isolation and purification of total lipids from animal tissues. *J. Biol. Chem.* **1957**, *726*, 497–509.
16. Dal Bosco, A; Mugnai, C; Ruggeri, S; Mattioli, S; Castellini, C. Fatty acid composition of meat and estimated indices of lipid metabolizm in different poultry genotypes reared under organic system. *Poultry Sci.* **2012**, *91*, 2039–2045.
17. Aristoy, M.C.; Toldrá, F. Concentration of free amino acids and dipeptides in porcine skeletal muscles with different oxidative patterns. *Meat Sci.* **1998**, *50*, 327–332.
18. Gil-Agustì, M.; Esteve-Romero, J.; Carda-Broch, S. Anserine and Carnosine Determination in meat samples by pure micellar liquid chromatography. *J. Chromat.* **2008**, *1189*, 444–450.
19. Martino, G.; Haouet, M.N.; Reali, C.; Olivieri, O.; Valfrè, F. Coenzime Q_{10} and its relationship to other nutritional components of animal products. *It. J. Food Sci.* **1995**, *1*, 19–25.
20. Rhee, K.S. Minimization of further lipid peroxidation in the distillation 2-thiobarbituric acid test of fish and meat. *J. Food Sci.* **1978**, *43*, 1776–1781.
21. Tarladgis, B.G.; Watts, B.M.; Yonathan, M. Distillation method for the determination of malonaldehyde in rancid foods. *J. Am. Oil Chem. Soc.* **1960**, *37*, 44–48.
22. *SAS® User's Guide*; SAS Institute Inc.: Cary, NC, USA, 2005.

23. Guy, J.H.; Burns, S.E.; Barker, J.M.; Edwards, S.A. Reducing post-mixing aggression and skin lesions in weaned pigs by application of a synthetic maternal pheromone. *Anim. Welf.* **2009**, *18*, 249–255.
24. Yonezawa, T.; Koori, M.; Takefumi, K.; Mori, Y. Appeasing pheromone inhibits cortisol augmentation and agonistic behaviors during social stress in adult miniature pigs. *Zool. Sci.* **2009**, *26*, 739–744.
25. Close, W.H.; Poorman, P.K. Outdoor pigs—Their nutrient requirements, appetiteand environmental responses. In *Recent Advances in Animal Nutrition*; Garnworthy, P.C., Cole, D.J. A., Eds.; Nottingham University Press: Loughborough, UK, 1993; pp. 175–196.
26. Noblet, J.; Ledividich, J.; Bikawa, T. Interaction between Energy-Level in the Dietand Environmental-Temperature on the Utilization of Energy in Growing-Pigs. *J. Anim. Sci.* **1985**, *61*, 452–459.
27. Schinkel, A.P. Describing the pig. In *A Quantitative Biology of the Pig*; Kyriazakis, I., Ed.; CABI Publishing: Wallingford, UK, 1999; pp. 9–38.
28. Bee, G.; Guex, G.; Herzog, W. Free range rearing of pigs during the winter. Adaptations in muscle fiber characteristics and effects on adipose tissue composition and meat quality traits. *J. Anim. Sci.* **2004**, *82*, 1206–1218.
29. Lebret, B.; Lefaucheur, L.; Mourot, J. La qualité de la viande de porc. Influence des facteurs d'élevage non génétiques sur les caractéristiques du tissu musculaire. *Prod. Anim.* **1999**, *12*, 11–28.
30. Lebret, B.; Massabie, P.; Granier, R.; Juin, H.; Mourot, J.; Chevillon. P. Influence of outdoor rearing and indoor temperature on growth performance, carcass, adipose tissue and muscle traits in pigs, and on the technological and eating quality of dry-cured hams. *Meat Sci.* **2002**, *62*, 447–455.
31. Bellizzi, M.C.; Franklin, M.F.; Duthie, G.G.; James, W.P.T. Vitamin E and coronary heart disease: The European paradox. *Eur. J. Clinic. Nutr.* **1994**, *48*, 822–831.
32. Yang, Z.H.; Miyahara, H.; Mori, T.; Doisaki, N.; Hatanaka, A. Beneficial effects of dietary fish-oil-derived monounsaturated fatty acids on metabolic syndrome risk factors and insulin resistance in mice. *J. Agric. Food Chem.* **2011**, *59*, 7482–7489.
33. Villamor, E.; Koulinska, I.N.; Furtado, J.; Baylin, A.; Aboud, S.; Manji, K.; Campos, H.; Fawzi, W.W. Long-chain n–6 polyunsaturated fatty acids in breast milk decrease the risk of HIV transmission through breastfeeding. *Am. J. Clin. Nutr.* **2007**, *86*, 682–689.
34. Yang, Z.H.; Miyahara, H.; Takemura, S.; Hatanaka, A. Dietary saury oil reduces hyperglycemia and hyperlipidemia in diabetic KKAy mice and in diet-induced obese C57BL/6J mice by altering gene expression. *Lipids* **2011**, *46*, 425–434.
35. Yang, Z.H.; Miyahara, H.; Takeo, J.; Hatanaka, A.; Katayama, M. Pollock oil supplementation modulates hyperlipidemia and ameliorates hepatic steatosis in mice fed a high-fat diet. *Lipids Health Dis.* **2011**, *10*, doi:10.1186/1476-511X-10-189.
36. Zhang, S.; Knight, T.J.; Stalder, K.J.; Goodwin, R.N.; Lonergan, S.M.; Beitz, D.C. Effects of breed, sex, and halothane genotype on fatty acid composition of pork longissimus muscle. *J. Anim. Sci.* **2007**, *85*, 583–591.

37. Chan, K.M.; Decker, E.A.; Chow, C.K.; Boissonneault, G.A. Effect of dietary carnosine on plasma and tissue antioxidant concentrations and on lipid oxidation in rat skeletal muscle. *Lipids* **1994**, *29*, 461–466.
38. Quinn, P.J.; Boldyrev, A.; Formazuyk, V.E. Carnosine its properties; Function and potential therapeutic applications. *Mol. Asp. Med.* **1992**, *13*, 379–444.
39. Cornet, M.; Bousset, J. Free amino acids and dipeptides in porcine muscles: Differences between 'red' and 'white' muscles. *Meat Sci.* **1999**, *51*, 215–219.
40. Seewell, D.A.; Harris, R.C.; Marlin, D.J.; Dunnett, M. Estimation of the carnosine content of different fiber types in the middle gluteal muscle of the thoroughbred horse. *J. Physiol.* **1992**, *455*, 447–453.
41. Abe, H.; Okuma, E. Discrimination of meat species in processed meat products based on the ratio of histidine dipeptides. *Nippon Shokuhin Kagaku Kogaku Kaishi* **1995**, *42*, 827–834.
42. Intarapichet, K.-O.; Maikhunthod, B. Genotype and gender differences in carnosine extracts and antioxidant activities of chicken breast and thigh meats. *Meat Sci.* **2005**, *71*, 634–642.
43. Essén-Gustavsson, B.; Lindholm, A. Fiber types and metabolic characteristics in muscles of wild boars, normal and halothane sensitive Swedish Landrace pigs. *Comp. Biochem. Physiol. A* **1984**, *78*, 67–71.
44. Battino, M.; Ferri, E.; Gorini, A.; Federico Villa, R.; Rodriquez Huertas, J.F.; Fiorella, P.; Genova, M.L.; Lenaz, G.; Marchetti, M. Natural distribution and occurrence of coenzyme Q homologues. *Memb. Biochem.* **1990**, *9*, 179–190.
45. Turunen, M.; Olsson, J.; Dallner, G. Metabolizm and function of coenzyme Q. *Biochim. Biophys. Acta* **2004**, *1660*, 171–199.
46. Min, B.; Ahn, D.U. Mechanism of lipid oxidation in meat and meat products—A review. *Food Sci. Biotech.* **2005**, *14*, 152–163.
47. Zhou, S.; Decker, E.A. Ability of carnosine and other skeletal muscle components to quench unsaturated aldehydic lipid oxidation products. *J. Agri. Food Chem.* **1999**, *47*, 21–55.
48. Cabaret, J. Animal health problems in organic farming: Subjective and objective assessments and farmers' actions. *Livest. Prod. Sci.* **2003**, *80*, 99–108.

Establishing Sprinkling Requirements on Trailers Transporting Market Weight Pigs in Warm and Hot Weather

Rebecca Kephart [1], Anna Johnson [1,*], Avi Sapkota [2], Kenneth Stalder [1] and John McGlone [2]

[1] Department of Animal Science, Iowa State University, Ames, IA 50011, USA; E-Mails: rkdavis@iastate.edu (R.K.); stalder@iastate.edu (K.S.)

[2] Departments of Animal and Food Science and Animal Care Services, Texas Tech University, Lubbock, TX 79409, USA; E-Mails: asapkota@purdue.edu (A.S.); john.mcglone@ttu.edu (J.M.)

* Author to whom correspondence should be addressed; E-Mail: johnsona@iastate.edu.

Simple Summary: Transport is an inevitable process in the modern, multi-site swine industry. Pigs do not have efficient physiological means (such as sweating) to cool themselves. Therefore, being transported in hot weather can cause heat stress and even death. Sprinkling the pigs and/or bedding may facilitate cooling, thereby improving well-being and survivability of pigs arriving at the plant.

Abstract: This study was conducted July of 2012 in Iowa, in WARM (<26.7 °C) and HOT (≥26.7 °C) weather. Four sprinkling methods were compared, with one treatment being randomly assigned to each load: control- no sprinkling (not applied in HOT weather), pigs only, bedding only, or pigs and bedding. Experiment 1 used 51 loads in WARM- and 86 loads in HOT weather to determine sprinkling effects on pig measures (surface temperature, vocalizations, slips and falls, and stress signs). Experiment 2 used 82 loads in WARM- and 54 loads in HOT weather to determine the sprinkling effects on transport losses (non-ambulatory, dead, and total transport losses). Experiment 1 found that, in WARM weather, there were no differences between sprinkling treatments for surface temperature, vocalizations, or slips and falls ($p \geq 0.18$). However, stress signs were 2% greater when sprinkling pigs- or bedding only- compared to control ($p = 0.03$). Experiment 2 found that, in WARM and HOT weather, sprinkling did not affect non-ambulatory, dead, or total transport losses ($p \geq 0.18$). Although the current study did not find any observed sprinkling effects for pig measures or transport losses it is extremely important to note that the inference space of this study is relatively small, so further studies should be conducted to see if these results are applicable to other geographical regions and seasons.

Keywords: market-weight pig; sprinkling; transport loss; well-being

---

1. Introduction

Transporting swine is essential to the multi-site pork production. Around 113 million pigs were marketed in 2012 in the U.S. [1]. For pigs, marketing is a combination of potentially novel (defined as the first exposure), unfamiliar (defined as more than one exposure that is infrequent), and physically exerting experiences that could be perceived as stressful [2]. The term "*transport losses*" refers to pigs that become non-ambulatory (unable to keep up with the group and may have a structural injury) or are dead on arrival [2]. Increased transport losses and decreased meat quality may result if the pig is unable cope with these stressors [3–5].

The conditions under which pigs are handled and transported can have a direct impact on the pigs' well-being. In the U.S., trailers rely on passive ventilation, meaning air flow is dependent upon thermal buoyancy, movement of the vehicle itself, and the wind speed. To control the internal trailer environment, the National Pork Board's Transport Quality Assurance (TQA) program recommends that pigs (>27 °C) and bedding (>15 °C) are sprinkled to facilitate evaporative cooling with the intention of reducing heat stress [6]. However, these recommendations are based on experiential information rather than scientific data [6]. Therefore, the objectives of these experiments were to compare the effects of sprinkling methods inside trailers on (1) market weight pig measures at the time of unloading and (2) transport losses at the plant.

2. Experimental Section

2.1. General Procedures for Both Experiments

The protocol for these experiments was approved by the Iowa State University Institutional Animal Care and Use Committee and data was collected during 3 weeks in July 2012.

2.1.1. Animals, Farms, and Handling

The company's loading crew sorted and moved market weight barrows and gilts from their home pen to the entrance of the loading ramp. The trucker moved the pigs up the loading ramp and onto the trailer. Both the loading crew and the trucker used a combination of sort boards, rattle paddles, and electric prods during loading (the number of times these devices were used was not recorded for these experiments).

Following TQA recommendations, any pig that became hot or stressed during loading would not have been loaded onto the truck. However, no pigs in these experiments met that criteria. The pigs were transported from commercial finishing facilities to a commercial processing plant, all located in Iowa. Transport occurred throughout the day and night. The trucker unloaded the pigs and plant personnel moved the pigs from the loading dock to the rest pens. During unloading, plant personnel and the trucker used paddles, rattles, and boards (the number of times these devices were used was not recorded for these experiments).

2.1.2. Treatments and Experimental Design

Treatment one (control) was defined as not sprinkling pigs or bedding on the trailer. Treatment two (pigs only) was defined as pigs being sprinkled after loading was completed for 6 to 8 min. Treatment three (bedding only) was defined as bedding being sprinkled 4 to 6 min before the start of loading. Treatment four (pigs and bedding) was defined as both pigs and bedding being sprinkled for 6 to 8 min. Due to concerns about pig well-being, the control treatment was not applied when the temperature was ≥26.7 °C. Therefore, two data sets will be presented: WARM (temperature <26.7 °C; 4 treatments) and HOT (≥26.7 °C; 3 treatments) All treatments were applied by the researchers and were randomly assigned to trailers.

2.1.3. Transport Trailers and Density

All pigs were transported on aluminum drop deck (pot belly) trailers 17 m in length with diamond plate flooring. These were owned and operated by drivers employed by trucking companies contracted through the plant.

All compartments in the trailer were stocked according to the industry's current standard operating procedure of 0.41 m^2/pig or ~171 pigs/load [6]. The plant provided data on the number of pigs/trailer and the average weight of pigs on a trailer. For these experiments a density value was calucated and added to the statistical model because previous work has found density is an important variable in affecting animal based measures and transport losses [7–9].

$$\text{Density} = [(\text{average pig weight per trailer}) \times (\text{pigs per trailer})] / (\text{m}^2 \text{ floor space in trailer})$$

2.1.4. Temperature Humidity Index

Ambient relative humidity and air temperature were measured at an airport 16.9 km from the plant. The airport data logger (1088 Hygrothermometer, Technical Service Laboratory, Fort Walton Beach, FL, USA) collected temperature and dew point. Relative humidity was then calculated from dew point and temperature measurements. The airport data logger was accurate for ambient temperature and for dew point ± 0.003 °C. Ambient temperature (T) and relative humidity (RH) were used to calculate a temperature humidity index (THI) using the following equation [10]:

$$\text{THI} = \text{T} - \{[0.55 - (0.0055 \times \text{RH}_{\text{decimal}})](\text{T} - 14.5)\}$$

This equation was found to fit the model of pig transport by Fitzgerald and others [7]. Additionally, other evidence suggests that it is important to consider both temperature and humidity when determining heat stress in pigs [11–13].

2.2. Experiment 1: Effects of Sprinkling Inside Trailers Transporting Market Weight Pigs During WARM and HOT Weather on Pig Measures and Bedding Moisture at Unloading

A total of 51 loads were used in WARM- and 86 loads were used in HOT weather. In WARM weather, the treatments were control (n = 24), pigs only (n = 13), bedding only (n = 7), and pigs and bedding (n = 7). In HOT weather, the treatments were pigs only (n = 41), bedding only (n = 18), and pigs and bedding (n = 27).

2.2.1. Pig Measures

Pig measures were collected on a random sample of pigs at unloading using live observation. A random sample of pigs was defined as ignoring the first ~10 pigs at the beginning of unloading, counting 50 pigs (group A), ignoring a further ~10 pigs, and counting another 50 pigs (group B). This provided 100 pigs/load. For groups A and B, the following pig measures were tallied: vocalizations, slips and falls, and stress signs. Vocalizations were defined as an extended sound of high amplitude and frequency produced with an open mouth [2]. Slips were defined as a knee or hock touching the ground; falls were defined as a pig's body touching the ground [14]. Slips and falls were tallied as a single measure. Stress signs were defined as open mouth breathing, muscle tremors, and red-blotchy skin [15]. Surface temperature was measured laterally near the midline on 5 randomly selected pigs from groups A and B (total of 10 pigs/load). Surface temperature was measured with a dual laser infrared thermometer (model 42570, Extech Instruments, Nashua, NH, USA) which was accurate to ±1 °C.

2.2.2. Bedding Moisture

A total of 8 fresh bedding samples and 140 used bedding samples were collected from trailers. Fresh samples (0 loads) were defined as bedding that had not been previously used for transporting pigs. A fresh bedding sample was ~45 g. After each trailer had unloaded at the plant, a used bedding sample, defined as bedding which had transported ≥ 1 trailer loads of pigs was collected. Half of the used bedding was collected from the bottom trailer deck and the remainder was collected from the top deck. Each used bedding sample was ~410 g. Bedding samples were stored in a cardboard box at room temperature (~21 °C) on the floor for no longer than 1 wk after trial completion.

Bedding moisture was determined following standard operating procedure for drying samples. A tin measuring 7.6 cm wide by 2.2 cm deep (model A90, Wilkinson Industries Inc., Fort Calhoun, NE, USA) was weighed. Each bedding sample was kneaded by hand inside the closed storage bag for ~30 s. Two, 3 to 6 g subsamples (subsample A and B) were removed from the bag using a spoon. Subsample A was placed in one tin and subsample B was placed in a second. The bedding subsample in its respective tin was weighed (accurate ± 0.03 mg; model AT261 DeltaRange, Metler-Toledo GmBh Laboratory and Weighing Technologies, Greifensee, Switzerland) to determine wet weight. Bedding subsamples were dried for ~20 to 24 h at 100 °C in a convection oven (model DKN810, Yamato Scientific America Inc., Santa Clara, CA, USA). After drying, subsamples were re-weighed; this was defined as the dry weight. Moisture percent for each subsample was calculated using the following equation [16]:

$$\text{Moisture percent} = [(\text{dry weight}) / (\text{wet weight})] \times 100$$

A standard deviation of moisture percentage between subsample A and subsample B and an average of the moisture percent of subsample A and subsample B were calculated. Between subsample A and subsample B, the coefficient of variation (CV) was calculated using the following equation:

$$CV = (\text{Standard deviation} / \text{average}) \times 100$$

If the CV ≥ 10 the sample was re-subsampled and dried a second time (n = 14). If the sample was still found to be too variable on the second drying, that samples were removed from the data set (n = 0). The data from bedding moisture will be presented descriptively separated by the number of loads on the bedding, ranging from 0 to ≥ 4 loads.

2.2.3. Transport Events

Researchers recorded the time that loading started and ended, the time the trailer left the farm, and the time that unloading started and ended. Processing plant records provided the arrival time of the trailer at the plant. Loading was defined as the time interval from the first pig's front foot stepped onto the trailer until the last pig's hind foot stepped onto the trailer. Wait time at the farm was defined as the time from when the last pig's hind foot stepped onto the trailer until the trailer left the farm. Transport was defined as the time interval from when trailer left the farm until the trailer arrived at the plant. Wait time at the plant was defined as the time interval from when the trailer arrived at the plant until the first pig's front foot stepped off the truck. Unloading was defined as the time interval from when the first pig's front foot stepped off the truck until the last pig's hind foot stepped off the truck. Total transit time was defined as the time from when the first pig's front foot stepped onto the trailer (start of loading) until the last pig's hind foot stepped off the trailer (end of unloading).

2.2.4. Bedding Level

The number of 0.2 m^3 (22.7 kg) bags of wood shaving bedding/trailer were recorded. Because trailers rely on passive ventilation, in the winter bedding is believed to insulate pigs from extreme cold. In the summer, less bedding is included as a means of providing traction and absorbing waste.

2.3. Experiment 2: Effects of Sprinkling Inside Trailers on Market Weight Pig Transport Losses During WARM and HOT Weather

A total of 82 loads were used in WARM- and 54 loads were used HOT weather to determine if sprinkling effected transport losses. In WARM weather, the treatments were control (n = 48), pigs only (n = 11), bedding only (n = 15), and bedding and pigs (n = 8). In HOT weather, the treatments were pigs only (n = 31), bedding only (n = 9), and bedding and pigs (n = 14).

Transport Losses at the Plant

Plant employees identified non-ambulatory (sum of fatigued and injured) [2] and dead (sum of euthanized- and dead on arrival), Total transport losses were defined as the sum of non-ambulatory and dead.

2.4. Statistical Analysis

For both experiments, data were evaluated for missing and erroneous values by using the filter feature in Excel (Microsoft Office 2010, Microsoft Redmond, WA, USA). The remaining analyses were completed using SAS software (SAS V 9.2 Institute Inc., Cary, NC, USA). Using the means and sort procedures data was checked for erroneous and potential outlier data points. Data that was identified as a potential outlier was checked against the original data. If correct it was simply highlighted in the excel data, if incorrect that value was substituted per the original data. Because all four treatments were only present when the temperature was <26.7 °C SAS was used to create two data sets from the single excel file data was originally entered (WARM and HOT data sets). $p < 0.05$ was considered significant for both experiments. $p \leq 0.10$ was considered tending for both experiments. For both experiments, each variable collected was evaluated on whether it should be present in the model. Variables that might have affected the pig measures were attempted in the model. Those variables that were found to be significant or were indicated by previous research to cause variation in pig transport were retained for the final model.

2.4.1. Experiment 1: Effects of Sprinkling Inside Trailers Transporting Market Weight Pigs During WARM and HOT Weather on Pig Measures and Bedding Moisture at Unloading

Because researchers sometimes counted more, or less than 50 pigs/group, data for vocalizations, slips and falls, and stress signs were analyzed as a percent of the pigs counted:

Percent pig measure = [(number of times a measure was counted) / (number pigs counted in that group)] × 100

Furthermore, the SAS program (SAS 9.3, SAS Institute Inc., Cary, North Carolina) was used to create a new variable from the percent of vocalizations, slips and falls, and stress signs from group A and group B of 50 (e.g., [percent stress signs group A + percent stress signs group B]/2). Surface temperature was analyzed as an average of the 10 pigs measured per load.

Data were analyzed using a mixed model (PROC MIXED, SAS 9.3 SAS, Institute Inc., Cary, NC, USA) where the response variables, surface temperature, vocalizations, slips and falls, and stress signs, were analyzed using sprinkling treatment and bedding level as fixed effects, THI at unloading and density as linear covariates, and farm, trucking company, and researcher at the plant as random effects.

2.4.2. Experiment 2: Effects of Sprinkling Inside Trailers on Market Weight Pig Transport Losses During WARM and HOT Weather

Analysis of non-ambulatory-, dead-, and total transport losses per trailer was performed using a generalized linear mixed model (GLIMMIX procedure, SAS 9.3 Cary, NC, USA). The data approximated a Poisson distribution and was log transformed by the GLIMMIX procedure (SAS 9.3 Cary, NC, USA) prior to statistical analysis. The model used sprinkling treatment as a fixed effect, THI at loading and density as linear covariates, and farm and trucking company as random effects. The ILINK option (SAS 9.3 Cary, NC, USA) was used to back-transform least squares means into their original unit of measure for ease of interpretation.

3. Results and Discussion

3.1. Experiment 1: Effects of Sprinkling Inside Trailers Transporting Market Weight Pigs During WARM and HOT Weather on Pig Measures and Bedding Moisture at Unloading

3.1.1. Sprinkling

In WARM weather, sprinkling treatment had no observed effect on surface temperature, vocalizations, or slips and falls ($p \geq 0.18$). However, stress signs were 2% greater for the bedding and pig treatment than control ($p = 0.03$; Table 1). In HOT weather, sprinkling method had no effect on surface temperature, vocalizations, slips and falls, or stress signs ($p \geq 0.19$; Table 1).

Table 1. Experiment 1. Effects of sprinkling [1] on pig measures [2] in market weight pigs in WARM [3] and HOT [4] weather.

	Sprinkling treatment					
WARM weather, measure	**Control n = 24**	**Pigs only n = 13**	**Bedding only n = 7**	**Bedding and pigs n = 7**	***p*-value**	**R^2**
Surface temperature, ° C	32.2 ± 0.5	32.7 ± 0.4	33.1 ± 0.6	32.3 ± 0.6	0.18	0.41
Vocalizations, % of pigs counted	2.4 ± 1.8	2.6 ± 1.8	2.7 ± 1.9	3.4 ± 1.9	0.65	0.04
Slips and falls, % of pigs counted	0.7 ± 0.2	0.5 ± 0.2	0.5 ± 0.3	0.2 ± 0.3	0.61	0.10
Stress signs, % of pigs counted	0.6 ± 0.4 [a]	0.5 ± 0.4 [a,b]	1.5 ± 0.6 [a,b]	2.6 ± 0.6 [b]	0.03	0.03
HOT weather	**n = 0**	**n = 41**	**n = 18**	**n = 27**		
Surface temperature, ° C	.	35.3 ± 0.3	34.8 ± 0.3	34.9 ± 0.3	0.19	0.37
Vocalizations, % of pigs counted	.	1.7 ± 1.2	1.7 ± 1.2	2.0 ± 1.2	0.63	0.01
Slips and falls, % of pigs counted	.	0.6 ± 0.4	0.9 ± 0.4	0.6 ± 0.4	0.51	0.05
Stress signs, % of pigs counted	.	7.2 ± 1.4	6.0 ± 1.6	5.7 ± 1.4	0.35	0.31

[1] Sprinkling methods, applied by researchers were: bedding only (bedding already being damp or being watered down by the researcher for 4–6 min before the start of loading), pigs only (pigs being watered after loading completed for 6–8 min when the bedding on the trailer was dry before loading started), pigs and bedding (both pigs and bedding being watered).

[2] Pig measures were: surface temperature (measured laterally near the midline with a dual laser infrared thermometer on 10 pigs/load), vocalizations (an extended sound of high amplitude and frequency produced with an open mouth [2], slips (a knee or hock touching the ground) and falls (a pig's body touching the ground [14]) and stress signs (open mouth breathing, muscle tremors, and red-blotchy skin [15]).

[3] Warm weather was defined as the temperature < 26.7 °C; based on 51 loads.

[4] Hot weather was defined as the temperature ≥ 26.7 °C; based on 86 loads.

[a,b,c] Values within the same row without common superscripts differed ($p \leq 0.05$).

Pig vocalizations are a non-invasive measure and which may indicate the distress [17–19]. Kiley [17] has described 13 different types of pig vocalizations being expressed at different ages and within a variety of situations, for example social-greeting or non-social-startle. Furthermore, studies have found that squeal type vocalizations are associated with unpleasant situations [17,18,20]. Although vocalizations were not different in the context of this study between bedding levels, they may still be a useful non-invasive measure when assessing how pigs are coping with the transport process.

The current study observed surface temperature ranging 29.3 °C to 36.2 °C in WARM weather and 30.1 °C to 38.7 °C in HOT weather (Figures 1 and 2). Although past research reported surface temperature for market weight pigs ranging between 38.6 °C to 39.5 °C [21,22], a review by Fox [23] in Canada reported that sprinkled pigs had 10% lower surface temperature than those pigs which were not sprinkled. Based on the surface temperatures seen in this study, it seems pigs in this study were not heat stressed and in turn this may indicate that the pigs' physiological responses combined with the sprinkling treatments could be effective at mitigating heat stress.

3.1.2. Bedding Moisture

Fresh bedding averaged ~5% moisture before any sprinkling treatments were applied. After sprinkling treatments had been applied and one load of pigs had been transported to the plant, bedding only and bedding and pigs sprinkling treatments had ~5% more moisture than pigs only or control treatments. However, when ≥2 loads had been transported, bedding moisture held constant at ~65% regardless of sprinkling treatment (Table 2).

Table 2. Experiment 1. Bedding moisture [1] by sprinkling method [2] combined WARM [3] and HOT [4] weather.

	Sprinkling treatment							
	Control		Bedding only		Pigs only		Bedding and pigs	
	Bedding moisture (%)							
Loads	**Mean**	**SD**	**Mean**	**SD**	**Mean**	**SD**	**Mean**	**SD**
0	5.5	1.5	3.7	.	7.6	5.3	4.5	.
1	63.3	6.2	68.8	8.2	62.5	15.2	70.6	8.7
2	63.2	5.4	65.4	5.2	63.6	11	73.1	9.4
3	62.5	4.2	59.4	6.4	70.1	9.4	62.8	8.3
≥4	60.6	2	61.7	7.3	70.7	5	68.4	5.3

[1] There were 27 samples collected from trailers given the control treatment: 0 loads, n = 2; 1 load, n = 14; 2 loads, n = 6; 3 loads, n = 2; and ≥4 loads, n = 3. There were 58 samples taken from trailers given the pigs only treatment: 0 loads, n = 1; 1 load, n = 26; 2 loads, n = 11; 3 loads, n = 11; and ≥4 loads, n = 6. There were 25 samples collected from trailers given the bedding only treatment: 0 loads, n = 1; 1 load, n = 6; 2 loads, n = 9; 3 loads, n = 5; and ≥4 loads, n = 4. There were 38 samples taken from trailers given the pigs and bedding treatment: 0 loads, n = 1; 1 load, n = 12; 2 loads, n = 10; 3 loads, n = 6; and ≥4 loads, n = 9. Bedding moisture was calculated by: [(dry bedding weight)/(wet bedding weight)] × 100.

[2] Sprinkling treatments were defined as: control (no water on pigs, bedding dry), pigs only (bedding dry, pigs watered for 6–8 min), bedding only (bedding already wet or bedding watered for 4–6 min), and bedding and pigs (both pigs and bedding wetted as previously described).

[3] WARM weather was defined as <26.7 °C; based on 50 loads.

[4] HOT weather was defined as ≥26.7 °C; based on 92 loads.

Lack of increasing moisture with subsequent loads suggests that only fresh bedding is effective at moisture absorbance. This study only observed trailers with wood shavings. Wood shavings are less absorbent than straw or corn stover (1.15 *vs.* 1.97 *vs.* 2.70 mean absorbency factor, respectively; [24,25]. Data from this study supports the TQA guidelines, suggesting trailers should be washed out and fresh bedding applied after every load [6], which may also help with better traction for the pigs [26], improve biosecurity [27] and may decrease stress [28–30]. However, individual company protocols vary on washout frequency and application of fresh bedding. Trailer wash out can range from \$15 to \$190 [31]. Annually, washing out trailers between each load and re-bedding the trailer has been estimated to cost ~\$8 to \$108 million annually [32]. However, this estimate does not include potential lost income to the driver while washing the trailer or environmental implications for water usage and bedding disposal. In addition, using three instead of six bags in warm weather (defined as temperature ranging 16.1 °C to 43.4 °C) has been estimated to save \$13 million [32]. Hence, adding the cost of washout, Kephart and others [32] found that using three bags/trailer and washing out after every load would cost between ~\$22 and \$121 million annually. A cost benefit analysis for using fresh bedding after every load, in relation to overall swine well-being improvements is suggested.

3.1.3. Transport Events

The mean loading times in this study (Table 3) were similar to previous studies by Gesing and others [15] and Brown and colleagues [33] at 38 min and 45 min respectively. Mean unloading time in the current study was also similar to Gesing and others [15] at 18 min. Transport time was about double for that reported by Gesing and others (59 min [15]), but comparable to Pilcher and others (107 min [34]). A possible explanation for this increased transport time in the current study was the distance between the farms and the plant (ranging from 74 to 296 km). The plant used by Gesing and others [15] was 85 km from the farm. The wait time at the plant observed in this study was longer than that reported by Gesing and others (9 min [15]). However, Pilcher and colleagues [34] and Gesing and colleagues [35] reported a mean wait time of ~21 min. Wait time can be affected by a variety of factors such as time of arrival and labor availability at the plant. A wait of ~20 min is very acceptable for the U.S. swine industry and within the context of this study was not detrimental to pig well-being. Transport event times will need to be carefully reviewed by trucking companies, processing facilities, and the truckers themselves due to changes made by the U.S. Department of Transportation (DOT). As of July 1st, 2013, the DOT hours-of-service safety regulation states that after 8 h of driving the trucker must take a 30 min break away from the truck [36]. For transportation of non-animate goods this will likely not be a challenge. However, if live animals are being transported, increased time when the trailer is stationary can result in an increased in both temperature and relative humidity [37].

Table 3. Experiment 1. Descriptive statistics for transport events [1] for sprinkling method in market weight pigs for both WARM [2] and HOT [3] weather.

WARM weather; Event, min	Mean	SD [4]	Min [5]	Max [6]
Loading	32	12	14	65
Wait time at farm	7	6	2	42
Transport	156	43	63	280
Wait time at plant	15	13	1	50
Unloading	15	6	5	36
Total time	230	52	126	390
HOT weather				
Loading	28	11	13	65
Wait time at farm	9	4	1	19
Transport	168	41	48	255
Wait time at plant	24	15	5	65
Unloading	24	15	5	65
Total time	238	62	56	369

1 Transport events were loading (the time from when the first pig stepped on to the trailer until the last pig stepped onto the trailer), wait time at the farm (the time from when the last pig stepped onto the trailer until the trailer left the farm), transport (the time from when the trailer left the farm was closed until the truck arrived at the plant), wait time at the plant was defined as the time from when the truck arrived at the plant until the first pig stepped off), unloading (the time from the first pig stepped off the trailer until the last pig stepped off the trailer the trailer).

2 WARM weather was defined as <26.7 °C; based on 50 loads.

3 HOT weather was defined as ≥26.7 °C; based on 92 loads.

4 SD abbreviation for standard deviation.

5 Min abbreviation for minimum.

6 Max abbreviation for maximum.

3.1.4. Temperature Humidity Index

In WARM and HOT weather, with increasing THI at unloading pig surface temperature increased ($p < 0.01$; Figures 1 and 2). In WARM weather, as THI increased from ~17 to 19, surface temperature increased ~7 °C. In HOT weather, as THI increased from ~20 to 24, surface temperature increased ~9 °C.

In WARM weather, no THI effects were observed at unloading on vocalizations, slips and falls, or stress signs ($p = 0.19$, $R^2 = 0.04$; $p = 0.15$, $R^2 = 0.10$; and $p = 0.44$, $R^2 = 0.03$, respectively; data not presented). In HOT weather, there were no THI observed effects on vocalizations or slips and falls ($p = 0.96$, $R^2 = 0.01$; $p = 0.40$, $R^2 = 0.05$; data not presented).

Figure 1. Experiment 1. Effects of temperature humidity index (THI) at unloading on surface temperature of market weight pigs at unloading in WARM weather (<26.7 °C; $p < 0.01$, $R^2 = 0.41$).

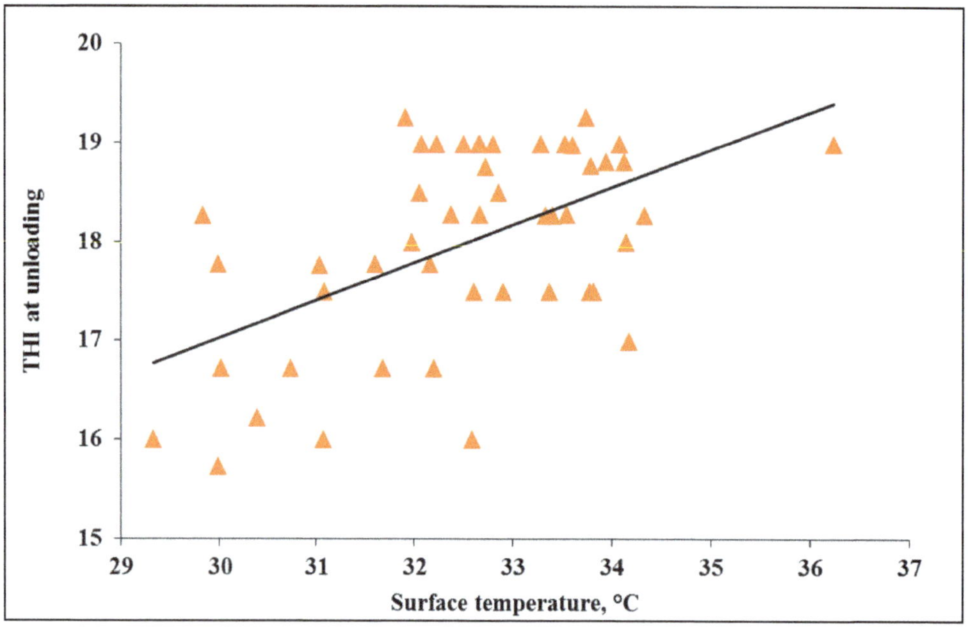

Figure 2. Experiment 1. Effects of THI at unloading on surface temperature of market weight pigs at unloading in HOT weather (≥26.7 °C; $p < 0.01$, $R^2 = 0.35$).

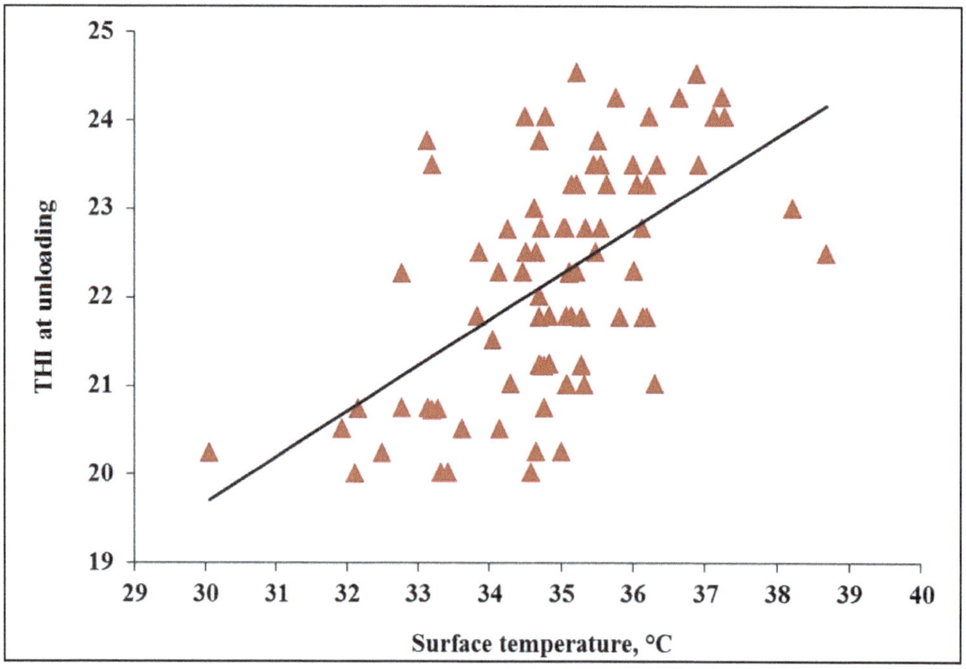

However, it was observed in HOT weather that as THI increased from ~20 to 24, stress signs at unloading increased ~27% ($p < 0.01$, Figure 3). Increased stress signs, such as open mouth breathing and red blotchy skin, could be explained by the pig's natural heat coping mechanisms. Although surface temperature ranges seen in this study are not reflective of severely heat stressed pigs this may simply mean that their physiological mechanisms were acting effectively. It is difficult to speculate as to why an increase in THI would increase slips and falls. It may be that pigs are motivated to exit the trailer quicker and hence lose their footing more because of the heat in the trailer. However, this theory would need to be further evaluated in controlled heat and behavioral studies.

Figure 3. Experiment 1. Effects of THI at unloading on stress signs of market weight pigs at unloading in HOT weather (≥26.7 °C; $p < 0.01$, $R^2 = 0.31$).

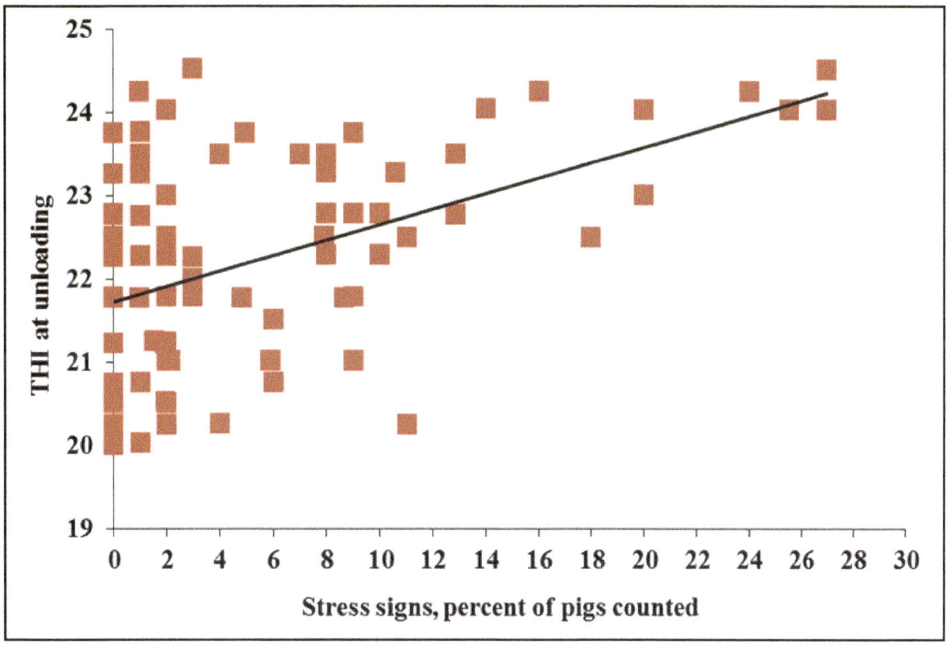

3.1.5. Density

In WARM weather, no density effects were observed on surface tempearture, vocalizations, slips and falls, or stress signs ($p = 0.45$, $R^2 = 0.41$ and $p = 0.39$, $R^2 = 0.04$; $p = 0.15$, $R^2 = 0.10$; and $p = 0.98$, $R^2 = 0.03$, respectively; data not presented). In HOT weather, no effects of density were observed on surface temperature or vocalizations ($p = 0.74$, $R^2 = 0.37$; and $p = 0.36$, $R^2 = 0.01$, respectively; data not presented).

In HOT weather as density increased from ~275 to 300 kg/m^2, slips and falls tended to decrease ~5% ($p = 0.07$, $R^2 = 0.10$; data no presented) and stress signs tended to also decrease ~27% ($p = 0.07$, $R^2 = 0.03$; data no presented). Pigs in the current study were transported at an average density of 297 and 294 m^2/pig in WARM and HOT weather respectively, but the density equation used factored in weight and number of pigs on the trailer and was presented as a continous variable. This may be why the stress results in the current work disagree with Ritter and others [9] who reported that pigs transported at 0.52 m^2/pig (~252 kg/m^2) had a higher incidence of skin discoloration than pigs transported at 0.39, 0.42, or 0.46 m^2/pig (~336, 312, and 285 kg/m^2 respectively). Direct comparisons for changes in pig surface temperature based on density have not been published. Ritter and others [38] reported that density on the trailer had no effect on rectal temperature between 265 kg/m^2 (0.39 m^2/pig) and 333 kg/m^2 (0.49 m^2/pig) kg/m^2 respectively. Chung and others noted as rectal temperature increased surface temperature increased in a linear manner [21]. This raises an interesting statistical discussion in regards to fixed effects and covariates, the use of both density and THI equations and in turn results, making comparison of these data sets challenging.

3.1.6. Bedding Level

In WARM weather, no effects of bedding were observed on surface temperature, vocalizations, slips and falls, or stress signs ($p \geq 0.12$; Table 4). In HOT weather, no effects of bedding were observed on vocalizations or slips and falls ($p \geq 0.28$; Table 4). However, in HOT weather, increasing bedding from two to three bags/trailer increased surface temperatures 0.6 °C and stress signs 2.5 % ($p \leq 0.05$; Table 4). This may indicate that in hot weather extra bedding may exacerbate heat stressed experienced by pigs on the trailer.

Table 4. Experiment 1. Effects of bedding level [1] on pig measures [2] in market weight pigs in WARM [3] and HOT [4] weather.

	Bedding level			
WARM weather; measures	**3**	**4**	***p*-value**	**R^2**
	n = 41	**n = 10**		
Surface temperature, °C	32.3 ± 0.4	32.9 ± 0.6	0.12	0.41
Vocalizations, % of pigs counted	3.0 ± 1.7	2.6 ± 1.8	0.59	0.04
Slips and falls, % of pigs counted	0.5 ± 0.2	0.4 ± 0.3	0.72	0.10
Stress signs, % of pigs counted	1.1 ± 0.3	1.5 ± 0.5	0.42	0.03
HOT weather	**n = 67**	**n = 19**		
Surface temperature, °C	34.7 ± 0.2	35.3 ± 0.3	0.05	0.37
Vocalizations, % of pigs counted	1.9 ± 1.2	1.7 ± 1.2	0.56	0.01
Slips and falls, % of pigs counted	0.7 ± 0.4	0.6 ± 0.4	0.77	0.05
Stress signs, % of pigs counted	5.1 ± 1.3	7.6 ± 1.6	0.03	0.31

1 Bedding level is the number of ~0.2 m^3 (22.7 kg) bags of wood shavings/trailer.

2 Pig measures were: surface temperature (measured laterally near the midline with a dual laser infrared thermometer on 10 pigs/load), vocalizations (extended sounds of high amplitude and frequency produced with an open mouth [2]), slips and falls (a knee, hock, or body touching the ground [14]), and stress signs (open mouth breathing, muscle tremors, and red-blotchy skin [15]).

3 WARM weather was defined as the temperature <26.7 °C; based on 48 loads.

4 HOT weather was defined as the temperature ≥26.7 °C; based on 88 loads.

3.2. Experiment 2: Effects of Sprinkling Inside Trailers on Market Weight Pig Transport Losses During WARM and HOT Weather

3.2.1. Sprinkling

In WARM weather, the one non-ambulatory pig was from a trailer allocated to the pigs and bedding sprinkling treatment. In WARM and HOT weather, no effect of sprinkling treatment was observed for non-ambulatory, dead, or total transport losses ($p \geq 0.18$; Table 5). It is important to note that total transport losses in the present study were ~0.17 pigs/trailer or ~0.10%. Additionally, when comparing the total transport loses percentages from the present study with losses on a national level, the estimated national average for total losses was 0.69% [38]. If a higher rate of losses were seen in this study there may have been bigger differences between the treatments allowing for significance.

Table 5. Experiment 2. Effects of sprinkling [1] on transport losses [2] in market weight pigs in WARM [3] and HOT [4] weather.

WARM weather; transport losses, pigs/trailer	Sprinkling Treatment				p-value	R^2
	Control n = 48	Pigs only n = 11	Bedding only n = 15	Pigs and bedding n = 8		
Non-ambulatory	.	.	.	.	.	.
Dead	0.06 ± 0.04	0.13 ± 0.11	0.11 ± 0.09	0.00 ± 0.00	0.76	0.01
Total transport losses	0.06 ± 0.04	0.24 ± 0.15	0.13 ± 0.10	0.00 ± 0.01	0.33	0.03
HOT weather	**n = 0**	**n = 31**	**n = 9**	**n = 14**		
Non-ambulatory	.	0.07 ± 0.04	0.00 ± 0.00	0.01 ± 0.02	0.28	0.32
Dead	.	0.37 ± 0.10	0.21 ± 0.14	0.16 ± 0.09	0.31	0.27
Total transport losses	.	0.45 ± 0.11	0.18 ± 0.12	0.19 ± 0.10	0.18	0.35

[1] Sprinkling methods, applied by researchers were: Control (no water sprinkled and bedding dry; not applied in HOT weather), bedding only (bedding already being damp or wetted for 4–6 min before the start of loading), pigs only (pigs being wetted after loading completed for 6–8 min when the bedding was dry), pigs and bedding (both pigs and bedding being watered).

[2] Transport losses were non-ambulatory (sum of fatigued and injured pigs), dead (sum of euthanized- and dead on arrival), and total transport losses (sum of non-ambulatory and dead).

[3] WARM weather was defined as the temperature <26.7 °C; based on 79 loads.

[4] HOT weather was defined as the temperature ≥26.7 °C; based on 49 loads.

3.2.2. Temperature Humidity Index

In WARM weather, the one non-ambulatory pig occurred when THI was 18. In WARM weather, no THI at loading effects were observed were observed on dead or total transport losses ($p = 0.94$, $R^2 = 0.01$; $p = 0.90$, $R^2 = 0.03$; data not presented). In HOT weather, no THI effects were observed at loading on non-ambulatory, dead, or total transport losses ($p = 0.66$, $R^2 = 0.32$; $p = 0.12$, $R^2 = 0.27$; $p = 0.19$, $R^2 = 0.35$; data not presented). Pigs in the current study were only transported in the summer months. This may explain why the results differ from Fitzgerald and colleagues [7] who observed more pigs than the current study in all seasons. Fitzgerald and colleagues reported [7] increased total transport losses as both THI and density increased. Additionally, they observed higher numbers of transport losses (1.41 total transport losses pigs/trailer) than were observed in the current study (in WARM 0.14 total transport losses pigs/load; in HOT weather 0.25 total transport losses pigs/load). It is difficult to compare the results found in the current study with other studies because other studies use temperature and relative humidity separately rather than in as an index [8,34,38,39].

3.2.3. Density

In WARM weather, the one non-ambulatory occurred on a trailer with a density of 291 kg/m^2. In WARM weather, no effects of density were observed on dead or total transport losses ($p = 0.86$, $R^2 = 0.01$; $p = 0.81$, $R^2 = 0.03$; data not presented). In HOT weather, no effects of density were observed on non-ambulatory pigs ($p = 0.01$, $R^2 = 0.32$; Figure 4). In HOT weather, decreasing density from ~300 to 265 kg/m^2 increased dead pigs/trailer by 2 ($p = 0.01$; Figure 5). In HOT weather, decreasing density from ~300 to 240 kg/m^2 increased total transport losses by four pigs/trailer

($p < 0.01$; Figure 6). However the relationship between both dead and total transport losses and density was weak ($R^2 = 0.27$ and $R^2 = 0.35$, respectively). It is difficult to explain why dead and total transport losses increased with decreasing density, but pigs in this study were transported at similar density ranges compared to previous studies [7–9].

Figure 4. Experiment 2. Effects of density on trailers on non-ambulatory pigs per trailer in market weight pigs at unloading in HOT weather (≥26.7 °C; $p = 0.01$, $R^2 = 0.32$).

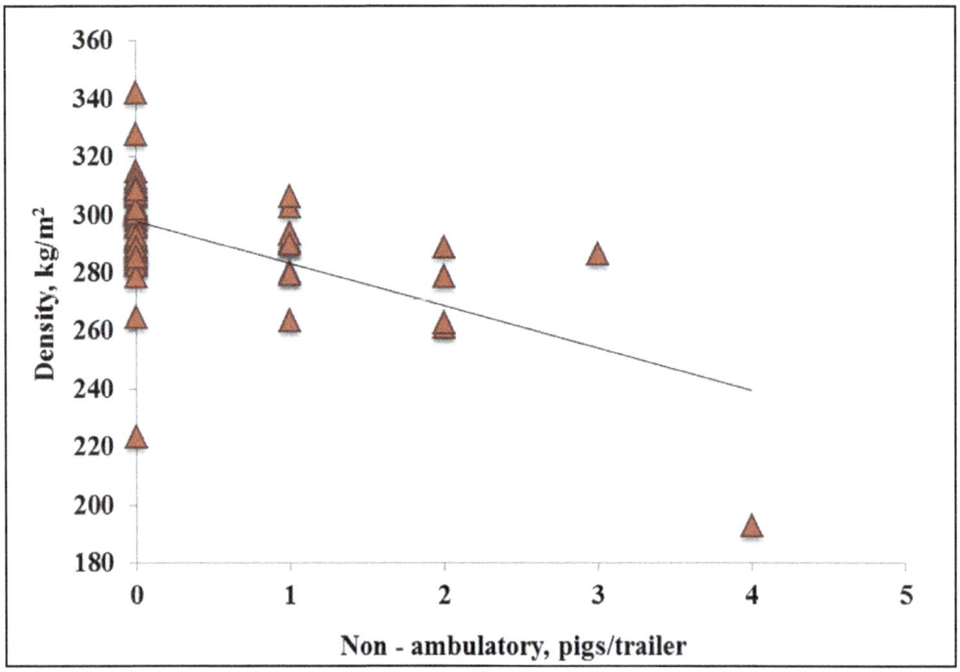

Figure 5. Experiment 2. Effects of density on trailers on dead pigs per trailer in market weight pigs at unloading in HOT weather (≥26.7 °C; $p = 0.01$, $R^2 = 0.27$).

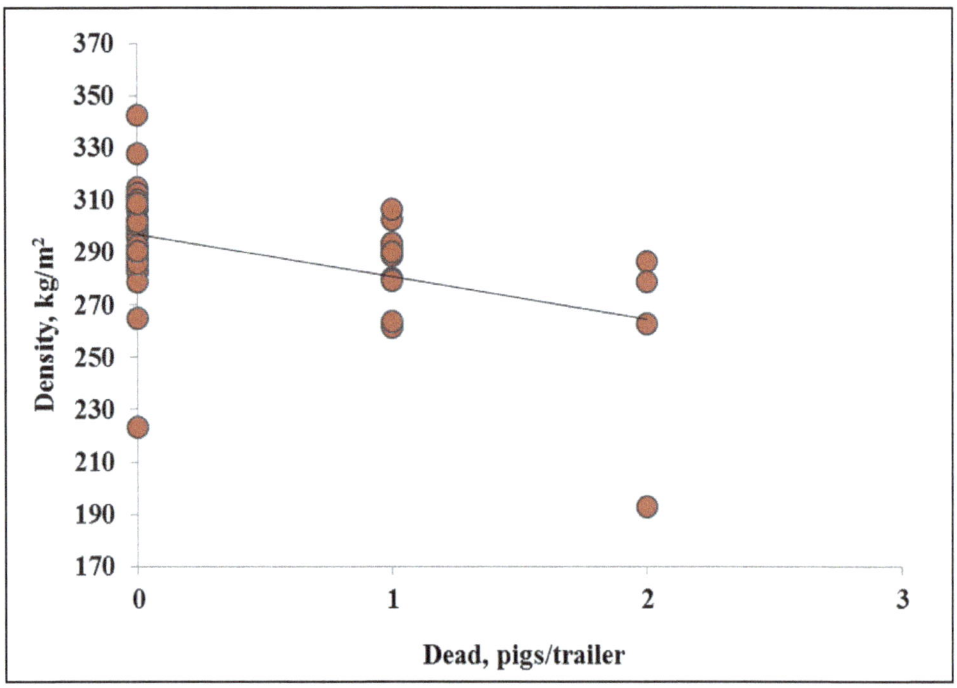

Figure 6. Experiment 2. Effects of density on trailers on total transport losses pigs per trailer in market weight pigs at unloading in HOT weather (≥26.7 °C; $p < 0.01$, $R^2 = 0.36$).

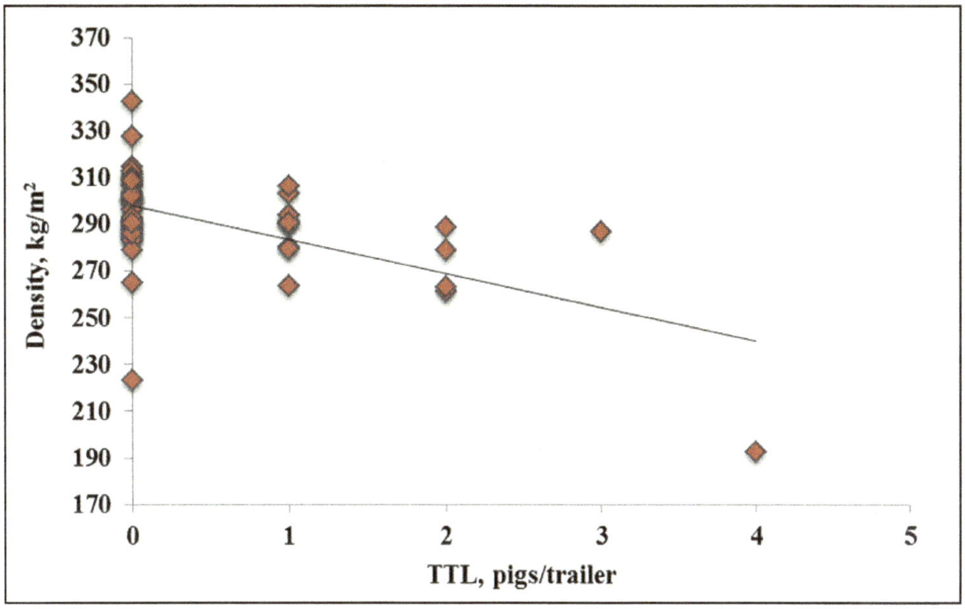

The current study reviewed a relatively small number of loads compared to past studies [7,8] and also observed a lower rate of transport losses [7–9] than previous work. This may explain why the results in the current study disagree with past studies. Pilcher and colleagues [34] found no effects of density on dead or total losses in pigs transported in November, December, May, and June. However, Pilcher and colleagues used density as a treatment and it was fixed rather than continous. Fitzgerald and colleagues [7] predicted that total transport losses would increase constantly as density increased. Ritter and colleagues [8] found that increasing density increased non-ambulatory and total transport losses. Ritter and others [9] reported increasing density increased non-ambulatory and total transport losses.

4. Conclusions

Stressors during transportation have been shown to be additive [7,40]. Therefore, reducing or preventing stressors may improve pig well-being. A variety of factors may influence animal based measures indicative of well-being and transport losses in the market weight pigs. Although the current study did not find any observed sprinkling effects for pig measures or transport losses it is extremely important to note that the inference space of this study is relatively small (July in Iowa), so further studies should be conducted to see if these results are applicable to other geographical regions and seasons.

Acknowledgments

Thank you to the plant and farms that participated, to the National Pork Board's Pork Checkoff program for funding, to Adrianne Kaiser, Avi Sapkota, David Smith, Jordann Wenzel, Kimberly Guay, and Rebecca Moest for data collection and to Nicholas Gabler for use of lab facilities and Martha Jeffery for assistance in the lab.

Author Contributions

J.M. and A.J. designed the experiment and had creative input into the writing. K.S. oversaw the statistical analysis and had creative input into the writing. R.K. collected the field data, conducted the statistical analysis and was the primary author on this paper. A.S. collected the field data and had creative input into the writing.

Conflicts of Interest

The authors declare no conflict of interest.

References and Notes

1. National Agriculture Statistics Service. Statistics by Subject: National Statistics for Hogs 2007–2012. 2013. Available online: http://www.nass.usda.gov/StatisticsbySubject/result.php?E9F60C8F-1297-3C82-AA04-BE07020602E&sector=ANIMALS%20%26%20PRODUCTS&group=LIVESTOCK&comm=HOGS (accessed on 15 June 2013).
2. Johnson, A.K.; Gesing, L.M.; Ellis, M.; McGlone, J.J.; Berg, E.; Lonergan, S.M.; Fitzgerald, R.; Karriker, L.A.; Ramirez, A.; Stalder, K.J.; Sapkota, A.; Kephart, R.; Selsby, J.T.; Sadler, L.J.; Ritter, M.J. Farm and pig factors affecting welfare during the marketing process. *J. Anim. Sci.* **2013**, *91*, 2481–2491.
3. Benjamin, M.E.; Gonyou, H.W.; Ivers, D.J.; Richardson, L.F.; Jones, D.J.; Wagner, J.R.; Seneriz, R.; Anderson, D.B. Effect of animal handling method on the incidence of stress response in market swine in a model system. *J. Anim. Sci.* **2001**, *79*, 279.
4. Hamilton, D.N.; Ellis, M.; Bertol, T.M.; Miller, K.D. Effects of handling intensity and live weight on blood acid-base status in finishing pigs. *J. Anim. Sci.* **2004**, *82*, 2405–2409.
5. Bertol, T.M.; Ellis, M.; Ritter, M.J.; McKeith, F.K. Effect of feed withdrawal and handling intensity on longissimus muscle glycolytic potential and blood measurements in slaughter weight pigs. *J. Anim. Sci.* **2005**, *83*, 1536–1542.
6. National Pork Board. Transport Quality Assurance Handbook, Version 4. Available online: http://www.pork.org/filelibrary/TQA/manual.pdf (accessed on 3 August 2011).
7. Fitzgerald, R.F.; Stalder, K.J.; Matthews, J.O.; Schultz-Kaster, C.M.; Johnson, A.K. Factors associated with fatigue, injured, and dead pig frequency during transport and lairage at a commercial abattoir. *J. Anim. Sci.* **2009**, *87*, 1156–1166.

8. Ritter, M.J.; Ellis, M.; Brinkmann, J.; DeDecker, J.M.; Keffaber, K.K.; Kocher, M.E.; Peterson, B.A.; Schlipf, J.M.; Wolter, B.F. Effect of floor space during transport of market-weight pigs on the incidence of transport losses at the packing plant and the relationships between transport conditions and losses. *J. Anim. Sci.* **2006**, *84*, 2856–2864.
9. Ritter, M.J.; Ellis, M.; Brinkmann, J.; DeDecker, J.M.; Keffaber, K.K.; Kocher, M.E.; Peterson, B.A.; Schlipf, J.M.; Wolter, B.F. Effects of distance moved during loading and floor space on the trailer during transport on losses of market weight pigs on arrival at the packing plant. *J. Anim. Sci.* **2007**, *85*, 3454–3461.
10. National Oceanic and Atmospheric Association. *Livestock Hot Weather Stress*; U.S. Government Printing Office: Washington, DC, USA, 1976.
11. Agricultural and Biosystems Engineering. 2002. Livestock/poultry heat stress index and recommended management actions. Available online: http://www3.abe.iastate.edu/livestock/heat_stress.asp (accessed on 16 July 2013).
12. Ingram, D.L. Stimulation of cutaneous glands in the pig. *J. Comp. Physiol.* **1967**, *77*, 91–113.
13. Ingram, D.L. Adaptations to ambient temperature in growing pigs. *Pflugers Archiv-Eur. J. Physiol.* **1977**, *367*, 257–264.
14. American Meat Institute. Recommended animal handling guidelines auditing guide: A systematic approach to animal welfare. 2012. Available online: http://www.animal handling.org/ht/a/GetDocumentAction/i/80009 (accessed on 1 November 2011).
15. Gesing, L.M.; Johnson, A.K.; Selsby, J.T.; Abrams, S.; Hill, H.; Whitley, A.; Faga, A.; Bailey, R.; Stalder, K.J.; Ritter, M.J. Effects of grow-finish group size on stress responses at loading and unloading and the effect on transport losses from market-weight pigs. *Prof. Anim. Sci.* **2011**, *27*, 477–484.
16. Peters, J.; Combs, S.M.; Hoskins, B.; Jarman, J.; Kovar, J.L.; Watson, M.E.; Wolf, A.M.; Wolf, N. *Recommended Methods of Manure Analysis*; Cooperative Extension Publishing Operations: Madison, WI, USA, 2003.
17. Kiley, M. The vocalizations of ungulates, their causation and functions. *Zeitschrift für Tierpsychologie* **1972**, *31*, 171–222.
18. Xin, H.; DeShazer, A.; Leger, D.W. Pig vocalizations under selected husbandry practices. *Trans ASAE* **1990**, *32*, 2181–2184. Available online: http://digitalcommons.unl.edu/cgi/viewcontent.cgi?article=1533&context= psychfacpub (accessed on 10 October 2013).
19. Manteuffel, G.; Puppe, B.; Schön, P.C. Vocalization of farm animals as a measure of welfare. *Appl. Anim. Behav. Sci.* **2004**, *88*, 163–182.
20. Tallet, C.; Špinka, M.; Maruščáková, I.; Šimeček, P. Human perception of vocalizations of domestic piglets and modulation by experience with domestic pigs (*Sus scrofa*). *J. Comp. Psyc.* **2010**, *124*, 81–91.
21. Chung, T.; Jung, W.; Nam, E.; Kim, J.; Park, S.; Hwang, C.Y. Comparison of rectal and infrared thermometry for obtaining body temperature of gnotobiotic piglets in conventional portable germ free facility. *Asian-Aust. J. Anim. Sci.* **2010**, *23*, 1364–1368.
22. Managing and treating the sick pig. 2013. Available online: http://www.thepigsite.com/pighealth/article/48/managing-and-treating-the-sick-pig (accessed on 5 November 2013).

23. Fox, J.L. The effect of water sprinkling market weight pigs transported during summer on pig behavior, gastrointestinal tract temperature, and trailer micro-climate. 2013. Available online: https://atrium.lib.uoguelph.ca/xmlui/bitstream/handle/10214/5279/Fox_Jessica_201301_Msc.pdf?sequence=3 (accessed on 29 July 2013).
24. Voyles, R.; Honeyman, M.S. Absorbency of alternative livestock bedding sources. 2006. Available online: http://lib.dr.iastate.edu/ans_air /vol652/iss1/59/ (accessed on 1 July 2013).
25. McGlone, J.J.; Pond, W.G. *Pig Production: Biological Principles and Applications*; Delmar Learning: Clifton Park, NY, USA 2002; p. 309.
26. Sutherland, M.A.; McDonald, A.; McGlone, J.J. Effects of variations in the environment, length of journey, and type of trailer on the mortality and morbidity of pigs being transported to slaughter. *Vet. Rec.* **2009**, *165*, 13–18.
27. Environmental Contamination on the Farm. 2002. Available online: http://www.thepigsite.com/pighealth/article/628/environmental-contamination-on-the-farm (accessed on 28 June 2013).
28. Amory, J.R.; Pearce, G.P. Alarm pheromones in urine modify the behavior of weaner pigs. *Anim. Welf.* **2000**, *9*, 167–175.
29. Grandin, T. Animal welfare in slaughter plants. In Proceedings of the 29th Annual Convention of the American Association of Bovine Practitioners, San Diege, CA, USA, 12–14 September 1996.
30. Wyatt, T.D. Pheromones and animal behavior. 2003. Available online: http://catdir.loc.gov/catdir/samples/cam033/2002024628.pdf (accessed on 15 July 2013).
31. Livestock Network. Livestock Washouts. 2013. Available online: http://www.livestocknetwork.com/Livestock_Washouts/ (accessed on 2 August 2013).
32. Kephart, R.K.; Johnson, A.K.; Stalder, K.J.; Huiatt, T.W.; Sapkota, A.; McGlone, J.J. Costs of Bedding on the Trailer, Trailer Wash out, and Transport Losses in Market Weight Pigs. **2014**, in preparation.
33. Brown, J.; Stevens, T.; Gonyou, H.W. Loading facilities for market hogs. Saskatchewan's top 10. Prairie Swine Centre Annual Report 2011. Available online: http://www.prairieswine.com/wp-content/uploads/2011/07/Annual-Report-2011.pdf (accessed on 20 May 2013).
34. Pilcher, C.M.; Ellis, M.; Rojo-Gómez, A.; Curtis, S.E.; Wolter, B.F.; Peterson, C.M.; Peterson, B.A.; Ritter, M.J.; Brinkmann, J. Effects of floor space during transport and journey time on indicators of stress and transport losses of market-weight pigs. *J. Anim. Sci.* **2011**, *89*, 3809–3818.
35. Gesing, L.M. Pre-sorting and pen size effects on the stress responses at loading and unloading and transport losses in market weight pigs. M.S. Thesis, Iowa State University, Ames, IA, USA, 2010.
36. United States Department of Transportation. http://www.fmcsa.dot.gov/rules-regulations/topics/hos/statement.aspx (accessed on 12 June 2013).
37. Ellis, M.; Wang, X.; Funk, T.; Wolter, B.; Murphy, C.; Lenkaitis, A.; Sun, Y.; Pilcher, C. *Development of Improved Trailer Designs and Transport Management Practices that Create the Optimum Environment for Market Weight Pigs During Transport and Minimize Transport Losses*; National Pork Board Pork Checkoff Animal Welfare Research Report; National Pork Board: Des Moines, IA, USA, 2008.

38. Ritter, M.J.; Ellis, M.; Anderson, D.B.; Curtis, S.E.; Keffaber, K.K.; Killefer, J.; McKeith, F.K.; Murphy, C.M.; Peterson, B.A. Effects of multiple concurrent stressors on rectal temperature, blood acid-base status, and longissimus muscle glycolytic potential in market-weight pigs. *J. Anim. Sci.* **2009**, *87*, 351–362.
39. Kephart, K.B.; Harper, M.T.; Raines, C.R. Observations of market pigs following transport to a packing plant. *J. Anim. Sci.* **2010**, *88*, 2199–2203.
40. Grandin, T.; Schultz-Kaster, C. Handling pigs. Available online: http://www.porkgateway.org/FileLibrary/PIGLibrary/Factsheets/a6635v1-0.pdf (accessed on 29 July 2013).

A Prototype Tool to Enable Farmers to Measure and Improve the Welfare Performance of the Farm Animal Enterprise: The Unified Field Index

Ian G. Colditz [1,*], Drewe M. Ferguson [1], Teresa Collins [2], Lindsay Matthews [3,4] and Paul H. Hemsworth [5]

[1] CSIRO Animal, Food and Health Sciences, FD McMaster Laboratory, Armidale, NSW 2350, Australia; E-Mail: Drewe.ferguson@csiro.au
[2] College of Veterinary Medicine, Murdoch University, Murdoch, WA 6150, Australia; E-Mail: T.Collins@murdoch.edu.au
[3] Lindsay Matthews & Associates Research International, Scerne Di Pineto, Teramo 64025, Italy; E-Mail: lindsay.matthews1@gmail.com
[4] Psychology Department, University of Auckland, Auckland 1020, New Zealand
[5] Animal Welfare Science Centre, The University of Melbourne, Parkville, VIC 3010, Australia; E-Mail: phh@unimelb.edu.au

* Author to whom correspondence should be addressed; E-Mail: ian.colditz@csiro.au.

Simple Summary: Benchmarking is a tool widely used in agricultural industries that harnesses the experience of farmers to generate knowledge of practices that lead to better on-farm productivity and performance. We propose, by analogy with production performance, a method for measuring the animal welfare performance of an enterprise and describe a tool for farmers to monitor and improve the animal welfare performance of their business. A general framework is outlined for assessing and monitoring risks to animal welfare based on measures of animals, the environment they are kept in and how they are managed. The tool would enable farmers to continually improve animal welfare.

Abstract: Schemes for the assessment of farm animal welfare and assurance of welfare standards have proliferated in recent years. An acknowledged short-coming has been the lack of impact of these schemes on the welfare standards achieved on farm due in part to sociological factors concerning their implementation. Here we propose the concept of welfare performance based on a broad set of performance attributes of an enterprise and describe a tool based on risk assessment and benchmarking methods for measuring and managing welfare performance. The tool termed the Unified Field Index is presented in a general form comprising three modules addressing animal, resource, and management factors. Domains within these modules accommodate the principle conceptual perspectives for welfare assessment: biological functioning; emotional states; and naturalness. Pan-enterprise analysis in any livestock sector could be used to benchmark welfare performance of individual enterprises and also provide statistics of welfare performance for the livestock sector. An advantage of this concept of welfare performance is its use of continuous scales of measurement rather than traditional pass/fail measures. Through the feedback provided via benchmarking, the tool should help farmers better engage in on-going improvement of farm practices that affect animal welfare.

Keywords: animal welfare; assessment; unified field index; benchmarking; welfare performance

---

1. Introduction

Recent decades have seen an increase in societal interest in the management and care of animals used to produce food and fiber. Concern about the quality of life of farm animals has led to an increasing onus on farmers and on food and fiber supply chains to demonstrate that the physical and mental needs of animals are satisfied. In response, a large body of science has addressed criteria for assessing the welfare of animals. Underpinning these issues of quality of life and welfare assessment are philosophical and ethical questions about the relationships between humans and animals. These underpinning issues influence what we understand animal welfare to be and what needs to be measured or assessed in order to draw inferences about the welfare status of farm animals [1].

Three common perspectives can be recognized amongst the many approaches that have been developed to describe and measure animal welfare [2–4]. These perspectives can be summarized as understanding and interpreting welfare in terms of:

- Biological functioning—as evidenced through measures of normality of behavioral, physiological, health, and production variables;
- Emotional states—as evidenced through measures of abnormal behaviors, affective states (positive and negative feelings), cognitive function, and suffering.
- Naturalness—as evidenced by attributes of the animal, in particular normal behavioral repertoires, and by attributes of its environment, in particular congruence between the production environment and a notional ideal environment for the species or class of animal.

An important feature of these perspectives for understanding animal welfare is that they provide multiple dimensions for describing welfare in terms of the animal's status and the environment it experiences. A comprehensive welfare assessment system is therefore likely to need measures that inform each of these perspectives. Definitions of animal welfare developed in recent years, such as the one recently endorsed by the 172 member countries of the office international des epizooties (OIE) [5], encompass aspects of these three perspectives: "Animal welfare means how an animal is coping with the conditions in which it lives. An animal is in a good state of welfare if (as indicated by scientific evidence) it is healthy, comfortable, well nourished, safe, able to express innate behaviour, and if it is not suffering from unpleasant states such as pain, fear, and distress. Good animal welfare requires disease prevention and veterinary treatment, appropriate shelter, management, nutrition, humane handling and humane slaughter/killing. Animal welfare refers to the state of the animal; the treatment that an animal receives is covered by other terms such as animal care, animal husbandry, and humane treatment".

There are generic challenges to choosing the measures to include in assessment systems that are not unique to animal welfare. For instance, in the design of methods for assessing agricultural sustainability, Binder *et al.* [6] have noted that assessment models should aim for parsimony and sufficiency, and account for interactions between indicators used in the model. Thus, simplicity in the type and number of measures included in an index (parsimony) needs to be balanced against adequacy of the chosen measures to capture critical information needed to make a valid assessment (sufficiency). These design requirements for an effective sustainability assessment tool apply equally to assessment of animal welfare. Thus parsimony and sufficiency can be considered important attributes of an efficient animal welfare assessment system.

The key elements of a welfare assessment system that emerge from the above considerations include:

- The conceptual and ethical perspectives for understanding and describing welfare
- The purpose for undertaking the welfare assessment
- The process for implementing and evaluating the assessment procedure.

In this paper, we describe an assessment tool for use by farmers to manage and improve the welfare performance of their farm animal enterprise. The tool is designed to be refined and managed by farm animal industries. It uses data from farm records to generate industry wide statistics on variables relating to animal welfare. It encourages farmers to consider many of these variables to be performance criteria that, analogous to production criteria like milk yield or growth rate, can be measured on a continuous scale and improved upon from year to year. It harnesses the experience of high performing farmers to identify strategies for ongoing improvement in these variables of welfare performance. It places ownership of welfare performance in the hands of farmers. It differentiates welfare performance measured via the tool from welfare standards implemented through welfare assessment schemes to ensure compliance with regulatory standards. Before describing the tool in more detail and addressing the specific purposes of the tool, we need to consider more generally the range of purposes for which welfare assessments are undertaken.

2. Purposes of Welfare Assessment

The need to apply objective methods to assess the welfare status of farm animals usually arises in one of three settings, which align to three specific purposes:

- *Compliance*: To determine compliance with policy, law, and regulatory standards;
- *Market assurance*: To assure both consumers and non-consumers that certain aspects of the welfare of animals, especially those not articulated within 1, are being met, for instance freedom to roam in an outdoor environment or absence of suffering;
- *Welfare management*: To assist owners and managers to monitor and improve the welfare of their livestock

These purposes can be summarized as compliance, market assurance, and welfare management. In fulfilling these purposes the assessment procedures require validity of the measures as indicators of welfare, congruence between the measures and the aspects of welfare under appraisal, and integrity of the assessment procedure. Schemes designed to address compliance and market assurance have a very high dependence on measures that have been validated through research or through processes that generate a consensus of expert opinion. The external focus of compliance and market assurance schemes towards the needs of regulators and consumers means the outcome of assessment is usually graded into various categories such as acceptable or unacceptable. A risk of presenting the outcome of assessment in this way is the failure to provide appropriate feedback, direction or incentive for farmers to continually improve the welfare status of animals on their farms (see [7] for a discussion of this dilemma). Thus, compliance and market assurance schemes might measure welfare status but not provide clear directions on how to improve animal welfare.

These limitations have been revealed in a number of studies. The impact of the Royal Society for the Prevention of Cruelty to Animals (RSPCA) Freedom Food scheme on the welfare of dairy cattle was studied and outcomes of measures compared between farms belonging to the Freedom Food scheme or other schemes [8]. The Freedom Food farms performed worse on some measures including hock injuries, lameness, and restrictions in rising behavior, but better on measures of mastitis, cleanliness, and body condition. Importantly, regardless of the scheme, welfare problems remained prevalent indicating that measuring compliance alone is insufficient to ensure good welfare [9]. The Scottish Agricultural College [10] compared the welfare of dairy cows in organic and conventional milk production systems and showed that levels of lameness and hock damage were lower on organic farms as a result of shorter winter housing periods and a higher age of first calving heifers which are both elements of the less intensive housing approach described in organic standards. Thus, while compliance with specific standards in farm assurance schemes may lead to some improvement in animal welfare [9] there is little compelling evidence that such schemes produce comprehensive or continuous advances in welfare.

2.1. The Need for Tools to Assist Farmers Manage and Improve Animal Welfare

The inadequacy of welfare assessment procedures that address compliance and market assurance purposes to lead to welfare improvements points to the need for a separate set of assessment tools to assist farmers in this task. Recognition of the need for such tools is not new and a number of well-developed aids are available to help farmers manage specific welfare and health risks. An example of the detail provided by such aids can be found in the cattle heat load toolbox [11] which enables managers of commercial beef cattle feedlots in Australia to use a combination of input and output measures to predict and manage heat stress events. By using a combination of observed local climatic conditions and animal responses to heat such as panting scores, feedlot managers can manage risks and implement strategies to reduce the impact of severe hot weather [12]. Additional indices, namely the heat load index (HLI) and the accumulated heat load (AHL) determine the animals' heat load balance taking into account the duration of daily heat exposure and the availability of natural cooling at night [12]. Using a web-based model that incorporates the HLI and AHL indices, feedlot managers can determine specific heat risk assessments for different cattle genotypes on a daily and pen-by-pen basis if required. This tool combines the well quantified physiological impact of heat stress on beef cattle with environmental data to establish criteria for intervention; however, as the impact of heat stress on the animal's experience and its affective state remain unknown [13], the extent to which the tool addresses the impact of heat load on the emotional dimension of animal welfare is not known. The web-based suite of programs named Paraboss [14], which was developed as an aid in the management of the major parasite risks to sheep in Australia, provides another example of health and welfare related tools addressing the needs of farmers.

2.2. Benchmarking as an On-Farm Tool for Welfare Assessment

Problems of communication and technology transfer are at the heart of the deficiencies in welfare assessment procedures undertaken for compliance and assurance purposes in addressing the needs of farmers [15]. In the 1970s, agricultural extension officers began exploring alternatives to top-down communication to farmers as a means of gaining better engagement. In particular, methods then under development for improving business management through benchmarking were trialed [16]. These methods involve learning from the practical experience of businesses by comparing performance between businesses to identify best practices. More recently, versions of benchmarking as an approach to helping farmers manage welfare of their animals have been explored through health and welfare planning programs on organic farms in Europe [15], dairy cow comfort in North America [17], pig tail health in Sweden [18], and road transport practices in North America [19]. In 2013, a program of benchmarking grazing best management practice was introduced for beef cattle producers in the Fitzroy river basin of central Queensland [20]. The voluntary program includes an animal health and welfare module and uses self-assessment of management practices against industry standards. In its simplest form, benchmarking compares performance between industries to describe in statistical terms the range and average of outcomes achieved. In more detailed studies, it also identifies business practices associated with superior performance as exemplars that lower performing business might adopt. Benchmarking programs in a range of cereal grains and horticulture industries have proven highly successful for identifying best practices used by leading producers that enable fellow producers to improve performance [16,21]. These successes in cropping industries illustrate the potential for benchmarking to deliver benefits to livestock welfare management.

2.3. A Role for Risk Assessment in Welfare Management

Another approach to the development of tools for on farm management of animal welfare has been the use of risk assessments of the hazards that pose potential threats to welfare [22,23]. This strategy adopts the standard methodology of risk assessment that starts with identification of hazards then involves quantification of their likelihoods and potential impacts in terms of intensity, duration, and prevalence, in order to establish the need for monitoring and managing the risks. The European Food Safety Authority has developed risk assessment systems for a number of farm animal species and production systems for the dairy, chicken, meat, pig, beef cattle, and fish farming industries. A recent trend in agricultural benchmarking programs has been the combination of standard benchmarking procedures with risk assessment and risk management practices to provide both an aid to farm managers for the improvement of on-farm practices and a system for market assurance of farm practices and product quality [21]. Documentation of risk assessments, farm practices and monitoring procedures are important components of benchmarking and assurance schemes and provides a basis for internal and external auditing of the schemes. Cereal and horticultural industries have preceded livestock industries in adoption of this approach [24,25]; although use of risk assessment in livestock management is expanding. For instance, assessment of heat stress risk is a requirement for accreditation of feedlots in Australia [26].

3. A Unified Field Index for Managing Animal Welfare Performance On-Farm

To address the apparent shortcomings of current animal welfare assessment processes to assist farmers to manage welfare, we propose an approach for on-farm welfare management built around risk assessment, across enterprise benchmarking of welfare performance outcomes and external auditing. What follows is a provisional framework designed with a broad scope that might be applicable to all livestock sectors. The framework consists of assessment on a suite of domains that together with a process constitutes a new tool for livestock managers to monitor and improve the welfare of animals in their care. In addition, the tool generates records for internal and external audits that could provide assurance of welfare performance on individual farms and across a whole livestock sector. Audits help ensure integrity of the assessment process. We describe the framework as a Unified Field Index (UFI) for assessing welfare performance in the field (*i.e.*, on farm). We envisage its implementation through three levels:

- Level 1—occurs within the enterprise and is conducted by the livestock manager. It entails risk assessment, identification of the need for corrective actions, and key variables that require monitoring and recording. Results undergo periodic (e.g., yearly) internal review and self-audit to establish the need for modification and refinement. This level of a benchmarking program typically requires training and workshops to provide participants with the necessary skills [16].
- Level 2—is an external process that undertakes across-enterprise data analysis. The data analysis provides the confidential feedback to participants in the scheme that lets them benchmark their welfare performance against that of other producers. The analysis also identifies the practices of leading producers that contribute to their superior performance. It is the heart of the benchmarking process whereby new information and knowledge of superior practices is generated from on-farm experiences. Important outcomes of this analysis are the generation of industry-wide welfare statistics, as well as the identification of welfare performance goals and strategies that lower performing producers can adopt.
- Level 3—market assurance of practices and welfare outcomes can be provided through external audit of procedures undertaken in Levels 1 and 2.

We propose three assessment modules for the UFI that address animal, resource, and management based factors that are key input contributors to, or provide outcome indicators of welfare performance. Within each module are a number of domains as listed in Table 1. The domains provide the entry point for the risk assessment and for the development of monitoring and management strategies at Level 1 of the implementation process. Implementation of the UFI is presented schematically in Figures 1 and 2.

Table 1. Assessment modules and domains of the Unified Field Index (UFI) for management of on-farm welfare performance with examples of classes and sub-classes within each domain. Classes and sub-classes need to be tailored to each particular species and production system.

Module	Domain	Class	Sub-class or measures
Animal	Behaviors	Abnormal	
		Social	Agonistic, Affiliative
		Self care	
	Health	Mortality	Number/rate, Causes, Number found dead, Number euthanized
		Morbidity	Numbers/rates, Causes
		Current status	Skeletal, Soft tissue, Coat/pelage, Demeanor
	Affect	Demeanor	Valence, arousal
		Avoidance behaviors	
	Production	Targets	Means, Variances
	Reproductive performance		
	Holistic attributes		
Resources	Feed	Food on offer	
		Quality	
	Water	Quality	
		Quantity	
	Climate	Risk of extremes	
	Social	Density	
		Group structure	
	Comfort	Bedding	
		Shelter	
	Hygiene	Housing	
		Floor	
		Animal body cleanliness	
		Health status of companions	
Management	Skills	Training/ experience	
		Attitudes	
	Husbandry practices	Methods	
		Analgesia	
		Euthanasia methods	
	Genetics management	Suitability of genetics for environment	
		Breeding objectives for welfare traits, disease resistance, temperament, conformation	Based on estimated breeding values
			Non-quantitative selection criteria
		Culling criteria	
	Records	Training	
		Husbandry	
		Vaccinations	
		Medications	
		Farm chemicals	
		Production	
		Health	
	Review and action protocols		

Figure 1. Level 1 (on farm) implementation of the UFI.

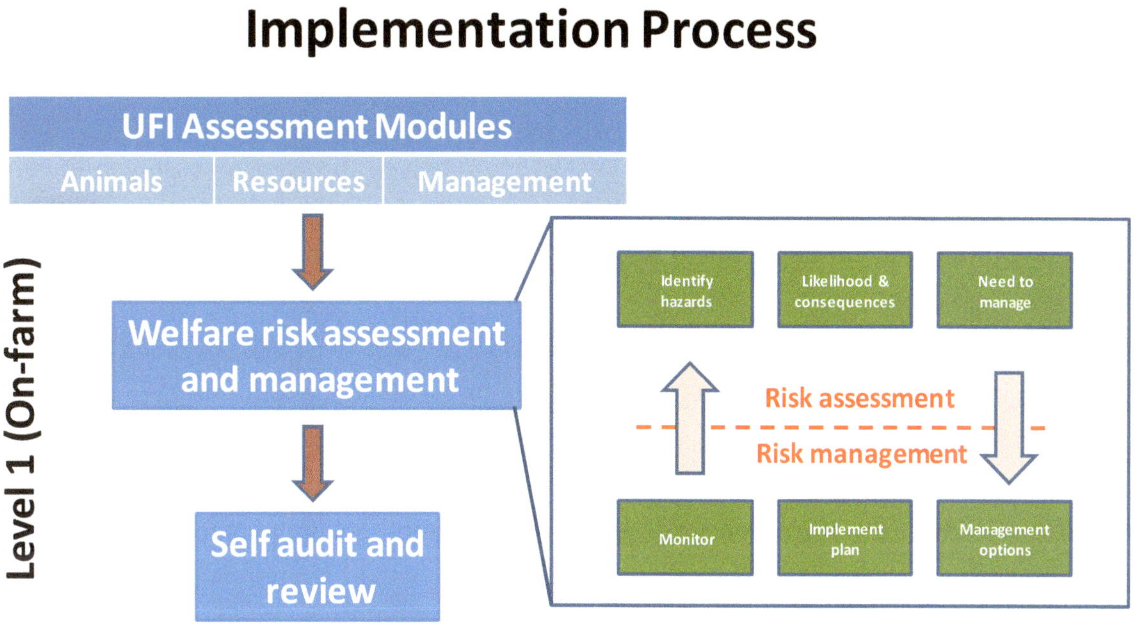

Figure 2. Schematic representation of implementation of the UFI.

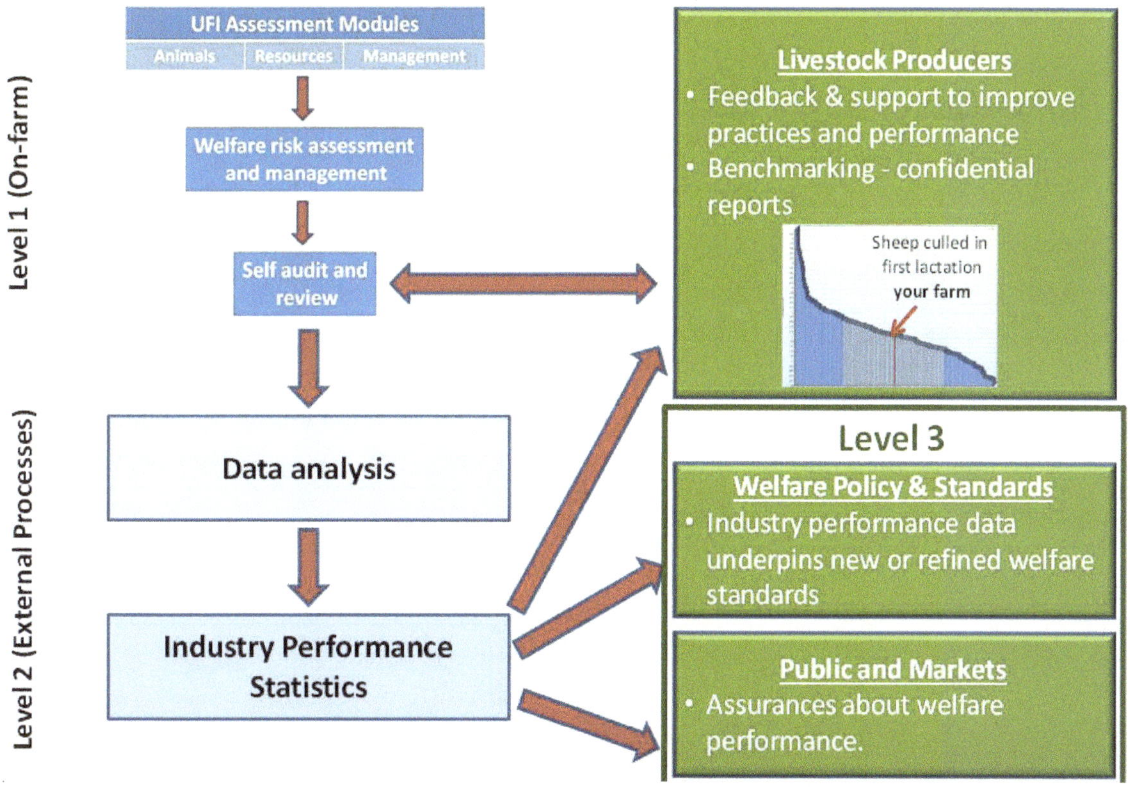

It is anticipated that co-ordination of a program for implementing the three levels of the UFI would require oversight by an industry body rather than by a regulatory authority. Indeed industry and farmer ownership of the tool and the outputs it generates is a key factor that differentiates the approach we propose here from conventional animal welfare assessments imposed on farmers though an authoritarian regulatory framework. Options for funding and management of such a program are not explored further in this paper.

4. Assessment Domains Included in the UFI

Our suggestion is that the assessment domains be largely consistent across species and production systems, although some minor modifications of the domains between species may be needed. Fine-tuning of the UFI to the nature of individual livestock species and their production systems would largely occur at the level of the class and sub-class of measures within each assessment domain. This tailoring to species and production system is analogous to the hierarchical design of the EU Welfare Quality program in which the four welfare principles (good feeding, good housing, good health, and appropriate behavior) are manifested through 12 welfare criteria which in turn are assessed through a suite of measures that are designed to be appropriate for each livestock species [27]. While the assessment domains in this general form of the UFI are broad in scope and number, it is anticipated that through the process of refinement at the industry level and implementation through the risk assessment procedure at the farm level, the number of domains to be monitored would be fine-tuned and reduced to the needs of each livestock industry, thus providing greater parsimony than is evident in the general form of the UFI. A limited number of measures would be required for each species or production system to ensure sufficiency of the process, especially to provide welfare performance statistics as described below. The use of the UFI as an assurance tool may involve meeting minimum standards within each domain. However, the integration of measures into one final score is not intended.

The domains are chosen to address the aspirational goals of the Five Freedoms [28] and the welfare principles and criteria of the EU Welfare Quality program. In addition, a number of management skills, management practices, and production criteria are included. These are described in a little more detail below. Electronic identification of individual livestock and the use of computerized records for individual animals are becoming widespread in livestock farming and create the opportunity for data collection and analysis to generate statistics of on-farm welfare performance in ways that have not been previously readily available to livestock managers. Many production variables are sensitive to stress and health status, and analysis of these variables across the whole flock or herd with particular emphasis on outliers and deviations from performance targets can provide information on welfare performance. Animal performance measures are therefore also included within the assessment domains of the UFI. The rapidly emerging electronic technologies for monitoring animals have the potential to assist farmers in the animal monitoring phase of Level 1.

4.1. Animal Module

4.1.1. Behavior Domain

Abnormal Behaviors: Animals display a range of abnormal behaviors when stressed or when exposed to adverse environmental conditions such as heat. Stereotypic (repetitive, rhythmic) behaviors are common in intensively-housed animals with impoverished environmental conditions. Fearfulness and other indicators of adverse reactivity of animals to the presence of humans that can be indicative of poor animal handling practices sit in this class.

Social behaviors: Social behaviors like mutual grooming and play are important indicators of the social health of social species like cattle, sheep, pigs, and chickens.

Self-care: Self-care is reduced in animals stressed by poor nutrition, ill health, and social bullying.

4.1.2. Health Domain

Mortality: Raw data on mortality can be criticized as being a worst case outcome of welfare management. Nonetheless, deaths do occur in well-managed livestock enterprises and the information that death rates provide about welfare management should not be ignored by livestock managers. Data on the numbers of animals found dead versus the number of animals euthanized is a valuable indicator of the level of monitoring and intervention to prevent suffering in moribund animals.

Morbidity: Disease compromises welfare, thus data on disease prevalence is central to effective disease control and good welfare management.

Current status: This domain provides the basis for visual assessment of the general health of the individual and the group. These measures are examples of ones that would be used in external audit for a snapshot of the flock or herd as well as during ongoing monitoring by the livestock manager.

4.1.3. Affect Domain

Qualitative behavioral assessment has been found to be a useful method for assessing affective states of livestock on farm [29–31]; however, the methodology is not currently suitable for application by individual observers such as livestock managers. Nonetheless, the assessment of demeanor or behavioral expression as used in clinical assessment of animals by veterinarians and by skilled livestock handlers such as pen riders in feedlots are two examples of visual assessments of behavior that most likely provide information on the emotional status of animals associated with ill health. Standardization and refinement of these measures and the development of new field-based measures of affect are needed.

4.1.4. Production Domain

Analysis of performance against production targets, especially the identification of the number of outlier animals, provides information on the level of management of the enterprise. Increased risk of disease and death in animals below the group mean for growth, body weight, and body condition is recognized in a range of species including lambs [32], dairy cows [33], pigs [34], and rainbow trout [35]. While performance against targets is not always informative of welfare, in combination with other measures, it can help provide a picture of welfare management of the enterprise. The value of these data is greatly enhanced through benchmarking. The domain does not equate good production with good welfare but recognizes that variation in production performance can be an indicator of potential welfare problems.

4.1.5. Reproductive Performance Domain

Reproductive performance is highly sensitive to stressors and diseases that affect welfare, as well as being fundamental to the profitability of the breeding enterprise, and is strongly influenced by the quality of management that animals receive and the suitability of the genotype for its environment. This class could be included with production, but is separated to emphasize the very high importance of good management of reproduction for achieving good welfare outcomes [36].

4.1.6. Holistic Domain

This assessment domain is a measure of naturalness and acknowledges philosophies which value "whole-of-animal" and "whole-of-production-system" attributes of welfare. Examples of holistic measures might include the ability of turkeys to reproduce by natural mating, and the opportunity for animals to express highly motivated behaviors such as nesting, rooting, and wallowing in pigs, dust bathing and scratching in poultry, and grazing in ruminants. It might be argued, however, that these examples are component measures that would be better captured in the behavioral domain than true holistic measures.

4.2. Resource Module

4.2.1. Feed Domain

Feed quality, quantity, ease of access, and suitability for the metabolic needs of the animals are important resources the animal needs.

4.2.2. Water domain

Includes quality, quantity, and ease of access.

4.2.3. Climate Domain

Includes the range of climatic variables animals are exposed to with particular emphasis on extremes.

4.2.4. Social Resources Domain

Social behaviors are listed within the animal module. This domain addresses social conditions imposed on the animal such as stocking density, group structure and access to companion animals.

4.2.5. Comfort Domain

This domain addresses indoor and outdoor infrastructure including bedding, availability of shelter, and protection from climatic extremes that affect comfort of animals.

4.2.6. Hygiene Domain

Hygiene conditions influence exposure to disease pathogens and environmental organisms that influence health and welfare. Management of diseased animals such as use of hospital pens in order to reduce exposure of an individual to infectious conspecifics is considered in this domain.

4.3. Management Module

While access for animals to the environmental resources listed above is controlled by management practices, the Management Module addresses non-resource aspects of animal management as well as business practices that impinge on animal welfare. It also addresses some of the process elements that are necessary for the program to be effective.

4.3.1. Skills Domain

Addresses whether stockpersons have appropriate skills training (or experience) and appropriate attitudes for working with animals.

4.3.2. Husbandry Practices Domain

This class addresses the methods used for husbandry practices, ages when the practices are performed, and whether analgesia is used for painful procedures. Methods used for euthanasia are documented also.

4.3.3. Genetics Management Domain

The impact of genetic practices on welfare of livestock has not been addressed in previous welfare assessment schemes, yet many livestock welfare problems are closely linked to the genetics of the animals [37]. So not only do genetic practices contribute to many welfare problems, they can also provide a partial solution to some of these problems. This domain addresses issues such as: (1) suitability of the genotype for the production environment; (2) ways animals are selected for breeding purposes including use of estimated breeding values (EBVs) and genetic tools such as the polled gene marker test in cattle [38]; (3) the weight given to welfare traits within quantitative multi-trait breeding objectives; and (4) non-quantitative criteria (e.g., visual classing criteria) used for selecting breeders. Culling criteria, culling numbers, and culling age can provide important information on welfare performance of the enterprise, as defects and poor performance of individuals that result in them being culled are often caused by or related to poor welfare.

4.3.4. Records Domain

Records are essential for self-audit and internal review, as well as for providing data for benchmarking and external audit, and are also required in many jurisdictions to substantiate compliance with regulations around use of agricultural and veterinary chemicals, product declarations and occupational health and safety.

4.3.5. Review and Action Protocols Domain

Success of the program depends on periodic internal review of data and of management processes. Review process, outcomes, and actions taken need to be documented.

5. What Is New with the Unified Field Index?

Current welfare assessment procedures undertaken for compliance and assurance purposes are largely based on the concept of standards that have been derived from research or consensus of expert opinion. Standards are accompanied by the risk that they are interpreted as all or nothing thresholds that only need to be exceeded but not continually improved upon [7]. In contrast, the UFI introduces the concept of welfare performance as a continuous trait (or suite of traits) or attributes of an enterprise that is measured through benchmarking of performance across enterprises within an industry. While yet to be substantiated by evidence, it is anticipated that feedback from benchmarking will create an incentive for continuous improvement in welfare performance and furthermore, that livestock farming industries will feel greater ownership of the methodology for monitoring welfare performance than of welfare standards imposed on them through top-down, authoritarian, external assessment schemes.

The UFI also utilizes data that are available through individual electronic identification of animals and computer based animal records to generate information on welfare performance from conventional livestock performance measures like growth rates, reproduction rates, culling statistics, and disease prevalence. Ideally, only relatively minor modifications would be needed to software currently used for managing livestock performance data in order to record additional welfare related variables. The UFI proposes that standardized industry-wide statistics of welfare performance be generated from this on-farm data for feedback through benchmarking processes to individual producers (Figure 2) and for public reporting of industry performance. While the suite of welfare performance statistics is likely to differ between industries, data on mortality and morbidity have been largely overlooked as measures of welfare by point-in-time welfare assessment programs such as Welfare Quality. Although death is recognized as a blunt measure of animal welfare, it nonetheless is a foundational measure of welfare performance of an enterprise. The science of medical statistics was born when John Graunt began analyzing the London Bills of Mortality during the Great Plague of London in 1665–1666. These types of statistics including the causes and numbers of deaths, illness, therapeutic treatments, and culling provide a starting point for the description of welfare performance of a livestock enterprise. Many of these statistics are currently estimated by livestock managers because they are important drivers of profitability. What is new in the UFI is the use of these statistics to measure welfare performance. Better defined statistics of welfare performance also have the potential to provide some new traits for genetic evaluation programs, although some welfare traits such as resistance to internal parasites based on worm egg counts are already well recognized and used in breeding programs [39]. It is anticipated that across-enterprise analysis of welfare performance will provide valuable knowledge to aid the development of regulatory standards for farming practices and animal welfare.

The UFI places greater emphasis on management practices than previous assessment schemes. Large bodies of scientific research have identified the impact of training, attitudes, husbandry practices, use of analgesics, euthanasia methods, and genetic practices on the welfare of animals; however on-farm assessment of these practices has previously focused on compliance with laws and regulations rather than recognizing the scope for farmers to adopt improved practices. Genetic practices are a particular case in point, where there is considerable scope for farmers to implement breeding programs such as selection for resistance to blow fly strike in sheep that improve welfare outcomes [40].

Through the use of self-assessment of welfare risks and self-monitoring of welfare performance, the UFI is largely non-prescriptive of the methods and practices farmers should use to achieve favorable welfare performance. Rather, through appropriate measurement and monitoring, it proposes farmers can generate their own understanding of good practices on their farm and learn from the achievements of similar enterprises. Indeed, benchmarking schemes and risk assessment protocols have the intent of being educational and informative for the user and at the same time empowering the user to be a better manager [16].

The UFI incorporates elements of each of the three perspectives for assessing animal welfare as noted in the introduction: biological functioning, emotional states, and naturalness. The first two share with the UFI a strong dependence on outcome measures based on animals, while the third has reliance both on outcome measures and input measures, especially environmental conditions that are predictors of adverse welfare outcomes. What the UFI may bring to the practice of welfare assessment is a stronger acknowledgment of the role of management practices as predictors of welfare outcomes and recognition of the role of dynamic management procedures in the continual improvement of welfare performance.

Thus, the UFI represents a change from the authoritarian imposition of animal welfare standards on farmers for compliance and some market assurance purposes on a number of counts. It is designed to provide a mechanism for farmers to improve the welfare of their livestock. It is non-prescriptive in the description of good welfare. Rather it sees knowledge and understanding of the levels of welfare achieved by industry as emerging from the data acquired from farming enterprises. It acknowledges the experience of farmers as a source of new knowledge on management practices that lead to superior welfare performance. It increases ownership and responsibility for welfare performance by farmers. In these respects, it follows the model for benchmarking of production performance used in many agricultural industries. Its primary purpose is to assist farmers to improve animal welfare outcomes in their businesses and the tool may, when further developed, be able to underpin some market assurance schemes. A potential outcome of this approach is the development of a stronger animal welfare culture within farm animal industries and an ability for the industries to demonstrate that they foster this culture. The UFI is not a competitor to welfare assessment procedures undertaken for compliance purposes, but a complementary approach to the more general goal of improving farm animal welfare.

6. Limitations of the UFI

As a prototype, the UFI is yet to be tested as a method of empowering livestock managers to achieve better welfare performance on their enterprises. The elements of self-assessment and self-monitoring may fail to satisfy consumers of the integrity of measures of welfare performance despite the proposed inclusion of external auditing processes. While the UFI may fail to fulfill market assurance purposes, the benchmarking and welfare management goals of Levels I and II on their own should be valuable. By introducing the concept of welfare performance, the UFI might face resistance from advocacy groups and consumers by being seen as an attempt to reframe the concept of welfare rather than as an attempt to introduce a new approach for improving the management of welfare. Some livestock industries might consider welfare performance statistics to be too sensitive or too readily subject to misinterpretation for public disclosure. On the other hand, a focus on statistics as a summary of welfare performance might overshadow for some farmers the importance of identifying and managing individual animals in a poor welfare state. In its present form, the UFI makes no attempt to combine or integrate measures across domains in order to generate an overall score or assessment of welfare performance and does not consider any trade-offs that might occur between measures in the assessment process. And finally, like other welfare assessment procedures, the UFI will remain encumbered by limitations in our knowledge of and ability to assess affective states of farm animals in the field.

Acknowledgments

The review was undertaken with the financial support of Australian Pork Limited, Australian Meat Processor Corporation, Dairy Australia, Meat & Livestock Australia, Australian Egg Corporation

Limited, Rural Industries Research and Development Corporation, Australian Government Department of Agriculture, and the authors' institutions on behalf of the Australian National Primary Industry Animal Welfare Research, Development and Extension Strategy. The valuable suggestions of journal reviewers are gratefully acknowledged.

Author Contributions

IC prepared the majority of the first draft. DF, TC, LM and PH contributed equally to subsequent revision and refinement of the paper.

Conflicts of Interest

The authors declare no conflict of interest.

References

1. Veissier, I.; Jensen, K.K.; Botreau, R.; Sandoe, P. Highlighting ethical decisions underlying the scoring of animal welfare in the Welfare Quality (R) scheme. *Anim. Welf.* **2011**, *20*, 89–101.
2. Appleby, M.C.; Sandoe, P. Philosophical debate on the nature of well-being: Implications for animal welfare. *Anim. Welf.* **2002**, *11*, 283–294.
3. Barnett, J.L.; Hemsworth, P.H. Welfare Monitoring Schemes: Using Research to Safeguard Welfare of Animals on the Farm. *J. Appl. Anim. Welf. Sci.* **2009**, *12*, 114–131.
4. Fraser, D.; Weary, D.M.; Pajor, E.A.; Milligan, B.N. A scientific conception of animal welfare that reflects ethical concerns. *Anim. Welf.* **1997**, *6*, 187–205.
5. Terrestrial Animal Health Code. Available online: http://web.oie.int/eng/normes/mcode/en_chapitre_1.7.1.htm (accessed on 10 March 2014).
6. Binder, C.R.; Feola, G.; Steinberger, J.K. Considering the normative, systemic and procedural dimensions in indicator-based sustainability assessments in agriculture. *Environ. Impact Assess. Rev.* **2010**, *30*, 71–81.
7. Anneberg, I.; Vaarst, M.; Sandoe, P. To inspect, to motivate—Or to do both? A dilemma for on-farm inspection of animal welfare. *Anim. Welf.* **2013**, *22*, 185–194.
8. Main, D.C.J.; Whay, H.R.; Green, L.E.; Webster, A.J.F. Effect of the RSPCA Freedom Food scheme on the welfare of dairy cattle. *Vet. Rec.* **2003**, *153*, 227–231.
9. Whay, H.R. On-farm animal welfare assessments and audits in the UK. In Proceedings of the 41st Annual Conference of the American Association of Bovine Practictioners, Charlotte, NC, USA, 25–27 September 2008; pp. 73–77.
10. The Welfare of Dairy Cows in Organic Milk Production Systems—AW1020. Available online: http://randd.defra.gov.uk/Default.aspx?Menu=Menu&Module=More&Location=None&Completed=0&ProjectID=12043 (accessed on 10 March 2014).
11. Cattle Heat Load Index. Available online: http://chlt.katestone.com.au/ (accessed on 10 March 2014).
12. Gaughan, J.; Mader, T.; Holt, S.; Lisle, A. A new heat load index for feedlot cattle. *J. Anim. Sci.* **2008**, *86*, 226–234.

13. Fisher, A.D.; Roberts, N.; Bluett, S.J.; Verkerk, G.A.; Matthews, L.R. Effects of shade provision on the behaviour, body temperature and milk production of grazing dairy cows during a New Zealand summer. *N. Z. J. Agric. Res.* **2008**, *51*, 99–105.
14. Paraboss. Available online: http://www.paraboss.com.au/ (accessed on 10 March 2014).
15. Leeb, C. The Concept of Animal Welfare at the Interface between Producers and Scientists: The Example of Organic Pig Farming. *Acta Biotheor.* **2011**, *59*, 173–183.
16. Lacy, J. Cropcheck: Farmer benchmarking participatory model to improve productivity. *Agric. Syst.* **2011**, *104*, 562–571.
17. Von Keyserlingk, M.A.G.; Barrientos, A.; Ito, K.; Galo, E.; Weary, D.M. Benchmarking cow comfort on North American freestall dairies: Lameness, leg injuries, lying time, facility design, and management for high-producing Holstein dairy cows. *J. Dairy Sci.* **2012**, *95*, 7399–7408.
18. Keeling, L.J.; Wallenbeck, A.; Larsen, A.; Holmgren, N. Scoring tail damage in pigs: An evaluation based on recordings at Swedish slaughterhouses. *Acta Vet. Scand.* **2012**, *54*, 32.
19. Gonzalez, L.A.; Schwartzkopf-Genswein, K.S.; Bryan, M.; Silasi, R.; Brown, F. Benchmarking study of industry practices during commercial long haul transport of cattle in Alberta, Canada. *J. Anim. Sci.* **2012**, *90*, 3606–3617.
20. Grazing BMP. Available online: http://www.bmpgrazing.com.au/#&panel1–7 (accessed on 2 April 2014).
21. Wilson, R.H.; Charry, A.A.; Kemp, D.R. Performance indicators and benchmarking in Australian agriculture: Synthesis and perspectives. *Ext. Farming Syst.* **2005**, *1*, 45–57.
22. Collins, L.M.; Part, C.E. Modelling Farm Animal Welfare. *Animals* **2013**, *3*, 416–441.
23. Paton, M.W.; Martin, P.A.J.; Fisher, A.D. Risk assessment principles in evaluation of animal welfare. *Anim. Welf.* **2013**, *22*, 277–285.
24. Freshcare. Available online: http://www.freshcare.com.au/ (accessed on 10 March 2014).
25. Australian Macadamia Society. Available online: http://www.australian-macadamias.org/about-us/the-ams?lang=en&r=1 (accessed on 10 March 2014).
26. Heat Stress Management in Feedlots. Available online: http://www.australiananimalwelfare.com.au/content/livestock-and-production-animals/heat-stress-management-in-feedlots (accessed on 26 May 2014).
27. Welfare Quality Assessment Protocols. Available online: http://www.welfarequalitynetwork.net/network/45848/7/0/40 (accessed on 26 May 2014).
28. Farm Animal Welfare Council. *Second Report on Priorities for Animal Welfare Research and Development*; Department for Environment, Food and Rural Affairs Publications: London, UK, 1993.
29. Brscic, M.; Wemelsfelder, F.; Tessitore, E.; Gottardol, F.; Cozzi, G.; van Reenen, C.G. Welfare assessment: Correlations and integration between a Qualitative Behavioural Assessment and a clinical/health protocol applied in veal calves farms. *Ital. J. Anim. Sci.* **2009**, *8*, 601–603.
30. Rousing, T.; Wemelsfelder, F. Qualitative assessment of social behaviour of dairy cows housed in loose housing systems. *Appl. Anim. Behav. Sci.* **2006**, *101*, 40–53.
31. Napolitano, F.; de Rosa, G.; Grasso, F.; Wemelsfelder, F. Qualitative behaviour assessment of dairy buffaloes (*Bubalus bubalis*). *Appl. Anim. Behav. Sci.* **2012**, *141*, 91–100.

32. Hatcher, S.; Eppleston, J.; Graham, R.P.; McDonald, J.; Schlunke, S.; Watt, B.; Thornberry, K.J. Higher weaning weight improves postweaning growth and survival in young Merino sheep. *Aust. J. Exp. Agric.* **2008**, *48*, 966–973.
33. Koeck, A.; Miglior, F.; Kelton, D.F.; Schenkel, F.S. Short Communication: Genetic association of body condition score with disease resistance in first lactation Canadian Holsteins. *Can. J. Anim. Sci.* **2012**, *92*, 285–289.
34. Fahmy, M.H.; Bernard, C. Causes of mortality in Yorkshire pigs from birth to 20 weeks of age. *Can. J. Anim. Sci.* **1971**, *51*, 351–359.
35. Janhunen, M.; Kause, A.; Jarvisalo, O. Costs of being extreme—Do body size deviations from population or sire means decrease vitality in rainbow trout? *Aquaculture* **2012**, *370*, 123–129.
36. Broom, D.M. Animal-Welfare—Concepts and Measurement. *J. Anim. Sci.* **1991**, *69*, 4167–4175.
37. Rodenburg, T.B.; Turner, S.P. The role of breeding and genetics in the welfare of farm animals. *Anim. Front.* **2012**, *2*, 16–21.
38. Mariasegaram, M.; Harrison, B.E.; Bolton, J.A.; Tier, B.; Henshall, J.M.; Barendse, W.; Prayaga, K.C. Fine-mapping the POLL locus in Brahman cattle yields the diagnostic marker CSAFG29. *Anim. Genet.* **2012**, *43*, 683–688.
39. Woolaston, R.R.; Baker, R.L. Prospects of breeding small ruminants for resistance to internal parasites. *Int. J. Parasitol.* **1996**, *26*, 845–855.
40. Greeff, J.C.; Karlsson, L.J.E.; Schlink, A.C. Identifying indicator traits for breech strike in Merino sheep in a Mediterranean environment. *Anim. Prod. Sci.* **2014**, *54*, 125–140.

12

Establishing Trailer Ventilation (Boarding) Requirements for Finishing Pigs during Transport

John McGlone [1,*], Avi Sapkota [1], Anna Johnson [2] and Rebecca Kephart [2]

[1] Animal and Food Sciences, Texas Tech University, Lubbock, TX 79409, USA; E-Mail: asapkota@purdue.edu

[2] Department of Animal Science, Iowa State University, Ames, IA 50011, USA; E-Mails: johnsona@iastate.edu (A.J.); rkdavis@iastate.edu (R.K.)

* Author to whom correspondence should be addressed: E-Mail: john.mcglone@ttu.edu.

Simple Summary: Transport is an inevitable process in the modern swine industry due to the multiple-site approach to raising pigs and transport can be a significant source of stress to the animals, which raises a welfare concern. Maintaining the environment inside the transport trailer is crucial for pig comfort. This study aims to determine the amount of ventilation, or varied side-wall boarding, required to keep pigs within their thermal comfort zone. Examination of 302 trailers transporting 48,143 pigs found that pig losses were highest when low boarding levels (open sides) were used in cold air temperatures (<5 °C). In mild air temperatures (5 to 26 °C), boarding levels had little impact on pig losses.

Abstract: Specifically, this study aimed to establish the effects on mortality and morbidity of boarding levels (amount of side-wall trailer ventilation) for finishing pigs in mild weather (8.80 ± 0.30 °C, 71.70% ± 1.12% humidity). Pigs from commercial finishing sites were transported in 302 pot-bellied trailers to commercial processing plants. Measures collected at the processing plant were rates of dead on arrival (DOA), non-ambulatory, non-injured (NANI), non-ambulatory, injured (NAI), and total dead and down (D&D). Boarding levels (% that side walls were closed off with inserted boards) were divided into 3 bins: low, medium, and high, and outside temperature was divided into 4 bins <5 °C, 5.10–10 °C, and 10.10–15 °C and >15 °C. Average rates of DOA, NANI, NAI, and D&D were approximately 0.30%, 0.12%, 0.04%, and 0.46%, respectively. The D&D was highest when boarding level was low with temperatures <5 °C ($p < 0.05$). However, variations in boarding level (medium and high boarding) in the temperature range of 5.10 °C to 23.30 °C did not affect pig losses.

Keywords: boarding; pig; transportation; ventilation; welfare

1. Introduction

Transportation has become an inevitable aspect of pork production in the U.S., with more than 113 million pigs transported annually [1]. In North America, trailers are used for commercial transport, resulting in a known multi-factorial stressor for swine. Transit losses may be influenced by: trailer micro-environment, loading density, transit time, wait time both at the farm (from loading to leaving) and plant (prior to unloading), and handling procedures [2,3]. Trailer microenvironment is characterized by temperature, humidity, air speed, air pressure, level of gases (ammonia, carbon dioxide), and the amount and condition of any bedding [4]. Pigs do not have an efficient method of coping with thermal stress [5–7]; therefore, external cooling methods are necessary while transporting pigs to maintain their optimal thermal comfort zone. Trailers used for commercial transport are not equipped with artificial ventilation, but rather rely on passive ventilation of air in and out of side vents to circulate air within the trailer. The Transport Quality Assurance (TQA) handbook was released in 2002 to provide guidelines for many aspects of swine transport [8]. As new information is released, the handbook is updated, with the most recent edition being published in 2008. The TQA handbook provides the following guidelines for side vent positioning during transport: 10% of air vents should be open when air temperature is <−12 °C; 25% at −12 to −7 °C; 50% at −6 to 4.40 °C; 75% at 4.50 to 9.40 °C; and 100% at >9.4 °C. These suggestions are based on professional judgment and experience, rather than scientific data. Boarding refers to the amount that the side walls of the trailer were closed by inserting boards. Zero boarding would be a trailer with no added boards and the sides as open as possible. Boarding at 100% would mean all air spaces were covered with boards. This study aimed to provide science-based suggestions for boarding at various levels during transport of finishing pigs in mild weather.

2. Experimental Section

2.1. General

The experimental protocol for this study was approved by Institutional Animal Care and Use Committee at Texas Tech University and Iowa State University. The study took place during the spring and fall of 2012. Gilts and barrows (*n* = 48,143) used in this study were of mixed commercial genetics and raised in commercial finishing sites in the Midwestern U.S., then transported to processing plants in 302 pot-bellied trailers. A power test performed by Lewis [9] shows that 250 trailers will yield significant results in this type of study. Approximately 51 different drivers participated in the study; with some drivers hauling multiple loads. The average number of finishing pigs per trailer was 158.40 ± 1.06. Trailers were bedded with wood shavings (1 bale = 22.70 kg, 0.20 m^3). Bedding level varied from 2 to 10 bales based on drivers' discretion. Observations were made as pigs were unloaded at the processing plants. The 2 participating processing plants wish to remain anonymous.

This study was a part of a multi-year series of experiments with many experiments. Details of trailers and general conditions of the study are found in another paper in this series [10]. Briefly, the work was conducted at 2 commercial abattoirs and over 1000 pig finishing barns and sites that feed these plants in the Midwestern USA. Trucks pulled trailers that were primarily pot-belly designs described in other papers [2,10]. Transport times ranged from 30 min to 12 h and were used as a covariate but were found to not impact our findings. Bedding levels were held constant. Most trailers contained mixes of barrows and gilts (so sex effects cannot be examined). Likewise, extremes in air temperature were not examined because boarding is held constant in cold weather (near 100% boarded) and in warm weather (no boarding, or 0% boarded). Therefore, this dataset is only during relatively mild air temperatures (not during cold or heat stress; see below). We know from our other work [10] that pig surface temperature varies little in the relatively mild conditions of this study. Finally, driver effects could not be evaluated because most data points were from a single driver and therefore a single experimental unit. We did not have the opportunity to evaluate replications of drivers with several boarding levels.

2.2. Treatments

Outside air temperature was logically divided into 4 bins: <5 °C, 5.1 to 10 °C, 10.10 to 15 °C, and >15 °C. Temperature ranges for <5 °C were −0.6 °C to 5.0 °C. Temperature ranges for >15 °C were 15.1 °C to 26.6 °C. Boarding levels, or the percent of plugs/panels used to close vents in the trailer, were divided into 3 bins: low (0–30%), medium (31–60%), and high (>61%). Higher boarding level percentages signify that fewer vents were left open. Table 1 shows the number of trailers with each boarding level across all temperature bins. Different boarding levels cause different levels of ventilation within the trailer, although we do not know how internal air speed changes with different boarding levels. In addition, boarding levels change the physical nature of the side panels and they change the insulation level of the side walls. Still, enough information on boarding levels is provided so others may replicate and extend this work in the future.

Table 1. Number of trailers represented in each boarding level by temperature bin.

Temperature	**<5 °C**			**5.1 to 10 °C**			**10.1 to 15 °C**			**>15.1 °C**		
Boarding level	Low	Med	High	Low	Med	High	Low	Med	High	Low	Med	High
n trailers	8	27	25	25	81	27	16	30	11	22	21	2

Drivers were requested to randomly assign boarding levels on each trailer at loading; these levels were confirmed by researchers when the truck arrived at the processing plant. Because of welfare concerns regarding low boarding levels in cold temperatures and high boarding levels in hot temperatures, these bins have smaller sample sizes than the others. Boarding levels given are representative of the boarding level in all compartments of the trailer. The researchers also tallied the number of transportation losses, confirmed the number of pigs on each trailer, and compared these numbers with plant records for quality control purposes.

Transport losses are classified as one of the following [11]:

- Dead on arrival (DOA): the animal dies during transit and arrives at the plant already deceased;
- Non-ambulatory, non-injured (NANI): the animal cannot move or walk, is fatigued, but does not show any obvious sign of injury, trauma, or disease; and may be standing, sitting or more commonly lying down; or
- Non-ambulatory, injured (NAI): the animal is injured during transport and shows obvious sign of injury, trauma, or disease;
- Total dead and down (D&D) is the sum of DOA, NANI, and NAI.

2.3. At the Processing Plant

Temperature and relative humidity (RH) were taken at the processing plants at the time of unloading (Kestrel 4500 Pocket Weather Tracker, Extech Instruments, Nashua, NH, USA). Because of personnel restrictions, temperature and RH were not recorded at the finishing site. Wait time at the plant was measured as the time between the arrival of the truck and the start of unloading. Trailers were unloaded in a random order depending on the preference of the driver. Order of unloading was not recorded. Skin surface temperature (SST) was measured on 5 random pigs selected from the first group and 5 random pigs selected from the second group. A random sample was considered as ignoring the first 10 pigs at the beginning of unloading, sampling 5 pigs within the next 50 unloaded (first group), ignoring another 10 pigs, and then sampling another 50 pigs (second group). Surface temperature was measured on the flank with an infrared thermometer with a sensitivity of 0.1 °C (Extech model 42570, Extech Instruments, Nashua, NH, USA).

2.4. Statistical Analyses

Primary model included effects of boarding level using trailers as experimental unit and outside air temperature and bedding level were covariates. All data were analyzed using SAS 9.2, using the General Linear Models procedures (SAS, 2010 SAS Inst., Cary, NC, USA). Average wait time, SST, and average rates of DOA, NANI, NAI, and D&D were calculated. Rates of losses in each temperature bin for each boarding level were calculated and least square means were compared in each bin. When comparing the means, p values <0.05 were considered significant.

3. Results and Discussion

Average air temperature at the plant was 8.80 ± 0.30 °C (−0.60 to 23.30 °C) and average RH was 71.70 ± 1.12% (19 to 100%). Average wait time at the plant for the trailers was 43.70 ± 1.74 min (range: 0 to 161 min; n = 234). Average skin surface temperature on the flanks of the pigs was 25.20 ± 0.22 °C (17.30 to 32.50 °C; n = 219).

Rates of DOA, NANI and NAI were not affected by boarding level when outside air temperature and bedding levels were used as covariates ($p > 0.05$); therefore, these factors were not considered in further data analysis. Average rates of DOA, NANI, NAI and D&D per trailer were 0.30 ± 0.04%, 0.04 ± 0.01%, 0.12 ± 0.02%, and 0.46 ± 0.05% respectively.

When pigs were transported at air temperature <5 °C and low level of boarding was used, rate of DOA was higher (0.57 ± 0.14%), compared to medium (0.11 ± 0.08%) and high (0.13 ± 0.08%), ($p < 0.05$). Figure 1 shows the rate of DOA across all temperature bins by boarding level.

Figure 1. Rate of dead on arrival (DOA) for each boarding level [1] across all temperature bins.

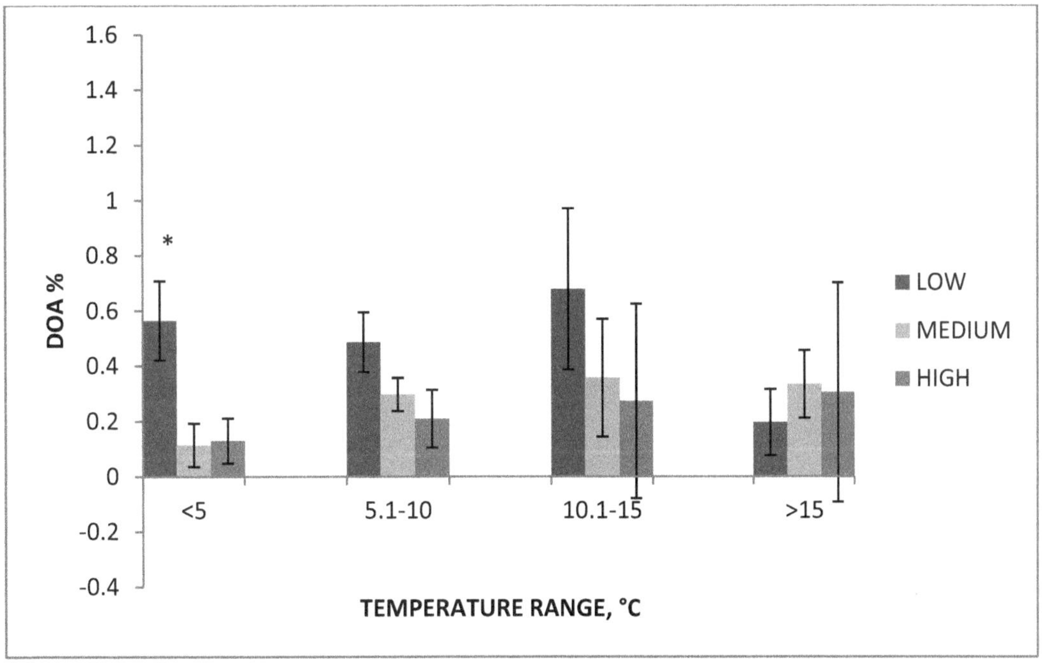

* $p < 0.05$ within temperature bin. [1] Low: boarding level <30%; medium: boarding level =31% to 60%; high: boarding level >60%.

Similar patterns were found for rates of D&D and NANI. Average rates of NANI at air temperature <5 °C while using low, medium and high boarding levels were 0.30% ± 0.05%, 0.02% ± 0.08% and 0.08% ± 0.04%, respectively. Figure 2 represents the rates of NANI by boarding level for each temperature bin.

Rates of D&D at air temperature <5 °C while using low, medium and high boarding levels were 0.94% ± 0.20%, 0.25% ± 0.11% and 0.21% ± 0.11%, respectively. Figure 3 represents D&D for each boarding level across all temperature bins.

Overall, low boarding levels resulted in the highest percentage of D&D across all temperature bins except for >15 °C. During transport in these colder temperatures, the air moving into the trailer may result in the pigs becoming too cold, especially if the bedding level is not appropriate. Too much bedding can accumulate moisture, which combined with cold air, may result in frostbite [10]. Another factor may be that the pigs exhaust themselves from shivering to maintain body heat. This study agrees with the TQA handbook's guidelines for boarding requirements during transport of swine based on the finding that between 5 °C and 15 °C, boarding levels of 25%, 50%, or 75% produced statistically similar levels of NANI and DOA.

Figure 2. Rate of non-ambulatory, non-injured (NANI) for each boarding level [1] across all temperature bins.

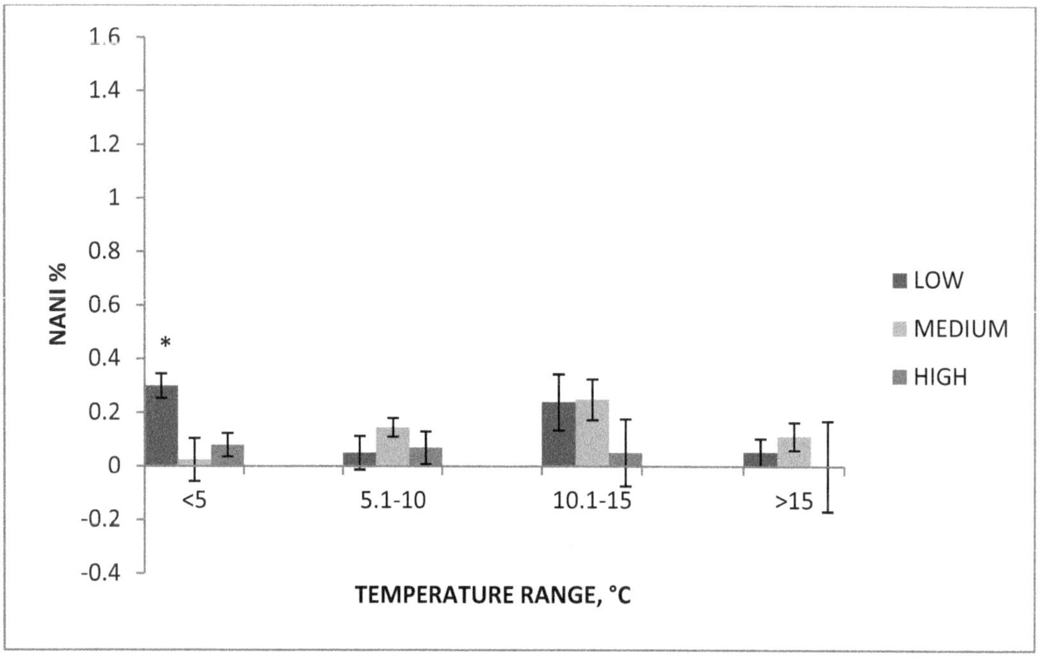

* $p < 0.05$ within temperature bin. [1] Low: boarding level <30%; medium: boarding level 31% to 60%; high: boarding level >60%.

Figure 3. Rate of total dead and down (D&D) for each boarding level across all temperature bins.

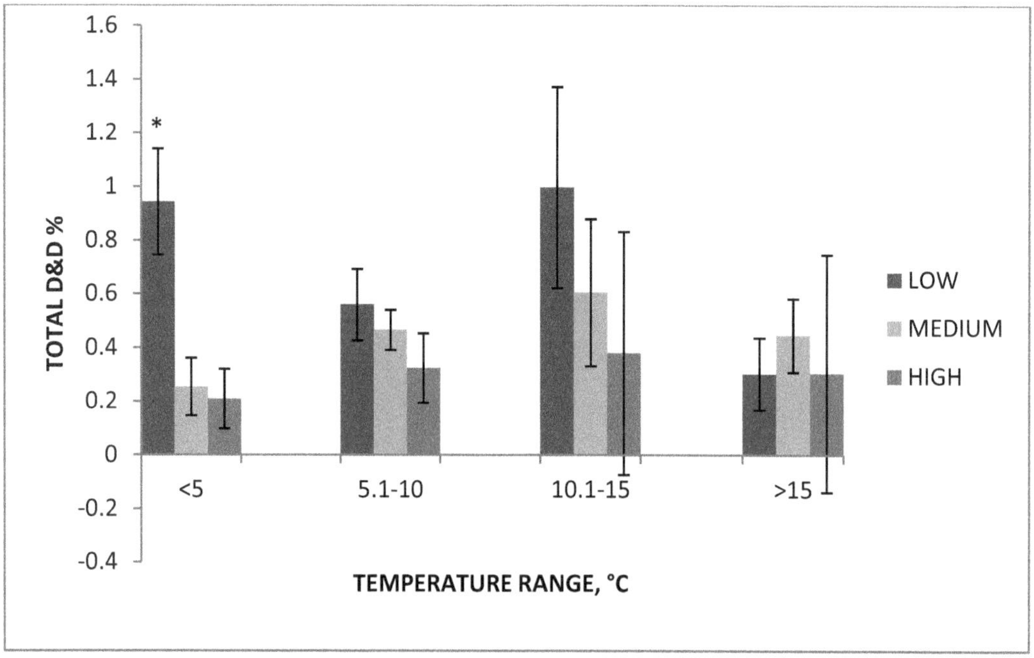

* $p < 0.05$ within temperature bin. [1] Low: boarding level <30%; medium: boarding level 31% to 60%; high: boarding level >60%.

Total transport losses are estimated to cost the US pork industry $50 to $100 million annually [12]. This figure includes direct cost due to loss of pigs and indirect costs due to labor and facilities required to handle D&D pigs. The same review estimates that annual DOA, NANI, NAI, and D&D rates average 0.25%, 0.37%, 0.05%, and 0.69%, respectively [11]. It should be noted that the results of this study show a higher proportion of NAI compared to NANI. Some plants do not differentiate between NAI and NANI, but rather list all non-ambulatory animals as "total down". These rates vary according to environmental conditions [2], management practices [13,14] genetic line [15,16], and transport facilities [17]. These figures represent not only a financial loss, but also an animal welfare concern. Sutherland [2] showed that rates of DOA increased at temperatures above 20 °C and rates of NANI increased as the temperature dropped below 5 °C. The findings of the present study agree with Sutherland's NANI finding [2]. In the same study, waiting time at the plant influenced rates of DOA, NANI, and D&D; DOA and D&D were highest when wait time exceeded 4 h. In the current study, wait time did not have an effect on losses, which may be because wait time in this study ranged from 0 to 161 min. In Sutherland's study, there was no difference in transport losses within this wait time range.

4. Conclusions

This study revealed that at outside air temperatures <5 °C, when less boarding was used average rates of DOA, NANI, and D&D increased. Below 5 °C, boarding levels should be above 30%. This indicates poor animal welfare and high economic loss. Using medium or high boarding levels at cold temperatures can reduce transportation losses. Boarding level should increase as outside air temperature decreases. Based on these results, the boarding level recommendations outlined in the TQA handbook are adequate for swine transport. Further evaluation needs to be done regarding proper ventilation in individual compartments and different types of trailers [18]. Also, this study needs to be conducted in different climates, such as the northeast U.S. Trailers with artificial ventilation are currently utilized in European countries, and still need to be tested in the U.S. [19].

Acknowledgments

We thank National Pork Board for funding this study. The cooperation of graduate and undergraduate farmers, trucking companies, and processing plants during data collection is greatly appreciated. Glenna Pirner helped with the preparation of this manuscript.

Author Contributions

Dr. John McGlone conceived the idea for this work and designed the experiments. Dr. Anna Johnson contributed to the experimental design. Avi Sapkota carried out the experiments, conducted data analysis, and drafted the article. Rebecca Kephart assisted with carrying out the experiments.

Conflicts of Interest

The authors declare no conflict of interest. This work was supported by the National Pork Board, Texas Tech University, and Iowa State University.

References

1. National Agriculture Statistics Service. Available online: http://usda01.library.cornell.edu/usda/nass/LiveSlau//2010s/2013/LiveSlau-01–24–2013.pdf (accessed on 21 August 2013).
2. Sutherland, M.A.; McDonald, A.; McGlone, J.J. Effects of variation in the environment, length of journey and type of trailer on the mortality and morbidity of pigs being transported to slaughter. *Vet. Rec.* **2009**, *165*, 13–18.
3. Peeters, E.; Driessen, B.; Steegmans, R.; Henot, D.; Geers, R. Effect of supplemental tryptophan, vitamin E, and a herbal product on responses by pigs to vibration. *J. Anim. Sci.* **2004**, *82*, 2410–2420.
4. Ellis, M.; Wang, X.; Funk, T.; Wolter, B.; Murphy, C.; Lenkaitis, A.; Sun, Y.; Pilcher, C. Development of improved trailer designs and transport management practices that create the optimum environment for market weight pigs during transport and minimize transport losses. 2008. Available online: http://www.pork.org/FileLibrary/ResearchDocuments/05–192-Ellis-UofILL.pdf (accessed on 6 August 2012).
5. Ingram, D.L. Stimulation of cutaneous glands in the pig. *J. Comp. Pathol.* **1967**, *77*, 93–98.
6. Ingram, D.L. Adaptations to ambient temperature in growing pigs. *Pflüg. Arch. Eur. J. Physiol.* **1977**, *367*, 257–267.
7. Hicks, T.A.; McGlone, J.J.; Whisnant, C.S.; Kattesh, H.G.; Norman, R.L. Behavioral, endocrine, immune, and performance measures for pigs exposed to acute stress. *J. Anim. Sci.* **1998**, *76*, 474–483.
8. National Pork Board. Transport Quality Assurance Handbook. 2008. Available online: http://www.pork.org/filelibrary/TQAAdvisor/TQA4Manual.pdf (accessed on 16 July 2012).
9. Lewis, C.R.G.; Krebs, N.; Hulbert, L.E.; McGlone, J.J. The use of a putative maternal pheromone during transport and the effect of trailer temperature on pig losses and welfare. *Anim. Prod. Sci.* **2010**, *50*, 1–9.
10. McGlone, J.; Johnson, A.; Sapkota, A.; Kephart, R. Establishing bedding requirements during transport and monitoring skin temperatures over seasons after transport for finishing pigs. *Animals* **2014**, *4*, 241–253.
11. Ritter, M.J.; Ellis, M.; Berry, N.L.; Curtis, S.E.; Anil, L.; Berg, E.; Benjamin, M.; Butler, D.; Dewey, C.; Driessen, B.; *et al.* Review: Transport losses in market weight pigs: I. A review of definitions, incidence, and economic impact. *Prof. Anim. Sci.* **2009**, *25*, 404–414.
12. Ellis, M.; McKeith, F.; Hamilton, D.; Bertol, T.; Ritter, M. Analysis of the current situation: What do downers cost the industry and what can we do about it? In Proceedings of the 4th American Meat Science Association Pork Quality Improvement Symposium, Columbia, MO, USA, 7 June 2003.
13. De Jong, I.C.; Prelle, I.T.; van de Burgwal, J.A.; Lambooij, E.; Korte, S.M.; Blokhuis, H.J.; Koolhaas, J.M. Effects of rearing conditions on behavioural and physiological responses of pigs to preslaughter handling and mixing at transport. *Can. J. Anim. Sci.* **2000**, *80*, 451–458.
14. Johnson, A.K.; Sadler, L.J.; Gesing, L.M.; Feuerbach, C.; Hill, H.; Faga, M.; Bailey, R.; Stalder, K.J.; Ritter, M.J. Effects of facility system design on the stress responses and market losses of market weight pigs during loading and unloading. *Prof. Anim. Sci.* **2010**, *26*, 9–17.

15. Geers, R.; Bleus, E.; van Schie, T.; Villé, H.; Gerard, H.; Janssens, S.; Nackaerts, G.; Decuypere, E.; Jourquin, J. Transport of pigs different with respect to the halothane gene: Stress assessment. *J. Anim. Sci.* **1994**, *72*, 2552–2558.
16. Weschenfelder, A.V.; Torrey, S.; Devillers, N.; Crowe, T.; Bassols, A.; Saco, Y.; Piñeiro, M.; Saucier, L.; Faucitano, L. Effects of trailer design on animal welfare parameters and carcass and meat quality of three Pietrain crosses being transported over a long distance. *J. Anim. Sci.* **2012**, *90*, 3220–3231.
17. Fitzgerald, R.F.; Stalder, K.J.; Matthews, J.O.; Schultz Kaster, C.M.; Johnson, A.K. Factors associated with fatigued, injured, and dead pig frequency during transport and lairage at a commercial abattoir. *J. Anim. Sci.* **2009**, *87*, 1156–1166.
18. Brown, J.; Samarakone, T.; Crowe, T.; Bergeron, R.; Widowski, T.; Correa, J.; Faucitano, L.; Torrey, S.; Gonyou, H. Temperature and humidity conditions in trucks transporting pigs in two seasons in Eastern and Western Canada. *Trans. ASABE* **2011**, *54*, 2311–2318.
19. Gilkeson, C.A.; Thompson, H.M.; Wilson, M.C.T.; Gaskell, P.H.; Barnard, R.H. An experimental and computational study of the aerodynamic and passive ventilation characteristics of small livestock trailers. *J. Wind Eng. Ind. Aerodyn.* **2009**, *97*, 415–425.

13

The Effects of Using a Ramp and Elevator to Load and Unload Trailers on the Behavior and Physiology of Piglets

John McGlone * and Avi Sapkota

Animal and Food Sciences, Texas Tech University, Lubbock, TX 79409, USA;
E-Mail: asapkota@purdue.edu

* Author to whom correspondence should be addressed; E-Mail: john.mcglone@ttu.edu.

Simple Summary: Transport is a routine practice in the modern swine industry. Loading the pigs into trailers can be a novel and stressful experience for the animals. This study compared behaviors and physiological variables during and after loading using a ramp or elevator to determine which method is the least stressful to the pigs. Loading pigs by ramp appears to cause more stress than loading by elevator.

Abstract: Transport is an inevitable process in the modern U.S. swine industry. The loading process is a novel and potentially stressful experience. This study uses behavior, heart rate and leukocyte counts to compare stress one hour before, during and after loading via ramp or elevator. Piglets were held in a home pen (control (CON)), walked up and down an aisle (handled (HAN)), or walked to a truck and loaded via elevator (ELE) or ramp (RAM). Sitting, feeding and blood parameters did not show a significant treatment by time effect ($p > 0.05$). Standing behavior did not differ between CON and HAN piglets nor between RAM and ELE piglets ($p > 0.05$); however, CON and HAN piglets stood more than RAM and ELE piglets during treatment ($p < 0.05$). After treatment, drinking behavior was increased in RAM piglets ($p < 0.05$). The heart rate of ELE piglets decreased 6.3% after treatment; whereas the heart rate of RAM piglets remained elevated 2.4% ($p < 0.05$). In terms of heart rate, loading by elevator appears to be less stressful than loading by ramp.

Keywords: elevator; piglets; ramp; welfare

---

1. Introduction

In the majority of swine production systems in the U.S., piglets are farrowed at sow farms and transported to grower-finisher sites at weaning. When the piglets are to be transported, they are handled and moved from their home pens, walked along an aisle, then loaded into the trailer. Trailers used to transport these piglets are usually pot-bellied or straight-deck designs [1]. Metal, wooden or concrete ramps of various angles are commonly used to load the piglets from the aisle to the trailer. Additionally, more ramps may be used within the trailer to move piglets from one deck to another. Trailers in the European Union (EU) may be equipped with hydraulic lifts to move pigs to the desired deck of the trailer, preventing the pigs from having to walk up a sloped ramp [2].

Handling prior to transportation contributes to the stress of the event. Handling stressors may include being moved from the home pen, mixing of conspecifics, use of handling aides (prods, boards, paddles, flags) and distance moved. During periods of physical or psychological stress, the body responds with the activation of the hypothalamic-pituitary-adrenal (HPA) axis. This results in secretion of cortisol from the adrenal glands [3]. A study done by Dhabhar *et al.* showed that cortisol secretion in rats experiencing 1 hour of acute physical stress was associated with decreased lymphocyte count and increased neutrophil count [4].

Parrott *et al.* found no significant differences in heart rate and plasma cortisol in ewes loaded by elevator and ramp [5]. It can be surmised that pigs would respond in a similar fashion, but there is limited literature regarding the use of elevators and swine stress and welfare. Two studies have shown that there was no difference in muscle pH between elevator and ramp loaded pigs and, therefore, no effect of loading stress on meat quality [6,7]. Another study found that loading via elevator reduced heart rate compared to loading via ramp [8]. While improving meat quality is an important aspect of the pork production process, it is also important to focus on animal welfare. Currently, improving animal welfare is a major concern to both the swine industry and the public; increasing animal welfare may decrease transport losses, improve meat quality and decrease economic losses. This study was designed to compare the use of a ramp and an elevator to load and unload piglets and to determine which method is the least stressful to the animals.

2. Experimental Section

2.1. General

This project was approved by the Texas Tech University Animal Care and Use Committee. All animals were housed in 2.1-m × 1.5-m pens with slatted floors at the Texas Tech Swine Research Farm near New Deal (Lubbock), Texas. Each pen contains 1 nipple waterer and a 3-hole feeder. Feed and water were provided *ad libitum* in the pens. Ventilation in the barn was via exhaust fan and ceiling louvers. A total of 120 weaned pigs of mixed commercial genetics, approximately 30 days of age, were used for this study. Pigs were randomly divided into 12 pens of 10 pigs each, 3 pens per treatment. Pigs were allowed to acclimatize to the new environment for 1 week before the study began. Four treatment groups were assigned: control (CON), handled (HAN), ramp (RAM) and elevator (ELE). CON piglets were not handled or moved from their pen. HAN pigs were moved out of the home pen, walked up and down the length of the aisle and then moved back into the home pen. HAN piglets were not held at the end of the aisle for any time period. RAM piglets were moved out of the home pen, walked down the aisle and then loaded onto the trailer using a ramp. ELE piglets were moved from their home pen, walked down the aisle and loaded onto the trailer using a hydraulic lift (Figure 1a,b). ELE and RAM piglets were held on the trailer (*i.e.*, not transported) for 1 hour and then moved back off the trailer via the treatment method and back to their home pens. Feed and water were available *ad libitum* in the home pens. Water was not available in the alley nor on the trailer. The movement of the pigs was facilitated by the use of sorting boards in accordance with the Transport Quality Assurance program guidelines [9]. Each treatment had 3 replications. Replications were performed on the same day, with at least 1 hour of rest between replications.

Figure 1. (**a**) Hydraulic lift elevator in the loading position. (**b**) Hydraulic lift elevator in the raised position.

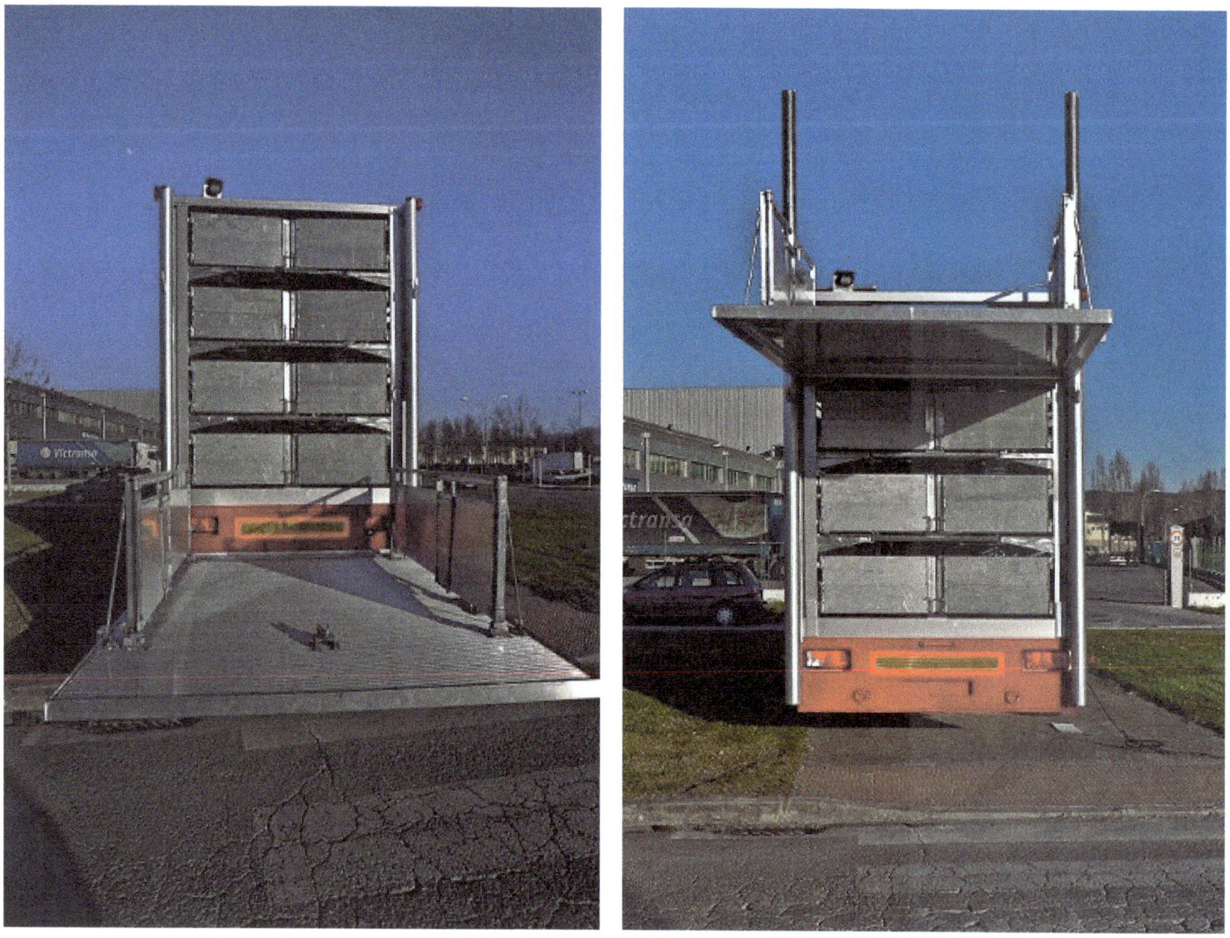

(**a**) (**b**)

2.2. Design of the Aisle, Ramp and Elevator

Pigs in the HAN, ELE and RAM groups walked a distance of 36 to 46 m inside the building in a 1.2 m-wide aisle.

The ramp was metal, 0.8 m wide with cleats 0.3 m apart to reduce slipping and falling. The ramp chute was solid on the sides, up to 0.9 m high and partially open above that. For RAM piglets, the ramp was 4.6 m long set at a 20° angle.

ELE piglets were moved along the same aisle, across the ramp (now adjusted to 0°) and onto the elevator floor. The floor was elevated to the desired deck using a remote control.

Holding pens on the trailer were 2.4 m by 2.1 m in dimension.

2.3. Heart Rate Data Collection

Two randomly selected piglets from each group wore a jacket fitted with a heart rate monitor (Jacketed External Telemetry (JET), Data Science International, St. Paul, MN, USA) and were allowed to be as near as possible to their pen mates (when placed in the same pen, other pigs tended to chew at the jacket, altering the results and causing more stress to the pig), while the heart rate data were collected for 30 minutes. Therefore, heart rate data were collected using only two pigs out of the pen. Heart rate data were collected first. Then, the pigs went back to their home pen, had at least 1 hour of rest, and the whole group was rerun for behavior and blood sample collection. The pigs used for heart rate were not used for blood sample collection, as they already had exposure to handling and treatments.

2.4. Blood Sample Collection

Blood samples were collected via the right side jugular vein using a vacutainer with ethylene diamine-tetraacetic acid (EDTA). Two piglets from each pen were randomly selected for blood collection. Five to 7 mL of blood were drawn at each time. Blood samples were placed on ice and transported back to the laboratory at the Department of Animal and Food Sciences, Texas Tech University. Blood parameters were measured by Cell Dyne (IDEXX Laboratories, Inc., Westbrook, ME, USA) for differential blood leukocyte count. Values of interest include total white blood cell count (WBC), neutrophil count (N), lymphocyte count (L) and N:L ratio.

2.5. Behavior

All piglets were observed by the same individual, and behavior was categorized into one of the following: standing, sitting, lying, drinking or feeding. Each pen was scan sampled every 5 minutes to record behaviors. Behavior was recorded as a percentage of piglets expressing each behavior.

2.6. Timeline for Data Collection

Timeline for heart rate (HR); A–D refer to periods:

	HR-A	HR-B	HR-C	HR-D
Acclimation near home pen	HR before treatment started	HR after pigs were walked on the aisle or loaded into trailer using ramp or elevator	HR after pigs were again walked on the aisle, unloaded from trailer using ramp or elevator	HR after pigs were back near to their home pen
5 min	10 min	10 min	10 min	5 min

Timeline for bleeding; A–D refer to blood sampling times:

BLEED-A	BLEED-B	BLEED-C	BLEED-D
Baseline, one hour before treatment	At the start of treatment	Immediately after treatments were initiated	After pigs were back in their home pen

Timeline for behavior (BEHAV); A–C refer to periods:

BEHAV-A	BEHAV-B	BEHAV-C
Before treatment started	During treatment	After treatment
1 hour	1 hour	1 hour

For HAN pigs, behavior Time Period B includes some time immediately after the pigs were returned to the home pen. For instance, if a group of pigs took 10 minutes to be moved up the alley and back into the home pen, the next 50 minutes are included in the 1-hour observation for Time Period B.

2.7. Data Analyses

Each pen consisted of 9 or 10 piglets; therefore, the number of piglets displaying each behavior was converted to a percent of total pigs present in the pen. Heart rate data were summarized first as beats per minute (bpm) and then averaged to calculate as A, B, C and D, as mentioned above. Blood variables were also calculated as A, B, C and D. Behavior data were collected every 5 minutes and later averaged per hour as A, B and C, as mentioned above. The number of pigs showing a behavior were counted at first and later converted into the percent of pigs showing the behavior at a particular time point in each pen. The percent data were used for analysis. The data were analyzed using the PROC GLM statement in SAS 9.2 (SAS, 2010 SAS Inst., Inc., Cary, NC, USA). The model included treatment, pen within treatment, time and treatment × time effects as independent variables. The mean square of the pen within-treatment effect was used as the error term to determine the significance of the time and treatment by time interaction. Least square means were used to compare individual adjusted means.

3. Results and Discussion

3.1. General

There were significant treatment × time interactions for standing, drinking and heart rate ($p < 0.01$). Lying behavior tended to show a significant treatment × time interaction ($p = 0.07$). Other behaviors (sitting, lying and feeding) and blood parameters did not show a significant treatment by time effect ($p > 0.05$). All blood, heart rate and behavior results are summarized and displayed in Table 1.

Table 1. Summary of the percentage of piglets displaying behaviors, the values of blood parameters and the heart rates of pigs in response to treatments before, during and after treatments.

	Control				**Handle**				**Elevator**				**Ramp**					*p*-value (TRT × TIME)
Period [a]	A	B	C	D	A	B	C	D	A	B	C	D	A	B	C	D	SE	
Sit [b] **(%)**	1.4	1.6	1.9	-	2.1	3.7	0.6	-	2.6	3.7	0.8	-	2.8	2.0	1.7	-	0.82	0.3
Stand [b] **(%)**	37.8	37.2	21.4	-	31.3	24.7*	9.4	-	40.0	75.8*	23.2	-	37.0	93.9*	22.0	-	6.94	<0.01
Lying [b] **(%)**	45.8	48.9	66.7	-	57.2	64.1	84.1	-	47.3	17.2*	57.0	-	50.9	4.1*	59.2	-	8.48	0.07
Drink [b] **(%)**	14.7	11.7	8.9	-	9.1	7.5	5.4	-	9.8	0.0*	13.9	-	8.9	0.0*	15.8	-	1.96	<0.01
Feed [b] **(%)**	0.3	0.5	1.1	-	0.3	0.0	0.6	-	0.3	0.0	1.7	-	0.5	0.0	1.4	-	0.38	0.6
WBC [c] **($\times 10^3$/μL)**	20.8	23.4	23.7	23.2	18.2	19.4	20.6	21.8	19.3	23.6	26.1	23.8	19.4	25.9	29.0	26.8	1.16	0.16
N [d] **($\times 10^3$/μL)**	5.7	9.3	12.3	11.2	7.9	8.7	10.8	10.7	7.8	11.4	16.3	13.7	7.8	10.0	16.5	15.4	0.98	0.12
L [e] **($\times 10^3$/μL)**	12.6	11.9	9.3	10.4	9.2	9.6	8.7	7.2	10.5	10.9	8.5	7.3	10.7	14.6	10.9	9.9	0.94	0.38
N:L RATIO [f]	0.5	0.8	1.3	1.1	0.9	0.9	1.3	1.7	0.8	1.1	1.9	2.3	0.7	0.7	1.5	1.6	0.23	0.58
HR [g] **(bpm)**	193.3	199.3	183.5	-	180.6*	183.2*	186.8	-	185.0	196.9	184.5	-	201.0	202.3	207.2*	-	3.1	0.02

* Indicates that treatment means are different than control means ($p < 0.05$); [a] A = one hour prior to treatment; B = immediately prior to treatment; C = immediately after treatment was initiated; D = one hour after treatment ended. [b] Behavior was observed every five minutes and averaged for each time period. Blank values indicate that data were not collected at that time period. [c] Total white blood cell count. [d] Neutrophil count. [e] Lymphocyte count. [f] Neutrophil:lymphocyte ratio. [g] Heart rate (HR): values were averaged over five minutes for Periods A and D and over 10 minutes for Periods B and C. Blank values indicate that data were not collected at that time period.

3.2. Behavior

A significant treatment × time interaction was observed for standing behavior during treatment (37.20 ± 6.94%, 24.70 ± 6.94%, 75.80 ± 6.94% and 93.90 ± 6.94% for CON, HAN, ELE and RAM, respectively; $p < 0.01$). Standing behavior did not differ among CON and HAN pigs ($p > 0.05$). ELE and RAM piglets showed greater frequency of standing behavior than did CON and HAN ($p < 0.05$); however, standing behavior among ELE and RAM piglets did not differ from each other during treatment. Figure 2 shows the percentage of piglets standing at each time point.

There was a tendency towards a significant treatment × time effect for lying behavior (48.9 ± 8.48%, 64.1 ± 8.48%, 17.2 ± 8.48% and 4.1 ± 8.48% for CON, HAN, ELE and RAM, respectively; $p = 0.07$). The percentage of piglets displaying lying behavior during treatment was not different for CON and HAN piglets ($p > 0.05$); however, a lesser percentage of ELE and RAM piglets displayed lying behavior during treatment. The ELE and RAM piglets did not differ from each other for lying behavior during treatment ($p > 0.05$). Figure 3 shows the percentage of piglets lying at each time point.

Figure 2. Percentage of pigs showing standing behavior an hour before (A), during (B) and after (C) each treatment (control, handling, ramp and elevator).

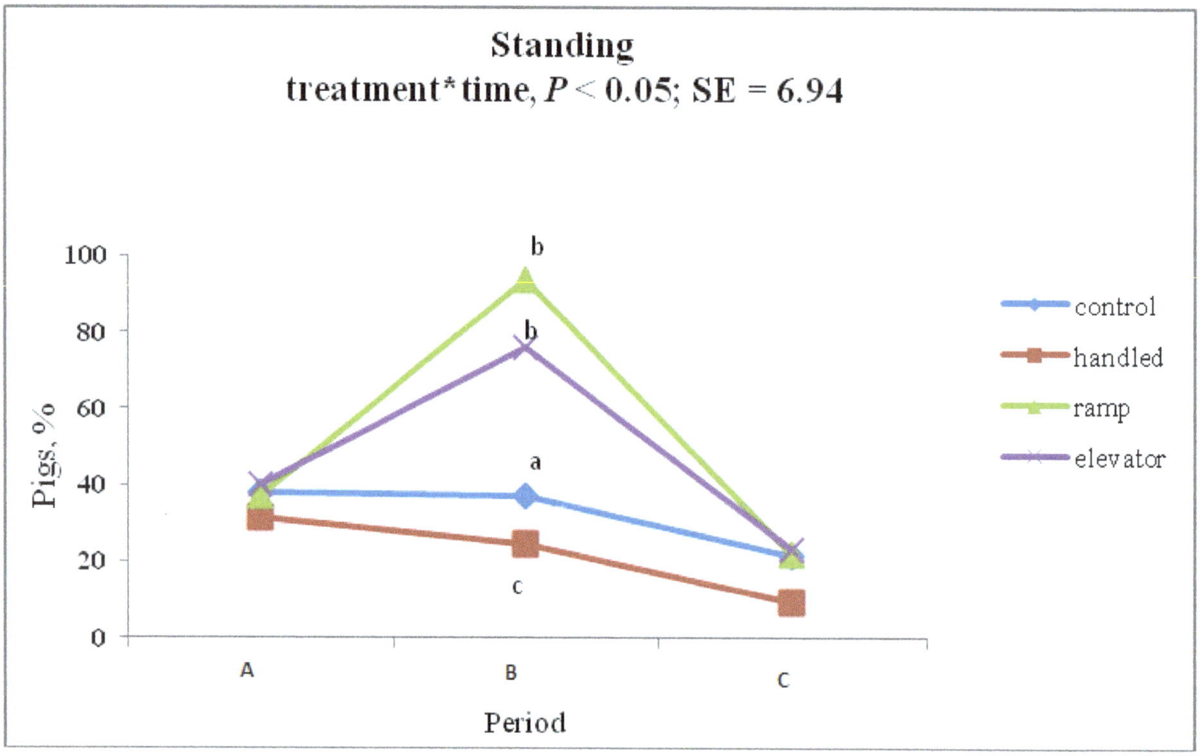

[a,b,c] Different superscripts within a period represent differences in standing behavior.

Figure 3. Percentage of pigs showing lying behavior an hour before (A), during (B) and after (C) each treatment (control, handling, ramp and elevator).

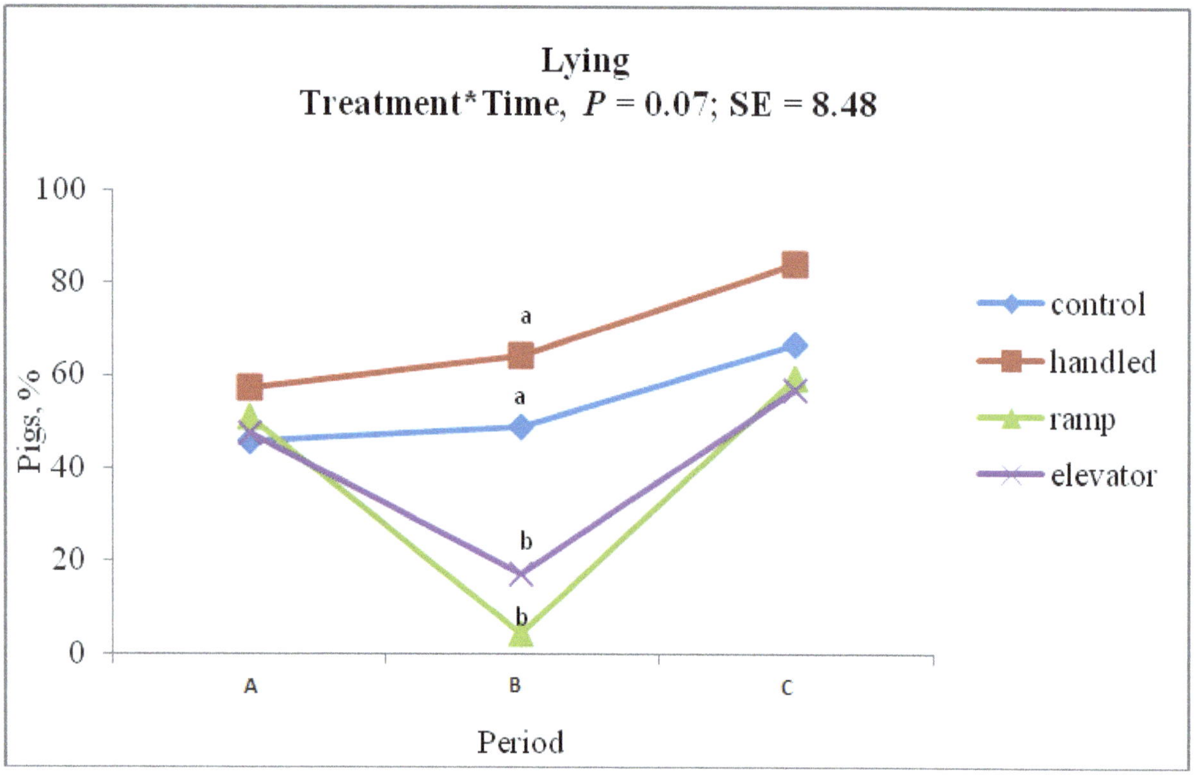

[a,b] Different superscripts within a period represent differences in lying behavior.

There was a significant time × treatment interaction for drinking behavior ($p < 0.01$). During the time of treatment, the percentage of CON (11.70 ± 1.96%) and HAN (7.50 ± 1.96%) piglets showing drinking behavior did not differ ($p > 0.05$). ELE and RAM piglets did not show any drinking behavior during the time of treatment. When piglets were brought back to the home pen, drinking behavior was higher in RAM (15.80 ± 1.96%) piglets compared to CON (8.90 ± 1.96%) and HAN (5.40 ± 1.96%) piglets ($p < 0.05$). The percentage of ELE piglets showing drinking behavior after treatment (13.90 ± 1.96%) was not different from CON, HAN and RAM piglets. Figure 4 shows the percentage of piglets drinking at each time point.

Figure 4. Percentage of pigs showing drinking behavior an hour before (A), during (B) and after (C) each treatment (control, handling, ramp and elevator).

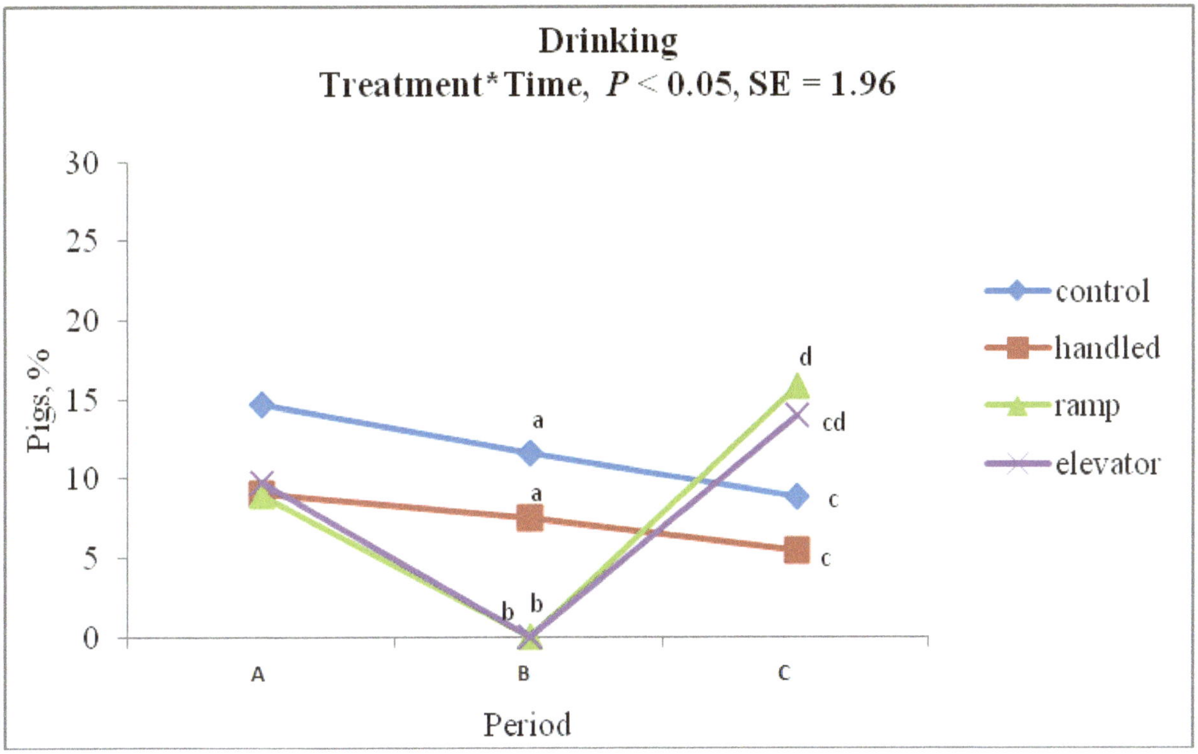

a,b,c,d Different superscripts within a period represent differences in drinking behavior.

3.3. Heart Rate

A significant treatment × time interaction was observed for heart rate ($p = 0.02$). The heart rate of ELE piglets decreased from 196.90 ± 3.10 bpm during treatment to 184.50 ± 3.10 bpm when piglets were placed back in the home pen ($p = 0.01$). The heart rate (bpm) of RAM piglets, on the other hand, increased from the "during" period (202.30 ± 3.10) to the "after" period (207.20 ± 3.10) ($p > 0.05$). Figure 5 shows the heart rate of piglets at each time point.

Figure 5. The heart rate (beats per min) of pigs an hour before, during and after each treatment (control, handling, ramp and elevator).

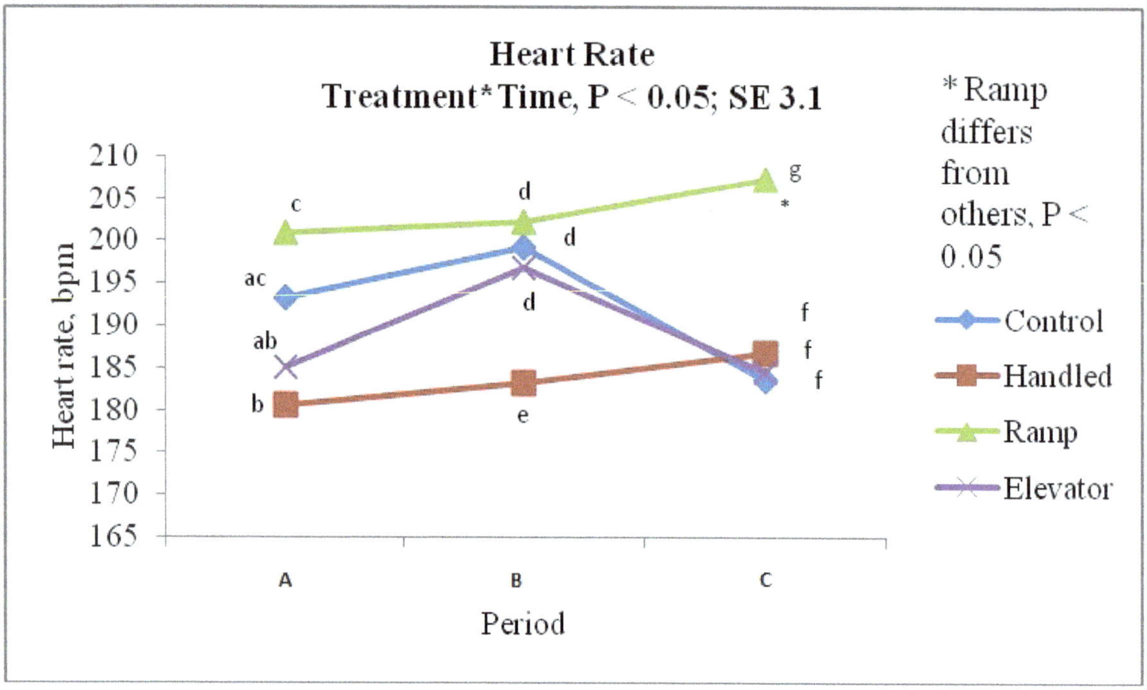

a,b,c,d,e,f,g Different superscripts within a period represent differences in heart rate.

4. Conclusions

The behavior of pigs can vary before, during and after a stressful event. In addition, physiological measures, such as temperature, respiratory rate, heart rate, blood parameters and immune measures, are affected by stress [10,11]. Sitting, standing, lying, feeding and drinking behaviors before, during and after piglets were loaded into the trailer either using a ramp or elevator were compared with control and handled piglets. The number of piglets showing standing behavior inside the trailer did not differ between ELE and RAM piglets, but these numbers were greater than the numbers of CON and HAN piglets showing standing behavior at this time point. This shows that piglets were more restless in the trailer, which may be due to the novelty and stress of being moved. Feeding and drinking behavior were null when the piglets were in the trailer, because feed and water were unavailable in the trailer.

The heart rate of ELE pigs decreased after the pigs were brought back to the home pen; on the other hand, the heart rate of RAM pigs remained elevated. The heart rates of RAM and ELE piglets did not differ during treatment. The heart rate is considered an indicator of stress, and it may have been elevated in these treatment groups, due to the novelty of the experiences. An analysis of cortisol concentrations is warranted in future studies to support other physiological changes indicative of stress. Brown [12] reported a lowered heart rate, but an elevated cortisol concentration when a modular system was used to load and unload pigs, showing that pigs might still be stressed even though the heart rate is not elevated. They also reported little difference between ramp and elevator use, which is inconsistent with the findings of this study.

Even though the blood parameters did not differ between the ELE and RAM piglets, handling intensity and use of handling aides (prods, boards, *etc.*) can influence skin lesions (due to slips and falls) and meat quality, therefore affecting the overall welfare and economic impact. Correa [13] showed that handling intensity and handling aides used while loading can affect the stress response and meat quality of pigs. Ramp angle is another factor to be taken into consideration. Grandin [2] recommended 15° as a maximum angle for ramps used to load and unload pigs. Warriss [14] reported that time to ascend or descend did not differ significantly when the ramp angle was between 0° and 20°; however, it took longer for pigs to climb steeper ramps.

Pigs are susceptible to stress and may become stressed when faced with having to adapt to any changes in their regular environments or novelty [15]. Pigs are typically unaccustomed to handling, walking long distances and using ramps [16]. Pigs are moved from their home pens usually when they are moved to a new facility, such as to nursery pens after weaning, to growers' buildings after the nursery and to processing plants when they reach market weight. Pigs are usually transported via trailer and are loaded and unloaded via ramps. Stress due to the novelty of these experiences can lead to increased transit losses [1,17,18]. The transport of pigs cannot be avoided in the current multi-site production systems utilized in the U.S. The results of the current study agree with the findings of previous studies [5,8]. After the event, the heart rate is lower in pigs loaded by elevator compared to that of pigs loaded by ramp. Using an elevator to load and unload pigs can potentially minimize stress to the animals, as the handlers do not have to handle the pigs as much as they do when using ramps. Nonetheless, both the ramp and the elevator are novel experiences for most pigs and result in some level of stress during loading.

Acknowledgments

We thank Texas Tech University's Laboratory of Animal Behavior, Physiology and Welfare (www.labpw.ttu.edu) for funding this study. The graduate and undergraduate cooperation during data collection is greatly appreciated. Glenna Pirner helped with the preparation of this manuscript.

Author Contribution

John McGlone conceived of the idea for this work and designed the experiments. Avi Sapkota carried out the experiments, conducted the data analysis and drafted the article.

Conflicts of Interest

The authors declare no conflict of interest.

References and Notes

1. Ritter, M.J.; Ellis, M.; Bertelsen, C.R.; Bowman, R.; Brinkman, J.; DeDecker, J.M.; Keffaber, K.K.; Murphy, C.M.; Peterson, B.A.; Schlipf, J.M.; Wolter, B.F. Effects of distance moved during loading and floor space on the trailer during transport on losses of market weight pigs on arrival at the packing plant. *J. Anim. Sci.* **2007**, *85*, 3454–3461.
2. Grandin, T. Design of loading facilities and holding pens. *Appl. Anim. Behav. Sci.* **1990**, *28*, 187–201.

3. Dallman, M.F.; Akana, S.F.; Cascio, C.S.; Darlington, D.N.; Jacobson, J.; Levin, N. Regulation of ACTH secretion: Variations on a theme of B. *Recent Prog. Horm. Res.* **1987**, *43*, 113–173.
4. Dhabhar, F.S.; Miller, A.H.; Stein, M.; Mcewen, B.S.; Spencer, R.L. Diurnal and acute stress-induced changes in distribution of peripheral blood leukocyte subpopulations. *Brain, Behav. Immunity* **1994**, *8*, 66–79.
5. Parrott, R.F.; Hall, S.J.G.; Lloyd, D.M. Heart rate and stress hormone responses of sheep to road transport following two different loading procedures. *Animal Welfare* **1998**, *7*, 257–267.
6. Barton Gade, P. Effect of different stocking densities during transport on welfare and meat quality in Danish slaughter pigs. *Meat Sci.* **1998**, *48*, 237–247.
7. Costa, L.N.; Lo Fiego, D.P.; Dall'Olio, S.; Davoli, R.; Russo, V. Influence of loading method and stocking density during transport on meat and dry-cured ham quality in pigs with different halothane genotypes. *Meat Sci.* **1999**, *51*, 391–399.
8. Augustini, C.; Fischer, K. Physiological reaction of slaughter animals during transport. In *Transport of Animals Intended for Breeding, Production, and Slaughter*; Moss, R., Ed.; Springer: The Hague, The Netherlands, 1982; pp. 125–135.
9. National Pork Board. Transport Quality Assurance Handbook. 2008. Available online: http://www.pork.org/filelibrary/TQAAdvisor/TQA4Manual.pdf (accessed on 16 July 2012).
10. McGlone, J.J.; Salak, J.L.; Lumpkin, E.A.; Nicholson, R.I.; Gibson, M.; Norman, R.L. Shipping stress and social status effects on pig performance, plasma cortisol, natural killer cell activity, and leukocyte numbers. *J. Anim. Sci.* **1993**, *71*, 888–896.
11. Hicks, T.A.; McGlone, J.J.; Whisnant, C.S.; Kattesh, H.G.; Norman, R.L. Behavioral, endocrine, immune, and performance measures for pigs exposed to acute stress. *J. Anim. Sci.* **1998**, *76*, 474–483.
12. Brown, S.; Knowles, T.; Wilkins, L.; Chadd, S.; Warriss, P. The response of pigs to being loaded or unloaded onto commercial animal transporters using three systems. *Vet. J.* **2005**, *170*, 91–100.
13. Correa, J.A.; Torrey, S.; Devillers, N.; Laforest, J.P.; Gonyou, H.W.; Faucitano, L. Effects of different moving devices at loading on stress response and meat quality in pigs. *J. Anim. Sci.* **2010**, *88*, 4086–4093.
14. Warriss, P.; Bevis, E.; Edwards, J.; Brown, S.; Knowles, T. Effect of the angle of slope on the ease with which pigs negotiate loading ramps. *Vet. Rec.* **1991**, *128*, 419–421.
15. Grandin, T. Assessment of stress during handling and transport. *J. Anim. Sci.* **1997**, *75*, 249–257.
16. Lewis, C.R.G.; Hulbert, L.E.; and McGlone, J.J. Novelty causes elevated heart rate and immune changes in pigs exposed to handling, alleys, and ramps. *Livestock Sci.* **2008**, *116*, 338–341.
17. Stephens, D.; Perry, G. The effects of restraint, handling, simulated and real transport in the pig (with reference to man and other species). *Appl. Anim. Behav. Sci.* **1990**, *28*, 41–55.
18. Ritter, M.; Ellis, M.; Bowman, R.; Brinkmann, J.; Curtis, S.; DeDecker, J.; Mendoza, O.; Murphy, C.; Orellana, D.; Peterson, B. Effects of season and distance moved during loading on transport losses of market-weight pigs in two commercially available types of trailer. *J. Anim. Sci.* **2008**, *86*, 3137–3145.

14

Productive and Economic Responses in Grazing Dairy Cows to Grain Supplementation on Family Farms in the South of Brazil

Luiz Carlos Pinheiro Machado Filho [1,*], Leandro Martins D'Ávila [1], Daniele Cristina da Silva Kazama [1], Lauana Luiza Bento [2] and Shirley Kuhnen [2]

[1] Lab of Applied Ethology and Animal Welfare (LETA), Departament of Zootechny and Rural Development, Federal University of Santa Catarina, Rod. Admar Gonzaga, 1346, Florianopolis, SC 88034-000, Brazil; E-Mails: davila27@gmail.com (L.M.D.); daniele.kazama@ufsc.br (D.C.S.K.)

[2] Lab of Animal Biochemistry, Department of Zootechny and Rural Development, Federal University of Santa Catarina, Rod. Admar Gonzaga, 1346, Florianópolis, SC 88034-000, Brazil; E-Mails: lauana@zootecnista.com.br (L.L.B.); shirley.kuhnen@ufsc.br (S.K.)

* Author to whom correspondence should be addressed; E-Mail: pinheiro.machado@ufsc.br.

Simple Summary: In the South of Brazil, as in many regions where dairy production is pasture-based, the use of concentrate to supplement cattle diet frequently does not follow technical guidelines. This may result in inefficient management, with increased cost of production and lower pasture intake. In this study, small amounts of an energy supplement proved to be more economically efficient than a high protein commercial concentrate, despite a decrease in milk productivity. The cows were able to compensate for the lower levels of protein in the supplement with selective grazing for high protein plants. The quality of the milk was unaffected by the treatment.

Abstract: Pasture-based dairy production has been a major source of income for most family farms in the south of Brazil. Increasing milk prices have spurred an increase in grain supplementation, which has been poorly implemented, resulting in low levels of efficiency. To evaluate the consequences of supplementation on milk production and composition, grazing behavior and economic return, the widely used grain management system (CC-commercial concentrate, containing 21% CP, offered at 1 kg per 3.7 L of milk) was compared with an energy supplement (GC-ground corn, with 9.5% CP, offered at 0.4% of live weight). Ten Holstein cows were paired into two groups, and subjected to the two treatments in a crossover design. The cows remained in the same grazing group, and the grain supplement was offered individually at milking time and consumed completely. Each experimental period lasted 14 days, with 10 days for diet adaptation and four days for data collection; individual milk production and samples were collected to determine levels of fat, protein, lactose, carotenoids, vitamin A and N-urea. Grazing behavior was observed (scans every 5 min) in the first 4 h after the morning milking, and chemical composition of hand plucked samples of forage were measured. The cost of the supplement and profitability per treatment were calculated. Cows supplemented with GC consumed herbage with higher crude protein (CP: 16.23 *vs.* 14.62%; $p < 0.05$), had higher biting rate (44.21 *vs.* 39.54 bites/min; $p < 0.03$) and grazing time (22.20 *vs.* 20.55 scans; $p < 0.05$) than when receiving CC. There were no differences in milk composition between treatments ($p > 0.05$). However, higher concentrations of β-carotene and total carotenoids were detected in the milk of cows at 70–164 days of lactation, compared to <70 days of lactation ($p < 0.05$). Milk production was higher (13.19 *vs.* 11.59 kg/day; $p < 0.05$) when cows consumed CC, but resulted in lower profitability compared to GC (US$ 4.39 *vs.* US$ 4.83/cow per day). Our results show that higher productivity does not necessarily improve profitability. Cows receiving supplement with lower levels of protein were able to adjust their grazing behavior to meet their protein needs and this level of diet modification did not alter milk composition.

Keywords: livestock sustainability; grazing behavior; milk composition; Voisin's Rational Grazing

---

1. Introduction

In Western Santa Catarina State, a major dairy producing region in South America, milk production is typically pasture-based, with the use of concentrate supplementation. Santa Catarina State is the fifth largest and fastest growing milk producing state in Brazil, with about 80% of the farms based on family farming [1]. The region is comprised of family farm units, with small herds (about 20 cows), relying on milk production as their main source of income [2]. A large number of producers in the region have adopted the pasture-based system coupled with the use of supplements, and there are a growing number of ecologically-based properties, some of which have obtained organic certification. Most organic farms use Voisin's Rational Grazing (VRG), but this system is also used to manage conventional herds [3]. We estimate that VRG is used equally by organic and semi-intensive dairy farms [4]. VRG is a rotational grazing system [5], where cows typically graze a new paddock after each milking.

Family dairy farms in Southern Brazil use concentrate or corn silage to supplement grazing, particularly during seasons of forage scarcity, such as the fall and the beginning of winter [2,4]. However, organic farms are less likely to use concentrate [3,6]. Besides feeding management based on pasture, agroecological production in Brazil, and other regions of the world, is characterized as having smaller and less productive herds. This lower level of productivity has been attributed to crossbred cows, but also to the limited use of concentrate [7,8].

The subtropical climate of the region is favorable for forage cultivation all year round, allowing the succession of tropical, subtropical and temperate species in the same grassland. The climate also allows for the establishment of multispecies permanent pasture, especially when pasture management is based on the ecology of the region. In these pastures, estimating the nutritional needs of cows with distinct productive potential and stages of lactation, is quite complex [9]. Most often, concentrate supplementation is used to compensate for possible nutritional deficiencies, without a proper evaluation by the farmer if the supplement is reducing cows' pasture consumption, and thus increasing costs. Furthermore, organic farmers are less likely than conventional farmers to use a nutritionist for ration and feeding advice [8]. Energy may be a restricting factor in dairy cow productivity at pasture, because the energy content of forage does not generally meet the productive milk potential needs of the cows [10,11]. Even at its optimal grazing point, the pasture may have high concentrations of protein, but may be deficient in non-structural carbohydrates [12]. In this case, the forage energy is insufficient to provide the potential for milk production given by the protein concentration, limiting the productivity of cows feeding exclusively on pasture. On the other hand, milk quality is positively affected by pasture feeding; the more fresh forage the animals consume, the higher the levels of carotenoids and other anti-oxidants present in the milk [13].

There is a positive response in milk yield, energy-corrected milk (ECM), fat and protein, to increasing amounts of supplement [14]. However, an excess of grain may compromise the sustainability of dairy production as the energy costs may be unsustainable. In conventional milk production, based on feeding Total Mixed Ration (TMR, a mix of cereals and forage), it is estimated that an input of 14 kcal of fossil energy is required to produce 1 kcal of milk protein. Even with lower energy costs than the production of meat and eggs, milk production could be more efficient if production was entirely based on pasture and hay [15]. In fact, some researchers have argued that to improve environmental performance in milk production, we must: (1) reduce the use of concentrated ingredients with high environmental impact; (2) reduce the use of concentrates per kilogram of milk; and (3) reduce the surplus of nutrients, improving the flow of nutrients from the farm [16]. Pasture-based feeding is financially and environmentally economical, as it reduces the input of fossil fuel energy into the system.

Feeding management may represent an important constraint in organic dairy production. The use of low cost supplementation from food sources readily available on the property, like corn meal, is preferable, as long as it does not compromise milk quality or productivity of the system. Thus, in order to assess the productive and economic responses of dairy cows to the supplementation of pasture-based feeding with grain, two management systems were assessed: the current standard quantity of concentrate was compared to an estimated quantity of energy supplement, ground corn.

2. Material and Methods

2.1. Location

The experiment was conducted on a 16.9 ha family farm located in the western region of Santa Catarina State, Brazil (26°26'04"S and 52°49'33"W), during the spring of 2011. The experiment was carried out in a 7 ha VRG system, implemented in 2009, consisting of 65 paddocks with an average area of 1,100 m^2 each. At the time of the experiment, the pasture was comprised predominantly of *Lolium multiflorum*, *Trifolium repens*, *Axonopus catarinensis* and *Hemartria altissima*. The paddocks were used at the optimum grazing point obeying the 1st law of rational grazing [5]. The time spent in each paddock was 24 h and the instant stocking rate was 167 AU (500 kg)/ha/day. The animals were placed in a new paddock after the morning milking.

2.2. Animals

Of the 24 lactating cows on the farm, 10 Holstein cows were selected and paired based on body weight, days in milk (DIM), parity, concentrate consumption and daily milk production immediately before the beginning of the experiment (2 days). A detailed description of the animals is shown in Table 1. All procedures involved in this experiment were approved by the Ethics Committee on the Use of Animals of the Federal University of Santa Catarina (UFSC), protocol number PP00673.

Table 1. Characteristics of the animals used in the experiment: group, animal identity (ID), body weight (BW), days in milk (DIM), parity, body condition score (BCS) and milk production two days prior to the beginning of the experiment, mean and standard errors.

Group	Animal ID	BW(Kg)	DIM	Parity	BCS	Milk Production (kg/day)
	73	425	40	4	4	19.5
	74	530	80	2	3	17.1
A	86	480	90	1	3	10.7
	19	360	30	1	4	14.2
	49	500	150	2	3	10.9
Mean ± SE		459 ± 30.1	78 ± 21.3	2 ± 0.5	3.4 ± 0.2	14.5 ± 1.7
	18	440	50	1	3	14.1
	57	510	60	3	3	16.1
B	54	500	120	3	3	13.3
	71	360	20	1	4	14.9
	41	440	130	1	3	12.9
Mean ± SE		450 ± 26.8	76 ± 21.1	1.8 ± 0.5	3.2 ± 0.2	14.3 ± 0.6

2.3. Experimental Design and Treatment Description

The experimental design was a crossover with two treatments, involving two experimental periods of 14 days, with 10 days for diet adaptation and four days for data collection. The treatments consisted of supplementing the animals' feed with: (a) Commercial Concentrate (CC) supplied based on the average quantity generally used in the region [4], resulting in 1 kg of feed for each 3.7 L of milk produced; and (b) ground corn (GC) offered in the proportion of 0.4% of body weight, or an energy supplement equivalent to 15% of the estimated total daily dry matter intake. The amount of supplement per animal per day was divided into two equal portions and a portion was offered during both the morning and afternoon milking in individual troughs. Whereas the estimated composition of the pasture was 14% crude protein (CP) and 53% total digestible nutrients (TDN) [9,17], the energy was the limiting factor in achieving the productive potential of pasture nutrients. During the entire experiment all animals were together in one single herd, along with 14 other lactating cows. Therefore, pasture, water, mineral mix, shade, social group and the distance between the paddock and milking parlor were equal for all cows; the only difference between the two experimental groups was the concentrate (treatment) individually assigned to the animals.

2.4. Bromatological Analyses of the Diet

Analyses of dry matter (DM) and crude protein (CP) in pasture and supplements were performed according to the AOAC Official Methods of Analysis [18]. For the analysis of neutral detergent fiber (NDF), the Van Soest method was used [19]. DM, NDF, and CP contents of ground corn and commercial concentrate are shown in Table 2. It is important to note that, based on our analysis, the CP level of the CC was 21.28%, which is greater than the level declared on the label of the concentrate (18%).

Table 2. Chemical composition of the commercial concentrate (CC) and ground corn (GC) used for animals.

Variables	CC	GC
Dry matter (%)	89.27	87.75
Neutral Detergent Fiber (%)	30.30	11.94
Crude Protein (%)	21.28	9.48

2.5. Behavioral Observations and Data Collection

Milk production was measured on the 12th and 14th day of each experimental period, in the morning and afternoon milking. Milk samples were collected and homogenized to compose one sample per animal per period and analyzed for fat, protein, lactose, total solids, urea-N, somatic cell count (SCC), total carotenoids, lutein, zeaxanthin, b-carotene and vitamin A.

On the 11th and 13th day of each experimental period, grazing behavior was observed, and pasture samples were collected after the morning milking. Pasture samples were collected using the grazing simulation technique [20]. Three sub-samples were taken per animal on each day of observation in the first hour, at 40 min intervals, resulting in two samples per animal per period (one amalgamated sample per observation day).

Grazing behavior of the experimental cows was also recorded on the 11th and 13th day in the morning (8:00 am–12:00 pm). Behaviors were recorded every 5 min using the instantaneous scan sampling technique [21,22]. Following the definitions adopted by the Laboratory of Applied Ethology and Animal Welfare (LETA) of the Federal University of Santa Catarina, observed behaviors included: grazing (animal with the mouth below or at the level of forage or grabbing forage, either stationary or moving forward), ruminating (animal chewing with lateral jaw movements with the head at the same level or above its body, lying or standing), walking (animal moving, with the head above the superior level of forage), drinking (animal with the lips immersed in water, with neck movements indicating water ingestion), idle (animal still, not engaged in any of the behaviors described above, lying or standing), and others (any other behavior not described above) [23].

Animals were watched continuously for four h by two observers. The observers were trained at the beginning of the experiment to ensure inter-observer reliability [21,22] and were located at least 15 m distance from the cows to avoid interference during the observation periods. Observers alternated themselves the groups observed in the two observation days. Animals were identified by ear tags and coat color. For data analysis, observation of the grazing behavior was divided into two periods of two hours each; period 1 refers to the first two hours after morning milking (8–10 am), and period 2 was from 10 am–12 pm. The biting rate was also recorded; biting was counted for 30 s three times over three 30 min intervals after the first hour of observation, totaling 9 records per animal. The average of these 9 records was used as the biting rate for each animal.

2.6. Milk Composition Analysis

Analyses of total solids, protein, fat, lactose and urea-N were conducted using infrared method [24] while the flow cytometry method was used to determine SCC [25]. For carotenoids and vitamin A, the methodology described by Hulshof *et al.* [26] was used. Extraction was performed using ammonium hydroxide and ethanol (2.5:6 *v/v*), followed by the addition of ethyl ether (0.0025% BHT) and petroleum ether (1:1 *v/v)*. The samples were then centrifuged (4,000 rpm, 4 min), and the supernatant evaporated under N_2 flow at 40 °C. The residue was saponified (5% KOH for 3 h at 37 °C, 200 rpm) and re-extracted with hexane. Aliquots of the concentrated sample were injected into a liquid chromatograph (Shimzadu LC-10A), equipped with a C18 reverse-phase column (Vydac218TP54, 250 mm × 4.6 mm × 5 μm), protected by a 5 μm C18 reverse-phase guard column (Vydac218GK54), and a UV-visible detector operating at 450 and 392 for carotenoids and vitamin A, respectively. The eluent was $MeOH:CH_3CN$ (90:10, *v/v*, 1 mL/min) and the identification of the compounds of interest was performed using retention times of standard compounds (Sigma-Aldrich, St. Louis, MO, USA).

2.7. Statistical Analyses

Statistical analyses were performed using the mixed procedure from SAS statistical package version 9.0, considering the model:

$$Y_{ijk} = \mu + P_i + T_j + e_{ijk}$$

where, Y_{ijk} is the value of the dependent variable, μ the average value, P_i the effect of period, T_j the treatment effect, and e_{ijk} the random error N (0, s^2). The means of each treatment were compared using Tukey's test, considering a 5% significance level.

3. Results and Discussion

The analysis of pasture samples collected through the grazing simulation technique (Table 3) show a higher concentration of crude protein in the diet selected by cows given the GC treatment ($p < 0.05$), the supplement with lower protein levels (Table 2). These results suggest that grazing cows can select pasture with different chemical composition to compensate for a nutrient shortage in the diet offered. In the present study, cows eating ground corn were consuming a smaller amount of protein due to both a lower concentration of protein in the supplement, as well as smaller quantity of the supplement. Previous research has demonstrated the ability of ruminants to modify one or more components of their ingestive behavior in order to minimize unfavorable feeding conditions and achieve the nutritional needs for maintenance and production [27,28].

Considering the experimental design, where all animals were given both treatments, it is interesting to note that animals were able to select a higher CP pasture diet when the supplement was poor in the nutrient. Combining corn—or any other energy supplement—with pasture that contains a significant amount of legumes would likely be a sustainable strategy as the protein in the pasture can fulfill the nutritional needs of lactating cows [11]. Relying on foraged sources of protein, such as white clover, to feed cattle can also reduce greenhouse gas emissions from pasture-based milk production, thus lowering the carbon footprint [29].

Table 3. Dry matter (DM), crude protein (CP) and Neutral Detergent Fiber (NDF) concentrations in pasture samples collected by the grazing simulation technique with cows fed either commercial concentrate (CC) or ground corn (GC).

Variables	Treatments			
	CC	GC	SE [1]	P [2]
DM (%)	27.62	28.69	0.523	0.19
NDF (%)	61.69	60.80	0.891	0.31
CP (%)	14.62	16.23	0.461	0.05

[1] SE = Standard error; [2] P = Probability.

The grazing frequency, recorded in 2 h periods, and the biting rate per min are shown in Table 4. The frequency of grazing was similar between treatments in the first observation period (8–10 am) after the morning milking, and different during the second observation period (10 am–12 pm). In this case, the animals that were fed ground corn extended their grazing into the fourth hour of observation while the CC group did not ($p < 0.05$). A higher biting rate was also detected during grazing for those animals given the GC diet ($p < 0.05$). These results suggest that, compared to those receiving ground corn, the animals that were fed the commercial concentrate reached a level of satiety more quickly, adjusting their grazing behavior to the condition of concentrate supplementation [11]. Flexibility in grazing behavior to achieve the same intake has been reported in other studies; different genotypes may adjust their ingestive behavior to achieve the same intake in a grazing situation [30].

Table 4. Grazing frequency (5 min interval) in two observation periods (Period 1, from 8 to 10 am; Period 2, from 10 am to 12 pm) and average biting rate of cows given either commercial concentrate (CC) or ground corn (GC).

Variables	CC		GC		SE [1]	P [2]
	Period 1	Period 2	Period 1	Period 2		
Grazing frequency	23.80 [a]	20.55 [c]	23.80 [a]	22.20 [b]	0.37	0.04
Biting rate (min^{-1})	39.54 [a]		44.21 [b]		1.19	0.03

[1] SE = Standard Error; [2]P = Probability. [a,b,c] Letters indicate statistical differences in the same row.

As the grazing frequency and biting rate suggest, the difference in DM intake from supplements may have caused differences in pasture intake due to a substitution of pasture with concentrate. Lactating cows reduce their grazing time with an increase in supplements from 0 to 3 or 6 kg of concentrate per day [14]. Likewise, Bargo *et al.* [31] found a reduction in grazing time by 12 min/day per kilogram of concentrate compared with a non-supplemented diet; however, in their study there was no change in biting rate (58 bites/min) or bite mass (0.47 g of DM/bite) related to supplementation. The authors suggest a substitution rate ranging from 0.2 to 0.6 kg of pasture DM per DM kg of supplement. In the case of our study, it was not possible to measure pasture intake; however, we can infer that there was a reduction in the intake of pasture due to shorter grazing frequency in the second observation period, which was associated with a lower biting rate.

The total production of milk, fat, protein, lactose and total solids was higher in cows given commercial concentrate ($p < 0.05$, Table 5). However, the contents of fat, protein, lactose and total solids of milk were not affected by treatment ($p > 0.05$). The higher amounts of milk production from animals receiving commercial concentrate can be related to a higher intake of TDN in this treatment. Beyond the differences in supplement composition, a greater portion of CC was fed to lactating cows than the GC portion. Thus, the expected higher milk production from cows in CC treatments is in accordance with studies showing increased production of grazing cows with greater amounts of supplements [11,32].

Table 5. Average production of 3.5% fat corrected milk (FCM) and milk composition of cows on pasture supplemented with commercial concentrate (CC) or ground corn (GC).

Variables	Treatments		SE [1]	P [2]
	CC	GC		
3.5% FCM, kg/d	13.19	11.59	0.818	0.01
Fat%	3.29	3.24	0.188	0.69
Protein%	2.95	2.94	0.083	0.88
Lactose%	4.60	4.57	0.057	0.19
Total Solids%	11.78	11.67	0.283	0.45
Fat kg/d	0.45	0.39	0.029	0.02
Protein kg/d	0.40	0.35	0.022	0.01
Lactose kg/d	0.64	0.55	0.373	0.01
Total solids kg/d	1.61	1.41	0.092	0.01
SCC[3] Log	2.00	1.81	0.266	0.29
N-urea mg/dL	14.46	13.41	0.589	0.25

[1] SE = Standard Error; [2] P = Probability; [3] SCC log = $\log_{10}$ of somatic cell counts.

The somatic cell count (SCC) values did not differ between groups ($p < 0.05$) and all samples met Brazilian legal standards, thus indicating the health of the herd. Similarly, the concentration of N-urea was not affected by treatments ($p < 0.05$) and ranged between 10 and 15 mg dL^{-1}, indicating appropriate levels of dietary CP [33].

We would expect higher levels of carotenoids in the milk from cows fed ground corn as compared to concentrate [34]. Likewise, a higher intake of pasture for animals of the GC group would also be expected. Pasture and ground corn are likely to increase the levels of vitamins and their precursors in milk. However, in this experiment, the dietary differences did not affect carotenoid levels in the milk ($p > 0.05$). An interesting result of our study is that the contents of total carotenoids, β-carotene, vitamin A and vitamin A equivalent differ between lactation periods up to 70 days and beyond 70 days, regardless of treatment (Table 6). Higher contents of total carotenoids and β-carotene ($p < 0.05$) were detected during the lactation period beyond 70 days. These results differ from those obtained by Winkelman *et al.* [35], which showed a decrease of β-carotene during lactation. Changes in the secretion of carotenoids in milk during lactation may be attributed to a decrease in milk production or to the animal's ability to capture these pigments from blood plasma [13,36]. In our study, the results corroborate the hypothesis that a decrease in milk production that occurs in the second lactation period, and consequently the total fat produced, might result in a higher concentration of β-carotene per unit of fat at this later lactation stage. However, a specific effect on the stage of lactation has not been clearly established, since this may be linked to the seasonality of the feed.

Table 6. Carotenoid and Vitamin A contents (μg/g of fat) of milk produced at the initial and median phase of lactation by cows on pasture supplemented with GC or CC.

Variables	Days in Milk		
	0 to 70 Days $n = 9$	**More than 70 Days $n = 11$**	***P***
Total carotenoids	7.77	10.12	0.05
β-carotene	4.88	7.40	0.02
Vitamin A	7.95	9.26	0.53
Vitamin A equivalent	9.84	11.48	0.50

The concentrations of β-carotene found in this study are similar to those produced in milk from cows receiving supplementation in the northern hemisphere during the grazing season [26,37]. However, they are below the values found for animals kept exclusively on pasture in the northern hemisphere, suggesting that concentrate supplementation has a negative impact on this bioactive constituent of milk, even for cows on pasture [37,38].

The cost and revenue estimates related to supplementation and milk production were calculated and are shown in Table 7. The gross revenue of the CC group was US$ 6.07; however, based on the daily cost of feeding, animal production and sale value, the group posted a net return of US$ 4.39. For the GC group, the net return was US$ 4.83. Thus, the greater amount of milk produced by the CC treatment was not accompanied by an economic advantage for the producer and these aspects need to be considered in dairy production management. Extrapolating these values to this property with 25 lactating cows, opting for a GC supplement would result in an increase of US$ 0.44/animal per day, or US$ 332.35/month. Adopting ecologically-based practices in pasture and cattle management appears to reduce the cost of production and improve revenue. Improved economic performance has been observed in Western Santa Catarina State properties, the majority of which have adopted agroecological pasture management. It was also observed that the greatest economic return was strongly correlated with a higher rate of adoption of agroecological practices for pasture management [39].

Table 7. Economic impact of supplementing grazing cows with commercial concentrate (CC) or ground corn (GC). All other costs considered the same.

Variables	CC	GC
Daily supplement intake	3.22 Kg	1.78 Kg
Price of supplement (US$/kg)	US$ 0.52 [1]	US$ 0.28
Daily cost	US$ 1.69	US$ 0.51
Daily production /cow	13.19 L	11.59 L
Milk price/L	US$ 0.46	US$ 0.46
Daily gross income from milk per cow	US$ 6.07	US$ 5.33
Daily net income from milk per cow	US$ 4.39	US$ 4.83

[1] US$ 1.00 = R$ 1.74, in October 2011.

4. Conclusions

This study shows that higher milk productivity does not necessarily improve profitability. Cows with fewer supplements were able to adjust their grazing behavior to meet their protein needs, and this type of dietary modification did not alter milk composition. Future studies should focus on the adequacy of supplementation, taking into account the nutritional requirements of the cows, stage of lactation and distinct quality of pasture throughout the year, in order to improve economic efficiency without jeopardizing the quality of the milk produced.

Acknowledgments

We are grateful to and John Tezza for allowing us to conduct the research on their property and to Sergio Acuña Ballesteros for technical assistance. This study was funded by CNPq (National Council on Scientific and Technological Development), through the Project Inter-institutional Network of the Agroecological Dairy Productive Chain, Project No. 562908/2010-2, Call 22/2010. L.C.P. Machado F° was also provided with financial support from CNPq (National Council for Scientific and Technological Development, Brazil). Finally, we would like to thank Evelyn Nimmo for editing the English of the manuscript.

Author Contributions

Leandro Martins D'Ávila developed the work under the supervision of Professor Luiz Carlos Pinheiro Machado Filho (first author). Nutritional analyses were conducted under the guidance of the Prof. Daniele C. Kazama. The carotenoid analyses were conducted by the third author (Launa Luiza Bento) under the supervision of Professor Shirley Kuhnen.

Conflicts of Interest

The authors declare no conflict of interest.

References

1. ICEPA (2009), Sintese Anual da Agricultura de Santa Catarina. Available Online: http://www.cepa.epagri.sc.gov.br/Publicacoes/SINTESE2001.PDF (accessed on 15 July 2014).
2. Costa, J.H.C.; Hötzel, M.J.; Longo, C.; Balcão, L.F. A survey of management practices that influence production and welfare of dairy cattle on family farms in southern Brazil. *J. Dairy Sci.* **2013**, *96*, 307–317.
3. Honorato, L.A.; Machado Filho, L.C.P.; Barbosa Silveira, I.D.; Hötzel, M.J. Strategies use by dairy family farmers in the south of Brazil to comply with organic regulations. *J. Dairy Sci.* **2014**, *97*, 1319–1327.
4. Balcão, L.F. Tipologia da atividade leiteira na região noroeste de Santa Catarina. Dissertação (Mestrado em Agroecossistemas). Universidade Federal de Santa Catarina, Florianópolis, Brazil 2012; p. 103.

5. Voisin, A. *Produtividade do Pasto*; Mestre Jou: São Paulo, Brazil, 1974; p. 520.
6. Kuhnen, S.; Moacyr, J.R.; Mayer, J.K.; Navarro, B.B.; Trevisan, R.; Honorato, L.A.; Maraschin, M.; Machado Filho, L.C.P. Phenolic content and ferric reducing-antioxidant power of cow's milk produced in different pasture-based production systems in southern Brazil. *J. Sci. Food Agric.* **2014**, doi:10.1002/jsfa.6654.
7. Sato, K.; Bartlett, P.C.; Erskine, R.J.; Kaneene, J.B. A comparison of production and management between Wisconsin organic and conventional dairy herds. *Livest. Prod. Sci.* **2005**, *93*, 105–115.
8. Stiglbauer, K.E.; Cicconi-Hogan, K.M.; Richert, R.; Schukken, Y.H.; Ruegg, P.L.; Gamroth, M. Assessment of herd management on organic and conventional dairy farms in the United States. *J. Dairy Sci.* **2013**, *96*, 1–11.
9. National Research Council. *Nutrient Requirements of Dairy Cattle*, 7th ed.; NRC National Academy Press: Washington, DC, USA, 2001.
10. Soder, K.J.; Rotz, C.A. *Impact of Utilizing a Total Mixed Ration in Pennsylvania Grazing Dairy Herds*; USDA/Agricultural Research Service, Pasture Systems and Watershed Management Research Unit: University Park, PA, USA, 2007.
11. Pulido, R.G.; Muñoz, R.; Lemarie, P.; Wittwer, F.; Orellana, P.; Waghorn, G.C. Impact of increasing grain feeding frequency on production of dairy cows grazing pasture. *Livest. Sci.* **2009**, *125*, 109–114.
12. Pulido, R.G.; Aguilera, P.; Daetz, R.; Wittwer, F.; Orellana, P. Effect of type of concentrate on milk production and composition of dairy cows: Joint Annual Meeting. American Dairy Science Association. *J. Dairy Sci.* **2004**, *87*, 224.
13. Nozière, P.; Graulet, B.; Lucas, A.; Martin, B.; Grolier, P.; Doreau, M. Carotenoids for ruminants: From forages to dairy products. *Anim. Feed Sci. Technol.* **2006**, *131*, 418–450.
14. Sheahan, A.J.; Kolver, E.S.; Roche, J.R. Genetic strain and diet effects on grazing behavior, pasture intake, and milk production. *J. Dairy Sci.* **2011**, *94*, 3583–3591.
15. Pimentel, D. Impacts of Organic Farming on the Efficiency of Energy Use in Agriculture. An Organic Center State of Science Review. The Organic Center, Ithaca, NY, USA p. 40. Available online: http://www.organicvalley.coop/fileadmin/pdf/ENERGY_SSR.pdf (accessed on 15 July 2014).
16. Thomassen, M.A.; van Calker, K.J.; Smits, M.C.J.; Iepema, G.L.; de Boer, I.J.M. Life cycle assessment of conventional and organic milk production in the Netherlands. *Agric. Syst.* **2008**, *96*, 95–107.
17. Freitas, E.A.G.; Dufloth, J.H.; Greiner, L.C. *Tabela de Composição Químico-Bromatológica e Energética dos Alimentos Para Animais Ruminantes em Santa Catarina*; EPAGRI: Florianópolis, SC, Brasil, 1994; p. 333.
18. AOAC. *Official Methods of Analysis*, 15th ed.; AOAC: Washington, DC, USA, 1990.
19. Van Soest, P.J.; Robertson, J.B.; Lewis, B.A. Methods for dietary fiber, neutral detergent fiber, and nonstarch polysaccharides in relation to animal nutrition. *J. Dairy Sci.* **1991**, *74*, 3583–3598.
20. Euclides, V.P.B.; Macedo, M.C.M.; Oliveira, M.P. Avaliação de diferentes métodos para se estimar o valor nutritivo de forragens sob pastejo. *Rev. Bras. Zootecnia* **1992**, *21*, 691–702.
21. Altmann, J. Observational study of behavior: Sampling methods. *Behavior* **1974**, *49*, 227–265.

22. Lehner, P.N. *Handbook of Ethological Methods*, 2nd ed.; Cambridge University Press: Cambridge, UK, 1996; p. 672.
23. Coimbra, P.A.D.; Machado Filho, L.C.P.; Hötzel, M.J. Effects of social dominance, water trough location and shade availability on drinking behavior of cows on pasture. *Appl. Anim. Behav. Sci.* **2012**, *139*, 175–182.
24. *Whole Milk—Determination of Milkfat, Protein and Lactose Content—Guidance on the Opeation of Mid-Infrared Instruments*; IDF Standard 141C; Canadian Dairy Information Centre: Ottawa, ON, Canada, 2000.
25. *Milk—Quantittative Determination of Bacteriological Quality—Guidance for Establishing and Verifying a Conversion Relationship between Routine Method Results and Anchor Method Results*; IDF Standard 196; Canadian Dairy Information Centre: Ottawa, ON, Canada, 2004.
26. Hulshof, P.J.M.; van Roekel-Jansen, T.; van de Bovenkamp, P.; West, C.E. Variation in retinol and carotenoid content of milk and milk products in The Netherlands. *J. Food Compos. Anal.* **2006**, *19*, 67–75.
27. Forbes, T.D.A. Researching the plant-animal interface: The investigation of ingestive behavior in grazing animals. *J. Anim. Sci.* **1988**, *66*, 2369–2379.
28. Rutter, S.M.; Orr, R.J.; Yarrow, N.H.; Champion, R.A. Dietary preference of dairy cows grazing ryegrass and white clover. *J. Dairy Sci.* **2004**, *87*, 1317–1324.
29. Yan, M.J.; Humphreys, J.; Holden, N.M. The carbon footprint of pasture-based milk production: Can white clover make a difference? *J. Dairy Sci.* **2013**, *96*, 857–865.
30. Vance, E.R.; Ferris, C.P.; Elliott, C.T.; Kilpatrick, D.J. A comparison of the feeding and grazing behavior of primiparous Holstein-Friesian and Jersey x Holstein-Friesian dairy cows. *Irish J. Agric. Food Res.* **2012**, *51*, 45–61.
31. Bargo, F.; Muller, L.D.; Kolver, E.S.; Delahoy, J.E. Invited review: Production and digestion of supplemented dairy cows on pasture. *J. Dairy Sci.* **2003**, *86*, 1–42.
32. Fike, J.H.; Staples, C.R.; Sollenberger, L.E.; Macoon, B.; Moore, J.E. Pasture forages, supplementation rate, and stocking rate effects on dairy cow performance. *J. Dairy Sci.* **2003**, *86*, 1268–1281.
33. Prates, E.R.; Mühlbach, P.R.F.; Patino, H.O.; Barcelos, O.J. *Novos Desafios Para Produção Leiteira do Rio Grande do Sul*; UFRGS: Porto Alegre, Brazil, 2000; p. 176.
34. Kuhnen, S.; Menel Lemos, P.M.; Campestrini, L.H.; Ogliari, J.B.; Dias, P.F.; Maraschin, M. Carotenoid and anthocyanin contents of grains of Brazilian maize landraces. *J. Sci. Food Agric.* **2011**, *91*, 1548–1553.
35. Winkelman, A.M.; Johnson, D.L.; MacGibbon, A.K.H. Estimation of heritabilities and correlations associated with milk color traits. *J. Dairy Sci.* **1999**, *82*, 215–224.
36. Jensen, S.K.; Johanssen, A.K.; Hermassen, J.E. Quantitative secretion and maximal secretion capacity of retinol, beta-carotene and alpha-tocopherol into cows' milk. *J. Dairy Res.* **1999**, *66*, 511–522.
37. Butler, G.; Nielsen, J.H.; Slots, T.; Seal, C.; Eyre, M.D.; Sanderson, R.; Leifert, C. Fatty acid and fat-soluble antioxidant concentrations in milk from high- and low-input conventional and organic systems: Seasonal variation. *J. Sci. Food Agric.* **2008**, *88*, 1431–1441.

38. Slots, T.; Butler, G.; Leifert, C.; Kristensen, T.; Skibsted, L.H.; Nielsen, J.H. Potentials to differentiate milk composition by different feeding strategies. *J. Dairy Sci.* **2009**, *92*, 2057–2066.
39. Wendling, A.V.; Ribas, C.E.D.C. Indice de conformidade do pastoreio racional Voisin (IC-PRV). *Rev. Bras. Agroecol.* **2013**, *8*, 26–38.

15

Refining Housing, Husbandry and Care for Animals Used in Studies Involving Biotelemetry

Penny Hawkins

Research Animals Department, Royal Society for the Prevention of Cruelty to Animals (RSPCA), Wilberforce Way, Southwater, West Sussex, RH13 9RS, UK; E-Mail: penny.hawkins@rspca.org.uk.

Simple Summary: Biotelemetry, the remote detection and measurement of an animal function or activity, is widely used in animal research. Biotelemetry devices transmit physiological or behavioural data and may be surgically implanted into animals, or externally attached. This can help to reduce animal numbers and improve welfare, e.g., if animals can be group housed and move freely instead of being tethered to a recording device. However, biotelemetry can also cause pain and distress to animals due to surgery, attachment, single housing and long term laboratory housing. This article explains how welfare and science can be improved by avoiding or minimising these harms.

Abstract: Biotelemetry can contribute towards reducing animal numbers and suffering in disciplines including physiology, pharmacology and behavioural research. However, the technique can also cause harm to animals, making biotelemetry a 'refinement that needs refining'. Current welfare issues relating to the housing and husbandry of animals used in biotelemetry studies are single *vs*. group housing, provision of environmental enrichment, long term laboratory housing and use of telemetered data to help assess welfare. Animals may be singly housed because more than one device transmits on the same wavelength; due to concerns regarding damage to surgical sites; because they are wearing exteriorised jackets; or if monitoring systems can only record from individually housed animals. Much of this can be overcome by thoughtful experimental design and surgery refinements. Similarly, if biotelemetry studies preclude certain enrichment items, husbandry refinement protocols can be adapted to permit some environmental stimulation. Nevertheless, long-term laboratory housing raises welfare concerns and maximum durations should be defined. Telemetered data can be used to help assess welfare, helping to determine endpoints and refine future studies. The above measures will help to improve data quality as well as welfare, because experimental confounds due to physiological and psychological stress will be minimised.

Keywords: Three Rs; refinement; reduction; biotelemetry; environmental enrichment; animal husbandry; surgery; ethical review; animal welfare; welfare assessment

---

1. Introduction

The ethical decision-making process for research projects or procedures involving animals rests on a harm-benefit assessment, in which the likely harms (pain, suffering or distress experienced by animals) are 'weighed' against the potential benefits of the project. This assessment may be conducted by a number of different individuals or bodies, including the regulator, an ethics committee, the researcher or a combination of these. A good harm-benefit assessment involves setting out the potential harms to animals throughout their lives, including not only scientific procedures and their after effects, but also other aspects that may cause suffering such as early 'weaning', transport, husbandry restrictions (e.g., singly housing social animals) and some killing techniques. This approach also identifies opportunities to implement refinement, one of the Three Rs (Replacement of animal experiments with humane alternatives, Reduction of animal numbers to the minimum needed for statistical significance, and Refinement of animal husbandry and procedures to reduce suffering and improve welfare). Refinement can significantly reduce harms to animals, which will clearly impact on the harm-benefit assessment and have implications as to the justification for the project. However, refining one aspect of a procedure may have repercussions that affect welfare in other ways, so it is essential to conduct a thoughtful review of the animal's broader life experience when making decisions about appropriate refinements and how these will be implemented.

One example of a refinement that can give rise to wider welfare issues is biotelemetry, which can be defined as the remote detection and measurement of a human or animal function, activity or condition [1]. The first physiological signal telemetered from a conscious animal was recorded in 1963, when aortic blood flow was successfully transmitted from an exercising boxer dog at the San Diego Zoo hospital [2]. Since then, the use of biotelemetry has expanded hugely within a wide range of biological disciplines including physiology, pharmacology and behavioural studies in both the laboratory and field [3]. Its use has become so well-established that some regulatory bodies require data that can only be obtained using biotelemetry [4].

The use of biotelemetry to transmit physiological or behavioural data is often cited as a way of implementing two of the Three Rs; reduction and refinement. Biotelemetry can indeed reduce animal numbers, by enabling the collection of more, better quality data from each animal, e.g., because data can be gathered over longer periods, or multiple parameters can be recorded from the same individual [3,5]. Removing the need for tethers and restraint during recording, so that animals can behave more normally, is a refinement in that it can significantly reduce stress during data collection [5].

However, despite these benefits, the application of biotelemetry can also be a source of harms to animals. Surgical procedures to implant internal devices can cause pain and distress, as can the fitting of external devices, and the size, shape and weight of the device can be a welfare issue in smaller species [5]. Recording multiple parameters may add to the burden on the animal (e.g., if multiple sensors are implanted), and holding animals in the laboratory in the long term is also a cause for concern and debate as to acceptable maximum durations. Animals may be singly housed, either during recordings or permanently, which is a significant welfare issue for social species or strains.

Taking all of this into account, the use of biotelemetry within each project should **in itself** be subject to a harm-benefit assessment, in common with all other invasive procedures. It is essential to recognise this and regard biotelemetry as a 'refinement that may need refining' rather than a panacea. With this in mind, the RSPCA set up an expert Joint Working Group on Refinement (JWGR) in 2003 to produce good practice guidance reports on procedures involving biotelemetry [5] and housing and care for animals used in such projects [6]. This was within the context of the Society's work to promote effective ethical review of animal use and implementation of the Three Rs.

Ten years on, the use of telemetry has continued to increase, as have developments in device technology. This paper provides an update on some of the topics addressed in the JWGR on housing, husbandry and care for animals involved in biotelemetry studies. It does not address device attachment or implantation, but assumes that these will be fully refined in accordance with legal requirements to minimise suffering by employing effective pain management [7] and current good practice approaches to surgery such as the Laboratory Animal Science Association (LASA) asepsis guidelines [8].

Also over the last decade, the level of debate has increased within the scientific community about the scientific validity and translatability of many animal 'models'. Concerns that have come to the fore include the validity of 'extrapolating' between species, standards of experimental design and reporting, and confounding effects due to physiological and psychological responses to housing, husbandry and care that does not cater for animals' species-specific needs [9–14]. All of these issues have profound ethical implications with respect to the actual 'benefits' of animal research, how funding resources are spent, and whether the needs of patient groups are properly addressed. Reducing stress to animals by employing the approach to housing and care set out in this document will thus not only help to improve welfare, but will also enhance scientific validity.

2. Housing, Husbandry and Care Issues Associated With Biotelemetry

A refined biotelemetry system should: allow animals to be housed in stable, compatible groups; not preclude environmental enrichment; be minimally invasive; and would not be interfered with by other animals in the group. In practice, however, internally and externally mounted devices currently both facilitate and present obstacles to these standards [5,6]. This is expanded upon in Sections 2.1 and 2.2 below, which explain how to provide group housing and enrichment for animals on biotelemetry studies. Some instrumented animals are reused and housed long term, which is addressed in Section 2.3, while Section 2.4 provides examples of how available telemetered data can be used for an additional purpose: to help reduce suffering and improve welfare.

2.1. Group Housing

It is generally accepted that social species, including many commonly used laboratory mammals, should be housed in stable, compatible groups [7,15]. This varies with species, strain and sex, for example there is debate over the benefits of group housing hamsters and some strains of male mice.

Singly housing social species or strains is likely to have significant negative consequences for animal welfare and will also affect data quality, if social isolation leads to physiological responses that affect results [16–21]. Despite this, a proportion of animals used in biotelemetry studies are still singly housed. The reasons that are given for this should always be challenged, as many of the perceived obstacles to group housing can be overcome, as explained below.

Reason 1: Devices all transmit on the same wavelength. Although considerable developments have been made in this area in recent years, many commercially available telemetry devices still transmit at the same frequency. It is obviously impossible to obtain meaningful data from several devices, on different animals, that are all transmitting at the same wavelength within the same pen or cage. If the use of single wavelength devices is unavoidable, solutions include:

(1) The 'buddy' system, in which an instrumented animal is group housed with one or more uninstrumented individuals [20,21]. The fate of the buddy (or buddies) can be planned for in advance. Potential options are: (i) rehoming; (ii) use in another study, provided that the animals are suitable (e.g., of an appropriate age); or (iii) humane killing at the end of the study. Both options (i) and (ii) may involve changing established groups, in which case advice from animal technologists or the attending veterinarian can help to reduce stress to the animals. Option (iii) is an ethical issue, although it need not be an animal welfare issue if the killing technique is properly refined. The animals' tissues or organs should be used in other studies or for training purposes where appropriate, or facilities may sell surplus, euthanased animals for use as food for rehabilitated wildlife, raptors or 'exotic' companion animals. Some establishments have set up programmes in which surplus animals can be certified fit and rehomed to responsible carers [22,23] and there is a legal framework to support rehoming in many countries, provided that it is in the animal's best interests [7].

(2) Devices that can be switched on and off with a magnetically actuated system *in situ*, *i.e.*, following implantation, and used one at a time in pair- or group-housed animals. This avoids the issue of deciding fates for 'ex-buddies', provided that recording data sequentially is compatible with the scientific protocol, or can be compensated for by the experimental design. Switching devices on and off can also extend battery life, thus facilitating reduction in animal numbers because more data can be gathered from each animal (but see Section 2.3 below).

(3) Instrumenting all animals, and then separating them for data recording sessions only. This allows data to be recorded at the same time from different individuals, but periods of social isolation (and being moved to a different enclosure, if applicable) will be highly stressful for some animals, with implications for welfare and data quality [20,21]. The suitability of this approach will depend upon factors such as the species, duration of isolation and whether animals can habituate to the protocol.

(4) Use of data logging devices instead of transmitters, where data are recorded onto a microchip and downloaded once the device has been retrieved from the animal. Data can be retrieved following each session if external loggers are used, but there will clearly be a longer wait in the case of implanted loggers. Also, device failure may not be detected until the download is attempted, meaning that studies would have to be repeated.

At the time of writing, biotelemetry device manufacturers are working on technical innovations that will further facilitate pair and group housing, so it is good practice to keep up to date with developments in multi-wavelength devices and other innovations that can reduce the impact of telemetry on animals, e.g., smaller or lighter devices. A wider range of dual frequency and multi-channel devices has become available; initially for large animals such as dogs, but some are now marketed as small enough for use in rats. However, there are currently no commercially available, implantable, multi-wavelength devices that are suitable for mice.

Reason 2: Animals have undergone implantation surgery and are singly housed in case they damage one another's wounds. Surgical wound failure is painful and distressing, affecting both health and welfare and requiring either repair surgery or the euthanasia of the animal. However, the negative welfare impact of changing from social to permanent single housing should not be underestimated for social species. To look at this another way; wound damage or failure may occur, but the psychological distress due to changing to single housing will occur. In light of this, the ideal is to re-establish animals in their social groups as soon as possible following any kind of surgery, and this should also be the default position for biotelemetry [6].

Different facilities employ a variety of protocols with respect to regrouping after implantation surgery, ranging from immediate regrouping to waiting for a period of several days. In general, animals can be successfully regrouped after 24 hours [5] if steps are taken to ensure that:

- The pair or group was well-established and stable before surgery. If groups are stable before surgery, there is a greater chance of achieving harmonious regrouping afterwards. Drawing pairs or groups from littermates is an obvious option, which should be possible whether animals are bred either in-house or externally. Good liaison with the breeder will be necessary if animals are sourced from outside the establishment (liaison with any external breeding facilities to ensure consistency in housing and care conditions is also good practice, although if there are differences then the aim should be to 'level up' and implement the better husbandry protocols at both).
- If animals have undergone transport to the facility, they have had an adequate settling-in period to enable both recovery from any transport stress and acclimatisation to environmental changes and new caretakers. Absolute minimum settling-in periods before surgery have been suggested of a week for rodents, two weeks for dogs, and a month for non-human primates [6]. Note that animals should be allowed a minimum post-implantation recovery period of two weeks before conducting further procedures [20,21].
- Surgical procedures represent best practice with respect to asepsis, surgical approach, the competence of the surgeon and effective welfare assessment and pain management [5,8,24]. All of these will facilitate a more rapid return to normal behaviour, including social behaviour.
- Animals have recovered from anaesthesia so that they are capable of interacting appropriately with others.
- Wound closure has been fully refined, for example by the use of intradermal sutures [24]. This, together with effective pain management and careful asepsis, will stop animals paying excessive attention to their own wounds, reducing the risk of drawing the attention of others *via* visual or olfactory cues.

- Housing and care are also refined, including the provision of sufficient space and enrichment, which will shift animals' attention from their own and others' wounds and allow them to retreat from one another [6].
- There is adequate supervision from carers in the initial regrouping period, and for as long as is necessary to ensure that there is no persistent discomfort or pain. Behavioural assessments should also check that animals are interacting in an acceptable way, e.g., hierarchies are appropriate and there is no bullying [5,25].

There may be concerns about wound breakdown and bullying if group housing has not been usual practice, or if there is a proposal to regroup animals earlier following surgery. In these cases, a carefully-supervised pilot study, with advice from the attending veterinarian, could be undertaken. This should include and address all of the points in the above list.

One approach to reducing any negative effects of single housing that might arise is 'living apart together', in which animals have no (or minimal) physical contact with one another but can see, hear and/or smell other animals. Visual and olfactory contact is recommended for other species such as non-human primates, rabbits and dogs when separately housed [6,26–28]. However, the benefits of this limited contact can vary between species and strains. For example, female C57BL/6JOlaHsd mice benefit most from social housing after surgery, but if they are separated, limited contact through a grid partition is more stressful than housing them individually [29]. The literature on the effects of social *vs*. individual housing, including behavioural studies to evaluate whether particular species and strains benefit from limited contact, should be regularly reviewed to ensure that protocols reflect current knowledge about animal behaviour and welfare.

> *If single housing really is unavoidable for justifiable scientific reasons, animals should not undergo implantation surgery unless they are able to tolerate being housed on their own. A trial period should be set up to assess how well animals can adapt before moving on with the study.*

Reason 3: Animals are wearing jackets or have exteriorised devices and are singly housed in case they interfere with these. Similar issues arise when group housing animals with devices that are partly or entirely external as when following surgery. Some species can be group housed while fitted with external devices without problems, but with other species there may be concerns that animals could damage one another's jackets or devices, or that stress or injuries could occur due to excessive attention to these. The basic approaches to overcoming this are the same as those for group housing post-surgery, *i.e.*, maintaining stable groups, refining housing and care, and ensuring appropriate supervision.

Other measures that can be undertaken to facilitate group housing for animals with jackets, harnesses or exteriorised devices include ensuring that animals are fully habituated to the device and/or attachment, are trained to accept it and are also accustomed to other animals wearing it. Animals may habituate to relatively large exteriorised devices if they are given the opportunity. For example, mice with headpieces measuring 15 by 20 mm have been successfully housed in groups of 12, with no injuries to the animals or significant damage to any of the devices. This was facilitated by forming and maintaining stable groups and by adding non-working devices to the cage for the mice to explore and manipulate. Although some of the mice tried to bite others' devices for a period of 15 to 20 minutes when first re-grouped after the headpieces were fitted, this was not sustained and the animals quickly lost interest [30].

For studies where jackets are required, trials can be conducted using old jackets and dummy devices to help with habituation. If the only problem lies with animals undoing fastenings, these can simply be made more robust. Some animals (e.g., some groups of dogs, particularly very young ones) may persist in damaging one another's jackets and/or devices, so that it really is impossible to group house them. In such cases, any welfare impact can be reduced by minimising the duration of single housing and implementing 'living apart together' for those species that will benefit from this (see above). It should also be possible to allow socialisation time for singly housed animals in a shared area, with adequate supervision and activities to distract from one another's jackets. Given the wide availability and increasing use of jacketed electrocardiogram (ECG) telemetry systems in large animals, achieving group housing for these animals is a very important goal for animal welfare.

Reason 4: Cage-type monitoring systems that can only record from singly housed animals are being used. Automated, cage-based monitoring systems are sometimes used for behavioural monitoring, for example in phenotyping screens or in neuroscience studies. These may operate using video, by recording food and water consumption, by recording and analysing an animal's movements within a cage placed on a sensor platform, or by a combination of these. Some of these monitoring systems cannot record from or track multiple animals, which necessitates single housing. It is somewhat paradoxical for a behavioural monitoring and characterisation system to require animal housing that is inherently stressful and liable to lead to confounding results, so the use of such systems should be critically questioned on both animal welfare and scientific grounds.

There are some cage-based monitoring systems already available that use transponder technology to recognise individuals, or that include software capable of distinguishing between animals. Where possible, these should be used in preference to those that only permit single housing. As with biotelemetry device technology, it is important to monitor ongoing developments and regularly check whether there is an alternative product or option that permits group housing for social animals.

2.2. Providing Environmental Enrichment

Animals with exteriorised devices are sometimes subject to restrictions on environmental enrichment for fear that they will become entangled or entrapped in some enrichment items (e.g., some nesting materials or refuges). Concerns that animals might hurt or injure themselves on some items can also result in reduced provision of enrichment for animals on biotelemetry studies.

Simply removing the enrichment item is not an appropriate solution, but in some cases there may be justification for adjusting enrichment protocols on veterinary and animal welfare grounds. For example, entanglement in nesting materials can be a real problem for rodents with head caps or cannulae, so some nesting materials would not be appropriate for them. However, it is often possible to cater for the animals' needs in other ways, such as providing non-tangling nesting material and refuges with wide entrances that are designed so that animals cannot climb on top of them and catch exteriorised devices on the cage roof (Figure 1).

Figure 1. This nest box is designed for rats with external devices. (**a**) The box has a wide entrance and is bolted to the cage lid so that the animal cannot move it. The corners are extended to meet the side of the cage at the front left and back right of the box to prevent animals from squeezing between the box and cage walls. (**b**) The adapted box *in situ*.

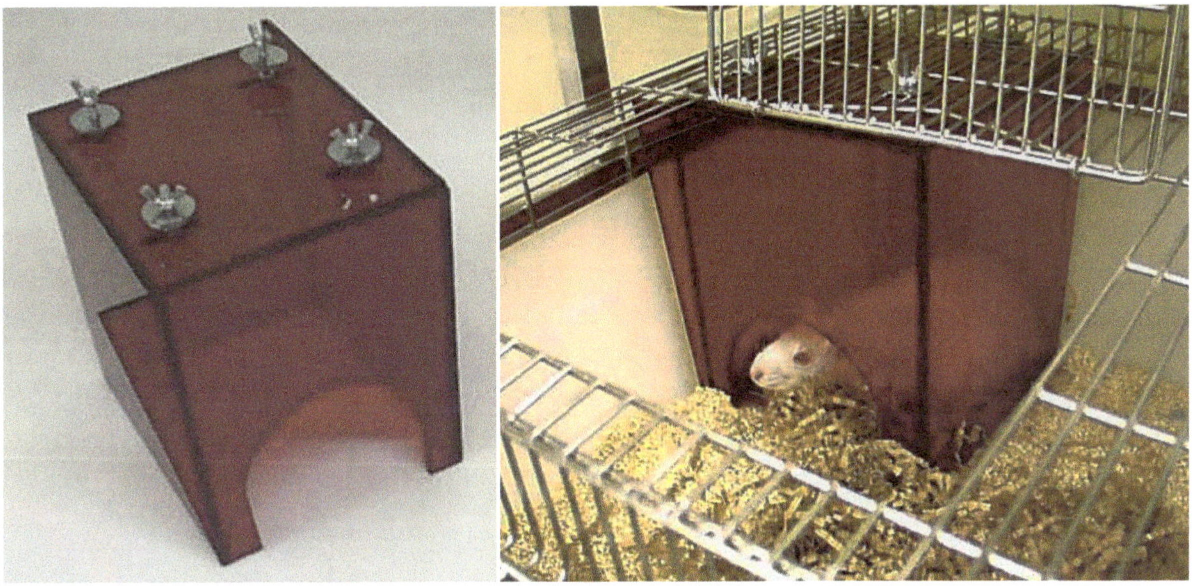

(**a**) (**b**)

Besides concerns about potential injury, some animals may be denied enrichment (including interaction sessions with carers) in case physiological responses to the stimulation will affect data quality [31]. This is unlikely to be the case; it is more likely that isolation and boredom will cause more stress and serious welfare problems [6,20,21], with negative effects on the science.

2.3. Long Term Housing in the Laboratory and Reuse

Instrumented animals are often reused in biotelemetry studies, for example in order to avoid conducting surgical procedures using naïve animals. As a consequence of this, larger species such as dogs and primates may be housed in the laboratory for some time (there are legal constraints on reuse in many countries, including Member States of the European Union. These include requirements relating to the severity of the previous procedures and the health and fitness of the animal [7]). Battery life is an inevitable constraint on the duration of an animals' stay in the laboratory, but the primary consideration should be animal welfare. Some facilities implement fixed time limits after which animals will no longer be reused, which may run to a couple of years or, exceptionally, six years or more. Others do not implement a fixed limit but regularly review the individual animals and how they respond to long term housing in the laboratory [31]. Regardless of whether time limits are in place, it is good practice to monitor animals for signs that they are becoming 'institutionalised' and losing the ability to cope with their environment. An appropriately tailored welfare assessment scheme, including indicators that animals are experiencing chronic adverse effects, is essential in this regard. Refining housing and care will also help to ensure that animals will be comfortable in their environment in the long term [6].

Enrichment is a husbandry refinement that can also supply additional indicators of an animal's welfare state; for example, animals who are becoming depressed or uncomfortable may stop making properly constructed nests, or climbing onto platforms, or they may generally become less interested in their enrichment items and one another. Welfare assessment protocols should be adequately tailored to animals on long-term studies and should ensure that subtle signs of suffering can be detected before more significant welfare problems occur [25].

There is also an ethical dilemma associated with long-term housing and reuse, in which the requirement to minimise the use of naïve animals has to be balanced against setting limits on the number of times animals are re-used, and on how long they should live in research facilities. The attending veterinarian, others with animal welfare expertise and well-informed ethics or animal care and use committees can play a useful role in considering and weighing these issues, e.g., by helping to decide on humane endpoints such as behaviours that indicate chronic distress, on absolute limits on the number of times animals are reused, or on the length of time that individuals stay at the facility. Input from the attending veterinarian is an essential part of the decision-making process, and is a legal requirement in many countries [7].

2.4. Using Telemetered Physiological or Behavioural Data to Help Assess Wellbeing

Many variables that are monitored and recorded in biotelemetry studies are also useful in assessing animal welfare. For example, heart rate, blood pressure and body temperature can all act as indicators that animals may be experiencing pain, suffering or distress, in conjunction with other criteria such as behaviour, body weight, *etc*. Physiological data can be obtained from animals with devices in place for scientific purposes (so there are no additional harms to experimental subjects) and used to evaluate the impact of disturbances (e.g., building work), or different housing and care protocols [5]. Some examples of ways in which practitioners are using biotelemetry to assess welfare include (on the basis of an online survey conducted by the author):

- using telemetered data to help determine humane endpoints;
- reusing implanted animals in welfare studies, e.g., to provide physiological correlates with behaviour;
- using telemetered data to assess stress due to restraint and transport;
- comparing responses to different housing, enrichments and interactions with humans;
- monitoring recovery from surgery using telemetered data; and
- using physiological data to help compare the effectiveness of different analgesic agents.

Opportunities to use telemetered data to reduce the suffering and improve the welfare of the animals on the study—or other animals—should be identified and taken up wherever possible. For example, discussion between the researcher and the ethics or animal care and use committee at the project planning stage may identify the potential to use the data in this way, or this may arise at mid-term or retrospective review of a project [31].

3. Recommendations

Whatever the species of animal, purpose of the study or nature of the biotelemetry system, the aim should be to provide a good standard of housing and care for animals on biotelemetry studies, as for any other project. Although biotelemetry can present some challenges to refining housing and care, many of these can be overcome by flexible thinking, keeping up to date with developments and being prepared to resource new equipment and approaches, as set out in the recommendations below.

- Recognise that although biotelemetry can facilitate reduction and refinement, the technique has the potential to cause suffering—it is a 'refinement that needs refining'. There is a need to apply a harm-benefit assessment to procedures involving biotelemetry and to ensure that these are fully refined.
- Keep up to date with technical developments such as wider availability of multi-frequency devices and smaller implants. If there are unmet technological needs that could help to refine the use of biotelemetry (e.g., multi-frequency, implantable devices for mice), communicate with device manufacturers to make them aware of the demand.
- Ensure that surgical procedures are conducted according to current good practice with respect to the competence of the surgeon, surgical approach, welfare assessment, pain management, wound closure and asepsis.
- Provide group housing for social animals used in biotelemetry studies as the default; ensure that animals are only singly housed if there is sound scientific or veterinary justification.
- If periods of single housing are unavoidable during data collection, keep these to a minimum and monitor animals carefully during reintroductions.
- Provide environmental enrichment as the default, thinking creatively about alternative approaches if some items would not be appropriate.
- Critically consider the pros and cons of automated observation systems that necessitate single housing, taking the welfare and scientific implications into account.
- Set a limit for maximum duration of laboratory housing for long term studies, with clear criteria for behavioural assessments and humane endpoints. Seek advice on this from the attending veterinarian, experienced animal technologists, and/or local ethics, animal care and use committee or animal welfare body as appropriate.

Acknowledgments

Many thanks to Dusty Karazan and Cindy Argue for a very helpful discussion; also to members of Compmed, the Laboratory Animal Refinement and Enrichment Forum (LAREF) and the LinkedIn Laboratory Animal Science Group for sharing information about their current practices with me. Thanks also to Maggy Jennings, Sophie Masneuf and Tony Webb for their helpful comments during the drafting of this paper.

Conflicts of Interest

The author declares no conflict of interest.

References

1. *Dictionary and Thesaurus – Merriam-Webster Online*. Available online: http://www.merriam-webster.com/ (accessed on 13 December 2013).
2. Sarazan, R.D.; Schweitz, K.T.R. Standing on the shoulders of giants: Dean Franklin and his remarkable contributions to physiological measurements in animals. *Adv. Physiol. Educ.* **2009**, *33*, 144–156.
3. Grenwis, J.E. Recent advances in telemetry promote further progress in reduction and refinement. NC3Rs Invited Articles, 2010. Available online: http://www.nc3rs.org.uk/news.asp?id=16 (accessed on 13 December 2013).
4. Anon. ICHS7A Safety Pharmacology Studies for Human Pharmaceuticals. 2000. Available online: http://www.ich.org/fileadmin/Public_Web_Site/ICH_Products/Guidelines/Safety/S7A/Step4/S7A_Guideline.pdf (accessed on 13 December 2013).
5. Morton, D.B.; Hawkins, P.; Bevan, R.; Heath, K.; Kirkwood, J.; Pearce, P.; Scott, L.; Whelan, G.; Webb, A. Refinements in telemetry procedures: Seventh report of the BVA(AWF)/FRAME/RSPCA/UFAW Joint Working Group on Refinement, Part A. *Lab. Anim.* **2003**, *37*, 261–299.
6. Hawkins, P.; Morton, D.B.; Bevan, R.; Heath, K.; Kirkwood, J.; Pearce, P.; Scott, L.; Whelan, G.; Webb, A. Husbandry refinements for rats, mice, dogs and non-human primates used in telemetry procedures: Seventh report of the BVA(AWF)/FRAME/RSPCA/UFAW Joint Working Group on Refinement, Part B. *Lab. Anim.* **2004**, *38*, 1–10.
7. European Commission. Directive 2010/63/EU of the European Parliament and of the Council of 22 September 2010 on the Protection of Animals used for Scientific Purposes. *Off. J. Eur. Union* **2010**, *L 276*, 33–79.
8. *Guiding Principles for Preparing for Undertaking Aseptic Surgery. A Report by the LASA Education, Training and Ethics Section*; Jennings, M., Berdoy, M., Eds.; Laboratory Animal Science Association (LASA): Tamworth, UK, 2010. Available online: http://www.lasa.co.uk/publications.html (accessed on 13 December 2013).
9. van der Staay, F.J.; Arndt, S.S.; Nordquist, R.E. Evaluation of animal models of neurobehavioral disorders. *Behav. Brain. Funct.* **2009**, *5*, doi:10.1186/1744-9081-5-11.
10. Kilkenny, C.; Parsons, N.; Kadyszewski, E.; Festing, M.F.W.; Cuthill, I.C.; Fry, D.; Hutton, J.; Altman, D.G. Survey of the quality of experimental design, statistical analysis and reporting of research using animals. *PLoS ONE* **2009**, *4*, doi:10.1371/journal.pone.0007824.
11. van der Worp, H.B.; Howells, D.W.; Sena, E.S.; Porritt, M.J.; Rewell, S.; O'Collins, V.; Macleod, M.R. Can animal models of disease reliably inform human studies? *PLoS Med.* **2010**, *7*, doi:10.1371/journal.pmed.1000245.
12. Editorial Staff of Annals of the New York Academy of Sciences. *Animal Models: Their Value in Predicting Drug Efficacy and Toxicity*; Wiley-Blackwell: Hoboken, NJ, USA, 2011; Volume 1245.
13. CAMARADES. *Why is CAMARADES Needed?* 2011. Available online: http://www.camarades.info/index_files/Why%20CAMARADES.htm (accessed on 29 January 2014).
14. Hawkins, P. Facts and demonstrations: Exploring the effects of enrichment on data quality. *The Enrichment Record* 2014, pp. 12–21. Available online: http://enrichmentrecord.com/current-issue/ (accessed on 18 February 2014).

15. National Research Council. *Guide for the Care and Use of Laboratory Animals*, 8th ed.; National Academies Press: Washington, DC, USA, 2011.
16. Pérez, C.; Canal, J.R.; Domínguez, E.; Campillo, J.E.; Guillén, M.; Torres, M.D. Individual housing influences certain biochemical parameters in the rat. *Lab. Anim.* **1997**, *31*, 357–361.
17. Späni, D.; Arras, M.; König, B.; Rülicke, T. Higher heart rate of laboratory mice housed individually *vs* in pairs. *Lab. Anim.* **2003**, *37*, 54–62.
18. Verwer, C.M.; van der Ven, L.T.M.; van den Bos, R.; Hendriksen, C.F.M. Effects of housing condition on experimental outcome in a reproduction toxicity study. *Reg. Tox. Pharmacol.* **2007**, *48*, 184–193.
19. Karelina, K.; Norman, G.J.; Zhang, N.; Morris, J.S.; Peng, H.; DeVries, A.C. Social isolation alters neuroinflammatory response to stroke. *PNAS* **2009**, *106*, 5895–5900.
20. Meijer, M.K.; Kramer, K.; Remie, R.; Spruijt, B.M.; van Zutphen, L.F.M.; Baumans, V. Effect of routine procedures on physiological parameters in mice kept under different husbandry procedures. *Anim. Welf.* **2006**, *15*, 31–38.
21. Meijer, M.K.; Sommer, R.; Spruijt, B.M.; van Zutphen, L.F.M. Influence of environmental enrichment and handling on the acute stress response in individually housed mice. *Lab. Anim.* **2007**, *41*, 161–173.
22. Laboratory Animal Science Association (LASA). *Laboratory Animal Science Association Guidance on the Rehoming of Laboratory Dogs. A Report Based on a LASA Working Party and LASA Meeting on Rehoming Laboratory Animals*; Jennings, M., Howard, B., Eds.; LASA: Tamworth, UK, 2004. Available online: http://www.lasa.co.uk/publications.html (accessed on 13 December 2013).
23. Hawkins, P.; Hubrecht, R.; Buckwell, A.; Cubitt, S.; Howard, B.; Jackson, A. *Refining Rabbit Care: A Resource for Those Working With Rabbits in Research*; RSPCA: Southwater, UK, 2008. Available online: http://www.rspca.org.uk/researchrabbits (accessed on 13 December 2013).
24. Wolfensohn, S.; Lloyd, M. Introduction to surgery and surgical techniques. In *Handbook of Laboratory Animal Management and Welfare*, 4th ed.; Wolfensohn, S., Lloyd, M., Eds.; Wiley-Blackwell: Chichester, UK, 2013.
25. Hawkins, P.; Morton, D.B.; Burman, O.; Dennison, N.; Honess, P.; Jennings, M.; Lane, S.; Middleton, V.; Roughan, J.V.; Wells, S.; Westwood, K. A guide to defining and implementing protocols for the welfare assessment of laboratory animals: Eleventh report of the BVA(AWF)/FRAME/RSPCA/UFAW Joint Working Group on Refinement. *Lab. Anim.* **2011**, *45*, 1–13.
26. Seaman, S.C. *Laboratory Rabbit Housing: An Investigation of the Social and Physical Environment*; A Summary of the Report to the UFAW Pharmaceutical Housing and Husbandry Steering Committee (PHHSC), Based on a Ph.D. Thesis, 2002. Available online: http://www.ufaw.org.uk/pdf/phhsc-schol1-summary.pdf (accessed on 13 December 2013).
27. Buchanan-Smith, H. Marmosets and tamarins. In *The UFAW Handbook on the Care and Management of Laboratory and Other Research Animals*, 8th ed.; Hubrecht, R., Kirkwood, J., Eds; Wiley-Blackwell: Chichester, UK, 2010; pp. 543–563.

28. MacArthur Clark, J.; Pomeroy, C.J. The laboratory dog. In *The UFAW Handbook on the Care and Management of Laboratory and Other Research Animals*, 8th ed.; Hubrecht, R., Kirkwood, J., Eds; Wiley-Blackwell: Chichester, UK, 2010; pp. 432–452.
29. Van Loo, P.L.P.; Kuin, N.; Sommer, R.; Avsaroglu, H.; Pham, T.; Baumans, V. Impact of 'living apart together' on postoperative recovery of mice compared with social and individual housing. *Lab. Anim.* **2007**, *41*, 441–455.
30. Masneuf, S. University of Zurich, Zurich, Switzerland. Personal observations, 2011.
31. LASA/RSPCA. *Guiding Principles on Good Practice for Ethical Review Processes*, 2nd ed.; 2010. Available online: http://www.lasa.co.uk/publications.html (accessed on 13 December 2013).

Effect of Transport Distance and Season on Some Defects of Fresh Hams Destined for DPO Production

Agnese Arduini [1,*], Veronica Redaelli [1], Fabio Luzi [2], Stefania Dall'Olio [1], Vincenzo Pace [3] and Leonardo Nanni Costa [1]

[1] Department of Agricultural and Food Science, School of Agriculture and Veterinary Medicine, University of Bologna, Via Fanin 50, 40127 Bologna, Italy; E-Mails: veronica.redaelli@unibo.it (V.R.); stefania.dallolio@unibo.it (S.D.); leonardo.nannicosta@unibo.it (L.N.C.)

[2] Department of Health, Animal Science and Food Safety, Faculty of Veterinary Science, University of Milan, Via Celoria 10, 20133 Milan, Italy; E-Mail: fabio.luzi@unimi.it

[3] OPAS, Pig Farmer Association, Strada Ghisiolo 57, 46030 San Giorgio, Mantua, Italy; E-Mail: vincenzo.opas@coopgsp.it

* Author to whom correspondence should be addressed; E-Mail: agnese.arduini@unibo.it.

Simple Summary: Transport to the slaughterhouse is a stressful event for pigs. Travel duration and conditions can negatively affect animal welfare and carcass quality. Some defects in fresh hams are strictly connected to pre-slaughter transportation. Journeys with short (<37 km) and long (>170 km) distances may increase damage in fresh hams and decrease Denomination Protected of Origin (DPO) Parma dry-cured ham production.

Abstract: Pre-slaughter handling is related to defects in fresh hams that result in exclusion from the DPO Parma chain, including hematomas, lacerations, microhaemorrhages and veining. To determine the effects of transport conditions on hams, we collected data on defects in 901,990 trimmed fresh hams from heavy pigs provided by 3,650 batches from slaughterhouse during 2012 and 2013. For all batches, transport distance (1–276 km) season and year of delivery were considered. A decrease of all defect occurrences was observed for increasing distance up to 170 km ($P < 0.05$). Above 170 km, however, all defects frequencies increased ($P < 0.05$). Season showed an effect on the incidence of defects, with an increasing of hematomas and lacerations in winter and autumn respectively ($P < 0.05$) and the highest percentage of veining and hemorrhages in spring

($P < 0.05$). Summer had the lowest incidence of defects on fresh hams. We concluded that the incidence of the examined defects and the subsequent rejection for DPO Parma ham production is lower in fresh hams transported 38–170 km during the summer.

Keywords: pigs; transport; distance; season; DPO Parma ham; pre-slaughter handling; defect

---

1. Introduction

Pre-slaughter is known to be a critical period for pigs [1,2], because several factors, *i.e.*, inadequate transport conditions, inappropriate handling [3] and length of the journey [4], can seriously affecting animals welfare both physically and psychologically. Additionally, carcass quality can be adversely affected by inadequate pre-slaughter conditions, such as rough practices of loading and unloading and inappropriate driving style of trucks and pigs that may lead to skin wounds, hemorrhages and hematomas [2]. Increased incidence of blood-splashed and skin damage was found in pigs handled roughly or driven by electric prods during pre-slaughter [5]. These injuries represent a significant economic loss, especially if they are located on the most valuable cuts such as hams, loins and shoulders. According to Von Borrell (2005) [6], transport is considered to be a major stressor might have deleterious effects on product quality. Previous research indicates that pig welfare is affected by both long and short journeys [7]. Mota-Rojas *et al.* [8] found that the percentage of bruised carcasses increases with journey duration, while Barton Gade and Christensen [9] reported an increased risk of skin damage during short transports (2–3 h), and Gispert *et al.* [10] found higher skin damage scores in short transports (<2 h) *vs.* long transports (>2 h).

The effect of the season on pig welfare and carcass quality have been also reported [11,12]. The frequency of skin blemishes, hematomas and blood splashing was shown to increase in winter, probably caused by slips and falls due to slippery icy floor [13–15].

Raw hams from heavy pigs (160–170 kg live weight) reared in Northern Italy are primarily processed to DPO (Denomination Protected Origin) dry-cured hams under the control of several consortia, of which Parma Consortium is largest, branding about 10 million dry-cured hams per year (PQI 2014, PQI 2013, Prosciutto di Parma.it) [16,17]. The Parma Quality Institute (PQI) [16] inspects fresh hams destined for the DPO dry-curing process for the presence of an inappropriate physical characteristics like lean-fat ratio or physical injuries, such as hematomas, microhaemorrhages, muscle lacerations and subcutaneous veining caused by pre-slaughter handling; these lesions lead to exclusion of the cuts from the DPO Parma chain. A study of more than 100,000 fresh hams monitored by PQI in 2013 found that 4.3 % of these were rejected for DPO dry-cured ham production due to hematomas, microhaemorrhages, muscle lacerations and subcutaneous veining. Extended to the annual production of fresh hams destined to DPO Parma dry-cured ham equal to 16 million, the total number of fresh hams rejected for pre-slaughter defects could reach 689,000 with an estimated economic loss around 7.6 million euro per year for the whole Parma Consortium and Italian Food Industry.

The aim of this study was to evaluate the effects of transport distance, in connection to the slaughter season, on the incidence of defects observed on fresh hams destined for processing to DPO dry-cured ham.

2. Experimental Section

2.1. Data Sampling

This study was carried out in 2012 and 2013 on data collected from 901,990 trimmed fresh hams of heavy pigs provided in 3,650 batches supplied by 411 farmers and slaughtered over 396 days in a single plant located in Northern Italy. Each batch contained 7–151 pigs with an average of 124 animals per batch. All pigs were 9 months old with live weights of kg 171.1 ± 6.1, as required by the Parma dry-cured ham Consortium [18].

2.2. Pre-Slaughter Conditions and Abattoir

Transportation distances from farm to slaughterhouse ranged from 1 to 276 km and average shipping speed based on motorway proximity and road conditions was estimated at 60 km/h. The deliveries were carried out using double trailer lorries with three hydraulic deck. The lorries had natural and mechanical ventilation system, with fans placed on the left side of the trucks. Stocking density during transport was estimated ranging 141–251 kg/m^2 and the journey duration ranged 0.25–5 h. The loading was done using the mobile ramp commonly present at the piggery (length m 6.0, width m 0.7, with solid side walls of m. 1.0 and adjustable height), while unloading at the slaughterhouse was carried out by a platform (length m 9.3, width m 2.7, solid side walls m 1.0) with adjustable height at the level of the lower deck. The vehicle was always unloaded before the rear trailer. Lairage time ranged between 30 min to 1.5 h. During this period, pigs were not mixed with unfamiliar animals. Averages and ranges of seasonal temperature and relative humidity during 2012 and 2013 in the area where pigs were transported are shown in Table 1.

Table 1. Temperature (°C) and Relative Humidity (%) in the slaughterhouse area during 2012 and 2013.

	Temperature (°C)						**Relative Humidity (%)**					
	2012			**2013**			**2012**			**2013**		
	Average	Range		Average	Range		Average	Range		Average	Range	
Winter	3	−2	9	4	0	8	81	58	100	85	69	100
Spring	17	11	23	16	10	21	70	44	100	73	50	100
Summer	24	17	32	23	16	30	66	39	100	70	42	100
Autumn	10	6	15	10	7	15	83	65	100	86	68	100

Pigs were driven with plastic sticks or rubber boards to resting pens, where they remained 0.5–4.0 h, with only a few batches resting overnight. After resting, pigs were showered and driven through a single chute to the stunning cage. Stunning was accomplished by electrical tongs (head only; 170 V, 1.3 A). Carcasses were then exsanguinated horizontally for 3 min and hanged vertically for 10 min before being immersed into the scalding tank. Carcasses were hot-boned and kept in the cooler (2–4 °C) overnight. The next day, hams were trimmed to the commercial shape, classified for damages and selected according to market criteria.

2.3. Defects Observed

Data on defects such as hematomas, lacerations, microhaemorrhages and superficial veining related to pre-slaughter practices were recorded on trimmed fresh hams. Hematomas are lumps formed by blood clots beneath the skin, typically associated with ruptured blood vessels, that can be produced by impacts against either the handling facilities or improperly used handling prods [3]. Lacerations are similar to dark hematomas distributed in the medial side of the ham and are caused by muscle tears, which may be related to slipping on wet floors during driving. Microhaemorrhages are characterized by pinpoint bleeding in the muscles due to capillary rupture and are generally attributed to rough handling, electrical stunning and vertical exsanguination [19–22]. Superficial veining is a subcutaneous venous lattice affecting the medial, or sometimes the entire, surface of the thigh. This ham defect appears several hours after slaughter, is particularly noticeable during the dressing process and is still evident at the end of the processing and seasoning [23]. The incidence and severity of the veining defect was found to be associated with the prolongation of pre-slaughter procedures (loading, transport and lairage time), with the use of CO_2 stunning methods and with the increase of time between the separation of ham from the hot carcass and chilling from 15 min to 60 min [23]; however, the causes remain largely unexplained [19].

Trimmed hams were classified on the basis of the presence of defects, according to PQI photographic standards, by two trained slaughterhouse operators and recorded in an electronic database according to batch and producer identity. Defects were calculated as percentage per batch.

2.4. Statistical Analysis

Batches were classified by distance between supplier and slaughterhouse using the FASTclust procedure of Statistical Analysis System (SAS 9.3 Cary, NC, USA, 2009). Data were assigned to four clusters based on the smallest Euclidean distance from the initial seed in the cluster. The number of batches assigned to each cluster and the respective mean distances, standard deviations (SD) and minimum (min) and maximum (max) distances are reported in Table 2. Slaughter days were grouped into seasons and were monitored over two years to evaluate defect incidence change from year to year. The distribution of batches and pigs between season and year is reported in Table 3. Defect incidences approximated a Poisson distribution and were log transformed by the GLIMMIX procedure (SAS 9.3 Cary, NC, USA) prior to statistical analysis. The model included cluster, season and year and their respective interactions as fixed effects, and farm within day of slaughter as random effects. The ILINK option was used to back-transform least squares means, and differences between least squares means were evaluated by Tukey-Kramer's test ($P < 0.05$).

Table 2. Distance and transport conditions for batches and pigs based on cluster.

Cluster (Distance)	**1 (11–37 km)**	**2 (38–86 km)**	**3 (89–170 km)**	**4 (199–276 km)**
No. of batches	1,573	990	347	740
No. of pigs	195,596	119,213	42,554	93,632
Average No. pigs/batch	124	120	123	127

Table 2. *Cont.*

Cluster (Distance)	**1 (11–37 km)**	**2 (38–86 km)**	**3 (89–170 km)**	**4 (199–276 km)**
Distance:				
-average (km)	21	50	121	237
-standard deviation (km)	10	9	18	12
-min (km)	1	38	89	199
-max (km)	37	86	170	276
Transport condition:				
-type of vehicle:				
single vehicle	298	246	74	112
double trailer	1,275	744	273	628
-estimated duration (h)	0.5	1–1.5	2–3	3–5
-average stocking density (kg/m^2)	213	206	207	218

Table 3. Distribution of batches and pigs based on season and year.

Cluster (Distance)	**1 (11–37 km)**	**2 (38–86 km)**	**3 (89–170 km)**	**4 (199–276 km)**
Season				
Winter				
No. of batches	384	200	103	172
No. of pigs	47,765	24,581	12,881	21,759
Spring				
No. of batches	401	266	87	190
No. of pigs	49,563	31,662	10,842	24,181
Summer				
No. of batches	415	256	71	176
No. of pigs	50,496	30,659	8,458	22,608
Autumn				
No. of batches	373	268	86	202
No. of pigs	47,772	32,311	10,373	25,048
Year				
2012				
No. of batches	780	433	202	373
No. of pigs	96,406	52,193	26,148	46,808
2013				
No. of batches	793	557	145	367
No. of pigs	99,190	67,020	16,406	46,824

3. Results and Discussion

In 2012, the incidence of hematomas, lacerations and microhaemorrhages observed in trimmed hams were 4.3%, 1.7% and 1.5%, respectively. In 2013, hematomas increased to 6.2%, while lacerations and microhaemorrhages showed very similar incidences equal to 1.7% and 1.6%, respectively. During the two years, PQI, detected in the whole Parma chain (around 4200 farms and 130 slaughter plants) about twice as much the incidence of these defects [16].

The results of variance analysis and the least-squares means of defects frequency by sources of variation are reported in Table 3. Distance, season and year showed to have a significant effect on the incidence of defects under study. Significant interactions between distance × season and between distance x year were found for hemorrhages, and for hemorrages and veining, respectively. Moreover, there was a significant season x year interaction for hemorrhages, veining and laceration. Incidence of defects decreased with increasing transport distance from Cluster 1 (11–37 km) to Cluster 3 (89–170 km) ($P < 0.05$). The higher incidence of defects associated with short transport distances may be due to the lack of time to lie down and recovery from loading stress. Also, a reduction of standing pigs and increasing journey duration could explain this result. Lambooij (2007) showed that the percentages of slaughter pigs standing during transport decreased with journey time, which leads to a reduction in risk of slips, falls and overlaps [2]. Additionally, these results could be the consequence of truck drivers working hurriedly to accomplish all planned transports for a given day, as well as the effect of the lower quality of rural roads, which represent the major part of the route in short journeys. Nevertheless, extending of transport distance above 170 km (Cluster 4) results in an increased incidence of defects, which reaches and exceeds the frequency recorded for Cluster 1. There were no differences in hematomas and veining between clusters 4 and 1, while lacerations and hemorrhages incidences were significantly higher ($P < 0.05$) in Cluster 4. Thus, the incidence of defects reported herein was not proportional to the increase of transport distance. Mota-Rojas *et al.* [8] observed an increase in pig carcass bruising prolonging the journey from 8 to 23 h. Gallo *et al.* [24] identified similar trends in slaughter beef transported for 36 h. The incidence of defects on fresh hams was also influenced by season of transport (Table 4). The percentage of hematomas was greatest ($P < 0.05$) in winter, decreasing in spring and summer ($P < 0.05$) and reaching the lowest incidence in autumn ($P < 0.05$). There are no differences between winter, spring and summer for lacerations, while the incidence of this defect was greater ($P < 0.05$) in autumn. Gosàlvez *et al.* [15] reported a higher incidence of bruised carcasses in pigs transported in winter and in autumn. Scheeren *et al.* [13] hypothesize that the greater proportion of skin damage in winter is linked to the tendency of pigs to stand during transportation to avoid making contact with the cold floor and walls of the trailer. Dalla Costa *et al.* [25] found that pigs were more difficult to handle in winter and need more coercion, which led to more handling-induced bruises. The higher incidence of lacerations observed in autumn could be related to the increase of live weight in this season, due to a restarting of feed intake for the decrease of temperature with respect to the summer. The average live weights recorded by the slaughterhouse during 2012 and 2013 confirms that in autumn there was an increase of more than one kg with respect to the summer (169.1 *vs.* 170.6 kg in 2012 and 169.4 *vs.* 170.9 kg in 2013). This seasonal increase of live weight of heavy pigs was also shown by the national slaughter statistics of heavy pigs [26].

The incidence of hemorrhages was greater ($P < 0.05$) in spring and in autumn while the veining defect was greater in spring. These results cannot easily be attributed to differences in seasonal conditions. The lowest occurrences of lacerations and hemorrhages were found in summer. Warmer temperatures recorded during this season probably lead to a more careful handling in order to reduce the risk of transport mortality [15,25,27]. It is well known that high environmental temperature is a risk factor for transport mortality [28,29].

A significant source of variation in the incidence of raw ham defects was found in studies over several years. The higher incidence of all defects was found in 2013, especially for hematomas and veining. Crisis-invested DPO dry-cured ham production became more important in 2013 with respect to the previous year. It is probably that the reduction of employees for reducing costs lead to an overworking of staff involved in transport and in pre-slaughter handling with a consequent reduction of its quality. The detrimental effect to animal welfare due to overworking of employees involved in animal handling was highlighted by Grandin [30].

Table 4. Results of variance analysis and least-squares means of defects incidence by sources of variation.

Sources of variation	Hematomas (%) P / Least squares mean	Lacerations (%) P / Least squares mean	Hemorrhages (%) P / Least squares mean	Veining (%) P / Least squares mean
Distance	**0.0079**	**<0.0001**	**<0.0001**	**<0.0001**
1 (11–37 km)	4.57 a	1.48 b	1.32 b	11.04 a
2 (38–86 km)	4.44 ab	1.31 c	1.34 b	11.14 a
3 (89–170 km)	4.08 b	1.30 bc	1.08 c	9.24 b
4 (199–276 km)	4.78 a	1.91 a	1.77 a	11.50 a
Pooled SEM(*)	0.11	0.06	0.05	0.22
Season	**<0.0001**	**<0.0001**	**<0.0001**	**<0.0001**
Winter	6.53 a	1.32 b	1.19 b	12.05 b
Spring	5.88 b	1.33 b	1.74 a	15.23 a
Summer	3.58 c	1.28 b	0.96 c	8.70 c
Autumn	2.87 d	2.13 a	1.71 a	8.18 c
Pooled SEM(*)	0.12	0.06	0.05	0.24
Year	**<0.0001**	**0.0359**	**<0.0001**	**<0.0001**
2012	3.70 b	1.42 b	1.24 b	9.73 b
2013	5.37 a	1.55 a	1.48 a	11.74 a
Pooled SEM(*)	0.08	0.04	0.04	0.04
Distance × season	**0.7421**	**0.3412**	**0.0352**	**0.5894**
Distance × year	**0.1526**	**0.7083**	**0.0137**	**0.0007**
Season × year	**0.1926**	**0.0056**	**<0.0001**	**<0.0001**

(*) SEM: Standard Error of Mean; Means in the same column without the same letter differ significantly ($P < 0.05$).

Interaction between distance and season (Table 5) affected the incidence of hemorrhages ($P < 0.05$). The defect increased markedly when distance increased above 170 km in spring and in autumn ($P < 0.05$). Differences between seasons were observed for less than 37 km distance (Cluster 1), with summer showing the lowest incidence of hemorrhages ($P < 0.05$). Above this distance, the lowest incidences of the defect were found in summer and in winter ($P < 0.05$).

Table 5. Effect of interaction between distance and season on the incidence of hemorrhages.

	Cluster (Distance)				Pooled SEM
	1 (11–37 km)	2 (38–86 km)	3 (89–170 km)	4 (199–276 km)	
Hemorrhages (%)					
Winter	1.36 ab x	1.14 ab y	0.87 b y	1.49 a y	0.0931
Spring	1.55 b x	1.71 b x	1.58 b x	2.16 a x	0.1096
Summer	0.98 ab y	1.00 ab y	0.65 b y	1.33 a y	0.0912
Autumn	1.48 b x	1.67 b x	1.52 b x	2.26 a x	0.1527

Least square means within a row with different letters (a–b) differ ($P < 0.05$); Least square means within a column with different letters (x–y) differ ($P < 0.05$).

Interaction between distance and year (Table 6) affected the frequencies of hemorrhages and veining. They increased both in 2012 and 2013 when distance increased above 170 km. The lowest incidences of these defects ($P < 0.05$) were found for cluster 3 (89–170 km) in 2012 only.

Table 6. Effect of interaction between distance and year on the incidence of hemorrhages and veining defects.

	Cluster (Distance)				Pooled SEM
	1 (11–37 km)	2 (38–86 km)	3 (89–170 km)	4 (199–276 km)	
Hemorrhages (%)					
2012	1.32 a	1.27 a	0.91 b	1.57 a x	0.0688
2013	1.33 b	1.42 b	1.28 b	1.99 a y	0.0796
Veining (%)					
2012	10.39 a x	10.63 a	7.63 b x	10.64 a x	0.2838
2013	11.73 y	11.68	11.17 y	12.42 y	0.3366

Least square means within a row with different letters (a–b) differ ($P < 0.05$); Least square means within a column with different letters (x–y) differ ($P < 0.05$).

Interaction between season and year (Table 7) affected the incidences of lacerations, hemorrhages and veining. No differences between years were observed for lacerations but these differences appeared for hemorrhages in summer and autumn and for veining in spring, summer and autumn. These results confirmed the effects of the season on the incidences of raw ham defects. With regards to the influence of the year, as stated before, its effect appears related to a reduction of the quality of animal handling.

Table 7. Effect of interaction between season and year on the incidence of lacerations, hemorrhages and veining defects.

	Season				Pooled SEM
	Winter	Spring	Summer	Autumn	
Lacerations (%)					
2012	1.19 b	1.31 b	1.16 b	2.23 a	0.0824
2013	1.47 b	1.35 b	1.41 b	2.04 a	0.0873
Hemorrhages (%)					
2012	1.28 b	1.71 a	0.71 c x	1.53 b x	0.0711
2013	1.11 b	1.76 a	1.30 b y	1.90 a y	0.0802
Veining (%)					
2012	11.40 b	17.55 a x	6.72 c x	6.60 c x	0.3040
2013	12.73 a	13.06 a y	11.27 ab y	10.14 b y	0.3369

Least square means within a row with different letters (a–c) differ ($P < 0.05$); Least square means within a column with different letters (x–y) differ ($P < 0.05$).

4. Conclusions

The study has examined the effects of travel distances from 1 to 276 km, showing that both short and long journeys may have adverse effects on fresh ham defects. The higher incidence of defects associated with short transport distances may be due to the lack of time to lie down and recovery from loading stress, but probably also to hauliers working quickly to accomplish all planned transports for a given day. Additionally, these results could be related to the lower quality of rural roads, which represent the major part of the route in short journeys. Extending the transport distance above 170 km results in an increased incidence of raw ham defects; the incidence of defects reported herein was not proportional to the increase of transport distance This research highlights the need for Italian pig industry to improve pre-slaughter handling in order to increase the quality of raw hams for DPO production, reducing the economic losses related to inadequate practices before slaughter and increasing the welfare of animals to make it as good as possible. However, additional research is necessary to understand seasonal influences on frequencies of defects on the fresh hams destined for the DPO process.

Acknowledgements

The authors wish to acknowledge the technical assistance of quality assurance staff of the abattoir for data collected at the slaughterhouse. This research was supported by Regione Lombardia, Programma di Sviluppo Rurale 2007–2013, Misura 124.

Thank you to authors that collaborated and helped with the preparation of this manuscript. All authors contributed equally to this work.

Conflicts of Interest

The authors declare no conflict of interest.

References and Notes

1. Gregory, N.G. Animal welfare at markets and during transport and slaughter. *Meat Sci.* **2008**, *1*, 2–11.
2. Lambooij, E. Transport of Pigs. In *Livestock Handling and Transport*, 3rd ed.; Grandin, T., Ed.; CABI Publishing: Wallingford, UK, 2007; pp. 228–244.
3. Grandin, T. Handling and Welfare of Livestock in Slaughter Plant. In *Livestock Handling and Transport*, 3rd ed.; Grandin, T., Ed.; CABI Publishing: Wallingford, UK, 2007; pp. 329–348.
4. Warris, P.D. The welfare of slaughter pigs during transport. *Anim. Welfare* **1998**, *7*, 365–381.
5. Correa, J.A.; Torrey, S.; Devillers, N.; Laforest, J.P.; Gonyou, H.W.; Faucitano, L. Effects of different moving devices at loading on stress response and meat quality in pigs. *J. Anim. Sci.* **2010**, *88*, 4086–4093.
6. Von Borell, E.; Schaffer, D. Legal requirements and assessment of stress and welfare during transportation and pre-slaughter handling of pigs. *Livest. Prod. Sci.* **2005**, *97*, 81–87.
7. EFSA Panel on Animal Health and Welfare (AHAW). Scientific Opinion Concerning the Welfare of Animals during Transport. *EFSA J.* **2011**, *9*, 1–125.
8. Mota-Rojas, D.; Becerril, M.; Lemus, C.; Sanchez, P.; Gonzalez, M.; Olmos, S.A.; Ramırez, R.; Alonso-Spilsbury, M. Effects of mid-summer transport duration on pre- and post-slaughter performance and pork quality in Mexico. *Meat Sci.* **2006**, *73*, 404–412.
9. Barton Gade, P.; Christensen, L. Effect of different stocking densities during transport on welfare and meat quality in danish slaughter pigs. *Meat Sci.* **1998**, *48*, 237–247.
10. Gispert, M.; Faucitano, L.; Oliver, M.A.; Guardià, M.D.; Coll, C.; Siggens, K.; Harvey, K.; Diestre, A. A survey of pre-slaughter conditions, halothane gene frequency, and carcass and meat quality in five Spanish pig commercial abattoirs. *Meat Sci.* **2000**, *55*, 97–106.
11. Torrey, S.; Bergeron, R.; Widowski, T.; Lewis, N.; Crowe, T.; Correa, J.A.; Brown, J.; Gonyou, H.W.; Faucitano, L. Transportation of market-weight pigs: I. Effect of season, truck type, and location within truck on behavior with a two-hour transport. *J. Anim. Sci.* **2013**, *91*, 2863–2871.
12. Ritter, M.J.; Ellis, M.; Bowman, R.; Brinkmann, J.; Curtis, S.E.; DeDecker, J.M.; Mendoza, O.; Murphy, C.M.; Orellana, D.G.; Peterson, B.A.; Rojo, A.; Schlipf, J.M.; Wolter, B.F. Effects of season and distance moved during loading on transport losses of market-weight pigs in two commercially available types of trailer. *J. Anim. Sci.* **2008**, *86*, 3137–3145.
13. Scheeren, M.B.; Gonyou, H.W.; Brown, J.; Weschenfelder, A.V.; Faucitano L. Effects of transport time and location within truck on skin bruises and meat quality of market weight pigs in two seasons. *Can. J. Anim. Sci.* **2014**, *94*, 71–78.
14. Correa, J.A.; Gonyou, H.W.; Torrey, S.; Widowski, T.; Bergeron, R.; Crowe, T.G.; Laforest, J.P.; Faucitano, L. Welfare and carcass and meat quality of pigs being transported for two hours using two vehicle types during two seasons of the year. *Can. J. Anim. Sci.* **2013**, *93*, 43–55.
15. Gosálvez, L.F.; Averós, X.; Valdelvira, J.J.; Herranz, A. Influence of season, distance and mixed loads on the physical and carcass integrity of pigs transported to slaughter. *Meat Sci.* **2006**, *73*, 553–558.
16. Prosciutto di Parma. *Dossier 2013*; Parma Quality Institute: Langhirano, Italy, 2014; pp. 5–38.

17. Technical Fact Sheet of Parma Ham. Available online: http://www.prosciuttodiparma.com/pdf/en_UK/14b_Technical_fact_sheet_Parma_ham_ENG.pdf (accessed on 25 August 2014).
18. Prosciutto di Parma (Parma Ham). Protected Designation of Origin. Available online: http://www.prosciuttodiparma.com/pdf/en_UK/disciplinare.28.11.2013.en.pdf (accessed on 25 August 2014).
19. Candek-Potokar, M.; Skrlep, M. Factors in pig production that impact the quality of dry-cured ham: a review. *Animal* **2012**, *6*, 327–338.
20. Velarde, A.; Gispert, M.; Faucitano, L.; Manteca, X.; Diestre, A. The effect of stunning method on the incidence of PSE meat and hemorrhages in pork carcasses. *Meat Sci.* **2000**, *55*, 309–314.
21. Velarde, A.; Gispert, M.; Faucitano, L.; Alonso, P.; Manteca, X.; Diestre, A. Effect of the stunning procedure and halothane genotype on meat quality and incidence of hemorrhages in pigs. *Meat Sci.* **2001**, *58*, 313–319.
22. Channon, H.A.; Payne, A.M.; Warner, R.D. Comparison of CO(2) stunning with manual electrical stunning (50 Hz) of pigs on carcass and meat quality. *Meat Sci.* **2002**, *60*, 63–68.
23. Russo, V.; Lo Fiego, D.P.; Nanni Costa, L.; Tassone, F. Study of some factors affecting the incidence of veining defect in thighs destined to dry-cured process of Parma ham. In Proceedings of the 5th International Symposium on the Mediterranean Pig, Tarbes, France, 16–19 November 2004; pp. 277–281.
24. Gallo, C.; Espinoza, M.A.; Gasic, J. Efectos del transporte por camión durante 36 horas con y sin período de descanso sobre el peso vivo y algunos aspectos de calidad de carne en bovinos. *Arch. Med. Vet.* **2001**, *33*, 43–53.
25. Dalla Costa, O.A.; Faucitano, L.; Coldebella, A.; Ludke, J.V.; Peloso, J.V.; dalla Roza, D.; Paranhos da Costa, M.J.R. Effects of the season of the year, truck type and location on truck on skin bruises and meat quality in pigs. *Livest. Sci.* **2007**, *107*, 29–36.
26. ISTAT - Istituto Nazionale di Statistica. Monthly Data on Red Meat 2012. Available online: http://agri.istat.it/sag_is_pdwout/jsp/dawinci.jsp (accessed on 25 August 2014).
27. Gregory, N.G. How climatic changes could affect meat quality. *Food Res. Int.* **2010**, *43*, 1866–1873.
28. Warris, P.D.; Brown, S.N. A survey of mortality in slaughter pigs during transport and lairage. *Vet. Rec.* **1994**, *134*, 513–515.
29. Riches, H.L.; Guise, H.J.; Penny, R.H.C.; Jones, T.A.; Cuthbertson, A. A national survey of transport conditions for pigs. *Pig J.* **1996**, *38*, 8–18.
30. Grandin, T. The Effect of Economic Factors on the Welfare of Livestock and Poultry. In *Improving Animal Welfare: A Practical Approach*; CABI Publishing: Wallingford, UK, 2010; pp. 214–226.

Permissions

All chapters in this book were first published in Animals, by MDPI; hereby published with permission under the Creative Commons Attribution License or equivalent. Every chapter published in this book has been scrutinized by our experts. Their significance has been extensively debated. The topics covered herein carry significant findings which will fuel the growth of the discipline. They may even be implemented as practical applications or may be referred to as a beginning point for another development.

The contributors of this book come from diverse backgrounds, making this book a truly international effort. This book will bring forth new frontiers with its revolutionizing research information and detailed analysis of the nascent developments around the world.

We would like to thank all the contributing authors for lending their expertise to make the book truly unique. They have played a crucial role in the development of this book. Without their invaluable contributions this book wouldn't have been possible. They have made vital efforts to compile up to date information on the varied aspects of this subject to make this book a valuable addition to the collection of many professionals and students.

This book was conceptualized with the vision of imparting up-to-date information and advanced data in this field. To ensure the same, a matchless editorial board was set up. Every individual on the board went through rigorous rounds of assessment to prove their worth. After which they invested a large part of their time researching and compiling the most relevant data for our readers.

The editorial board has been involved in producing this book since its inception. They have spent rigorous hours researching and exploring the diverse topics which have resulted in the successful publishing of this book. They have passed on their knowledge of decades through this book. To expedite this challenging task, the publisher supported the team at every step. A small team of assistant editors was also appointed to further simplify the editing procedure and attain best results for the readers.

Apart from the editorial board, the designing team has also invested a significant amount of their time in understanding the subject and creating the most relevant covers. They scrutinized every image to scout for the most suitable representation of the subject and create an appropriate cover for the book.

The publishing team has been an ardent support to the editorial, designing and production team. Their endless efforts to recruit the best for this project, has resulted in the accomplishment of this book. They are a veteran in the field of academics and their pool of knowledge is as vast as their experience in printing. Their expertise and guidance has proved useful at every step. Their uncompromising quality standards have made this book an exceptional effort. Their encouragement from time to time has been an inspiration for everyone.

The publisher and the editorial board hope that this book will prove to be a valuable piece of knowledge for researchers, students, practitioners and scholars across the globe.

List of Contributors

Masashi Hasegawa
Azabu University School of Veterinary Medicine, 1-17-71, Fuchinobe, Chuo-ku, Sagamihara, Kanagawa 252-5201, Japan
Animal Life Solutions, Inc., 16-6, Ibukino, Midori-ku, Yokohama,Kanagawa 226-0028, Japan

Nobuyo Ohtani
Azabu University School of Veterinary Medicine, 1-17-71, Fuchinobe, Chuo-ku, Sagamihara, Kanagawa 252-5201, Japan

Mitsuaki Ohta
Azabu University School of Veterinary Medicine, 1-17-71, Fuchinobe, Chuo-ku, Sagamihara, Kanagawa 252-5201, Japan

Kirrilly Thompson
Appleton Institute, Central Queensland University, 44 Greenhill Road, Wayville, Adelaide, SA 5034, Australia

Danielle Every
Appleton Institute, Central Queensland University, 44 Greenhill Road, Wayville, Adelaide, SA 5034, Australia

Sophia Rainbird
Appleton Institute, Central Queensland University, 44 Greenhill Road, Wayville, Adelaide, SA 5034, Australia

Victoria Cornell
Faculty of Medicine, Nursing and Health Sciences, Flinders University, Adelaide, SA 5001, Australia

Bradley Smith
Appleton Institute, Central Queensland University, 44 Greenhill Road, Wayville, Adelaide, SA 5034, Australia

Joshua Trigg
Appleton Institute, Central Queensland University, 44 Greenhill Road, Wayville, Adelaide, SA 5034, Australia

Hannah E. Flint
Department of Population Medicine, Ontario Veterinary College, University of Guelph, 50 Stone Rd E., Guelph, ON, N1G 2W1, Canada

Karen S. Schwartzkopf-Genswein
Agriculture and Agri-Food Canada, Lethbridge, AB, T1J 4B1, Canada

Ken G. Bateman
Department of Population Medicine, Ontario Veterinary College, University of Guelph, 50 Stone Rd E., Guelph, ON, N1G 2W1, Canada

Derek B. Haley
Department of Population Medicine, Ontario Veterinary College, University of Guelph, 50 Stone Rd E., Guelph, ON, N1G 2W1, Canada

John McGlone
Department of Animal and Food Sciences, Texas Tech University, Lubbock, TX 79409, USA

Anna Johnson
Department of Animal Science, Iowa State University, Ames, IA 50011, USA

Avi Sapkota
Department of Animal and Food Sciences, Texas Tech University, Lubbock, TX 79409, USA

Rebecca Kephart
Department of Animal Science, Iowa State University, Ames, IA 50011, USA

Ellen C. Jongman
Animal Welfare Science Centre, The Melbourne School of Land and Environment, University of Melbourne, Parkville, VIC 3010, Australia

Kym L. Butler
Animal Welfare Science Centre, The Melbourne School of Land and Environment, University of Melbourne, Parkville, VIC 3010, Australia
Biometrics Group, Department of Environment and Primary Industries (Victoria), Werribee, VIC 3030, Australia

Brizio Di Donfrancesco
The Sensory Analysis Center, Department of Human Nutrition, Ice Hall, Kansas State University, Manhattan, KS 66506, USA

Kadri Koppel
The Sensory Analysis Center, Department of Human Nutrition, Ice Hall, Kansas State University, Manhattan, KS 66506, USA

Marianne Swaney-Stueve
The Sensory Analysis Center, Department of Human Nutrition, Ice Hall, Kansas State University, Manhattan, KS 66506, USA

Edgar Chambers IV
The Sensory Analysis Center, Department of Human Nutrition, Ice Hall, Kansas State University, Manhattan, KS 66506, USA

Jorge A. Correa
F. Ménard Inc., Ange Gardien, QC, J0E 1E0, Canada
Département de sciences animales, Université Laval, Quebec City, QC, G1K 7P4, Canada
Present address: Canadian Meat Council, Ottawa, ON, K1Z8P9, Canada

Harold Gonyou
Prairie Swine Centre, Saskatoon, SK, S7H 5N9, Canada

Stephanie Torrey
Dairy and Swine and Development Research Centre, Agriculture and Agri-Food Canada,
Department of Animal and Poultry Science, University of Guelph, Guelph, ON, N1G 2W1, Canada

Tina Widowski
Department of Animal & Poultry Science, University of Guelph, Guelph, ON, N1G 2W1, Canada

Renée Bergeron
University of Guelph, Alfred Campus, Alfred, ON, K0B 1A0, Canada

Trever Crowe
Department of Mechanical Engineering, University of Saskatchewan, Saskatoon, SK, S7N 59, Canada

Jean-Paul Laforest
Département de sciences animales, Université Laval, Quebec City, QC, G1K 7P4, Canada

Luigi Faucitano
Dairy and Swine and Development Research Centre, Agriculture and Agri-Food Canada, Sherbrooke, QC, J1M 0C8, Canada

Kadri Koppel
Sensory Analysis Center, Department of Human Nutrition, Kansas State University, 1310 Research Park Drive, Manhattan, KS 66502, USA

Michael Gibson
Department of Grain Science and Industry, Kansas State University, Manhattan, KS 66506, USA

Sajid Alavi
Department of Grain Science and Industry, Kansas State University, Manhattan, KS 66506, USA

Greg Aldrich
Department of Grain Science and Industry, Kansas State University, Manhattan, KS 66506, USA

Giuseppe Martino
Faculty of Biosciences and Agro-Food Technologies and Environmental, University of Teramo, via C. Lerici 1, 64023, Mosciano S.A., Italy

Cecilia Mugnai
Faculty of Biosciences and Agro-Food Technologies and Environmental, University of Teramo, via C. Lerici 1, 64023, Mosciano S.A., Italy

Dario Compagnone
Faculty of Biosciences and Agro-Food Technologies and Environmental, University of Teramo, via C. Lerici 1, 64023, Mosciano S.A., Italy

Lisa Grotta
Faculty of Biosciences and Agro-Food Technologies and Environmental, University of Teramo, via C. Lerici 1, 64023, Mosciano S.A., Italy

Michele Del Carlo
Faculty of Biosciences and Agro-Food Technologies and Environmental, University of Teramo, via C. Lerici 1, 64023, Mosciano S.A., Italy

Francesca Sarti
Department of Agricultural, Food and Environmental Science, University of Perugia, Borgo XX Giugno, 74, 06121, Perugia, Italy

Rebecca Kephart
Department of Animal Science, Iowa State University, Ames, IA 50011, USA

Anna Johnson
Department of Animal Science, Iowa State University, Ames, IA 50011, USA

Avi Sapkota
Departments of Animal and Food Science and Animal Care Services, Texas Tech University, Lubbock, TX 79409, USA

Kenneth Stalder
Department of Animal Science, Iowa State University, Ames, IA 50011, USA

John McGlone
Departments of Animal and Food Science and Animal Care Services, Texas Tech University, Lubbock, TX 79409, USA

Ian G. Colditz
CSIRO Animal, Food and Health Sciences, FD McMaster Laboratory, Armidale, NSW 2350, Australia

Drewe M. Ferguson
CSIRO Animal, Food and Health Sciences, FD McMaster Laboratory, Armidale, NSW 2350, Australia

Teresa Collins
College of Veterinary Medicine, Murdoch University, Murdoch, WA 6150, Australia

Lindsay Matthews
Lindsay Matthews & Associates Research International, Scerne Di Pineto, Teramo 64025, Italy
Psychology Department, University of Auckland, Auckland 1020, New Zealand

Paul H. Hemsworth
Animal Welfare Science Centre, The University of Melbourne, Parkville, VIC 3010, Australia

John McGlone
Animal and Food Sciences, Texas Tech University, Lubbock, TX 79409, USA

Avi Sapkota
Animal and Food Sciences, Texas Tech University, Lubbock, TX 79409, USA

Anna Johnson
Department of Animal Science, Iowa State University, Ames, IA 50011, USA

Rebecca Kephart
Department of Animal Science, Iowa State University, Ames, IA 50011, USA

John McGlone
Animal and Food Sciences, Texas Tech University, Lubbock, TX 79409, USA

Avi Sapkota
Animal and Food Sciences, Texas Tech University, Lubbock, TX 79409, USA

Luiz Carlos Pinheiro Machado Filho
Lab of Applied Ethology and Animal Welfare (LETA), Departament of Zootechny and Rural Development, Federal University of Santa Catarina, Rod. Admar Gonzaga, 1346, Florianopolis, SC 88034-000, Brazil

Leandro Martins D'Ávila
Lab of Applied Ethology and Animal Welfare (LETA), Departament of Zootechny and Rural Development, Federal University of Santa Catarina, Rod. Admar Gonzaga, 1346, Florianopolis, SC 88034-000, Brazil

Daniele Cristina da Silva Kazama
Lab of Applied Ethology and Animal Welfare (LETA), Departament of Zootechny and Rural Development, Federal University of Santa Catarina, Rod. Admar Gonzaga, 1346, Florianopolis, SC 88034-000, Brazil

Lauana Luiza Bento
Lab of Animal Biochemistry, Department of Zootechny and Rural Development, Federal University of Santa Catarina, Rod. Admar Gonzaga, 1346, Florianópolis, SC 88034-000, Brazil

Shirley Kuhnen
Lab of Animal Biochemistry, Department of Zootechny and Rural Development, Federal University of Santa Catarina, Rod. Admar Gonzaga, 1346, Florianópolis, SC 88034-000, Brazil

Penny Hawkins
Research Animals Department, Royal Society for the Prevention of Cruelty to Animals (RSPCA), Wilberforce Way, Southwater, West Sussex, RH13 9RS, UK

Agnese Arduini
Department of Agricultural and Food Science, School of Agriculture and Veterinary Medicine, University of Bologna, Via Fanin 50, 40127 Bologna, Italy

Veronica Redaelli
Department of Agricultural and Food Science, School of Agriculture and Veterinary Medicine, University of Bologna, Via Fanin 50, 40127 Bologna, Italy

Fabio Luzi
Department of Health, Animal Science and Food Safety, Faculty of Veterinary Science, University of Milan, Via Celoria 10, 20133 Milan, Italy

Stefania Dall'Olio
Department of Agricultural and Food Science, School of Agriculture and Veterinary Medicine, University of Bologna, Via Fanin 50, 40127 Bologna, Italy

Vincenzo Pace
OPAS, Pig Farmer Association, Strada Ghisiolo 57, 46030 San Giorgio, Mantua, Italy

Leonardo Nanni Costa
Department of Agricultural and Food Science, School of Agriculture and Veterinary Medicine, University of Bologna, Via Fanin 50, 40127 Bologna, Italy